MR Imaging of the Genitourinary System

Editor

ERSAN ALTUN

MAGNETIC RESONANCE IMAGING CLINICS OF NORTH AMERICA

www.mri.theclinics.com

Consulting Editors
SURESH K. MUKHERJI
LYNNE S. STEINBACH

February 2019 • Volume 27 • Number 1

ELSEVIER

1600 John F. Kennedy Boulevard • Suite 1800 • Philadelphia, Pennsylvania, 19103-2899

http://www.mri.theclinics.com

MRI CLINICS OF NORTH AMERICA Volume 27, Number 1
February 2019 ISSN 1064-9689, ISBN 13: 978-0-323-65473-9

Editor: John Vassallo (j.vassallo@elsevier.com)
Developmental Editor: Meredith Madeira

Magnetic Resonance Imaging Clinics of North America (ISSN 1064-9689) is published quarterly by Elsevier Inc., 360 Park Avenue South, New York, NY 10010-1710. Months of issue are February, May, August, and November. Business and Editorial Offices: 1600 John F. Kennedy Blvd., Ste. 1800, Philadelphia, PA 19103-2899. Customer Service Office: 3251 Riverport Lane, Maryland Heights, MO 63043. Periodicals postage paid at New York, NY and additional mailing offices. Subscription prices are $404.00 per year (domestic individuals), $736.00 per year (domestic institutions), $100.00 per year (domestic students/residents), $437.00 per year (Canadian individuals), $959.00 per year (Canadian institutions), $545.00 per year (international individuals), $959.00 per year (international institutions), and $275.00 per year (international and Canadian students/residents). International air speed delivery is included in all *Clinics* subscription prices. All prices are subject to change without notice. **POSTMASTER:** Send address changes to *Magnetic Resonance Imaging Clinics*, Elsevier Health Sciences Division, Subscription Customer Service, 3251 Riverport Lane, Maryland Heights, MO 63043. Customer Service (orders, claims, online, change of address): Elsevier Health Sciences Division, Subscription **Customer Service, 3251 Riverport Lane, Maryland Heights, MO 63043. Tel:1-800-654-2452 (U.S. and Canada); 314-447-8871 (outside U.S. and Canada). Fax: 314-447-8029. E-mail: journalscustomer service-usa@elsevier.com (for print support); journalsonlinesupport-usa@elsevier.com (for online support).**

Reprints. For copies of 100 or more of articles in this publication, please contact the Commercial Reprints Department, Elsevier Inc., 360 Park Avenue South, New York, NY 10010-1710. Tel.: 212-633-3874; Fax: 212-633-3820; E-mail: reprints@elsevier.com.

Magnetic Resonance Imaging Clinics of North America is covered in the *RSNA Index of Imaging Literature, MEDLINE/PubMed (Index Medicus),* and *EMBASE/Excerpta Medica.*

Contributors

CONSULTING EDITORS

SURESH K. MUKHERJI, MD, MBA, FACR
Professor and Chairman, Walter F. Patenge
Endowed Chair, Department of Radiology,
Michigan State University, Chief Medical
Officer and Director of Health Care Delivery,
Michigan State University Health Team, East
Lansing, Michigan, USA

LYNNE S. STEINBACH, MD, FACR
Professor of Radiology and Orthopaedic
Surgery, Department of Radiology and
Biomedical Imaging, University of California,
San Francisco, San Francisco, California,
USA

EDITOR

ERSAN ALTUN, MD
Assistant Professor, Department of Radiology,
Abdominal Imaging Section, The University of
North Carolina at Chapel Hill, Chapel Hill, North
Carolina, USA; Associate Professor of
Radiology, Turkey

AUTHORS

ERSAN ALTUN, MD
Assistant Professor, Department of Radiology,
Abdominal Imaging Section, The University of
North Carolina at Chapel Hill, Chapel Hill, North
Carolina, USA; Associate Professor of
Radiology, Turkey

HINA ARIF-TIWARI, MD, DNB
Associate Professor of Body Imaging, Director,
Department of Medical Imaging, Abdominal
Imaging Fellowship Director, South Campus
Hospital, University of Arizona College of
Medicine, Tucson, Arizona, USA

JASPREET K. BISLA, MD
Assistant Professor, Department of Medical
Imaging, University of Arizona College of
Medicine, Tucson, Arizona, USA

ARITRICK CHATTERJEE, PhD
Department of Radiology, University of
Chicago, Chicago, Illinois, USA

JOÃO CRUZ, MD
Department of Radiology, Hospital Garcia
de Orta, Almada, Portugal; Department
of Radiology, Hospital da Luz, Setúbal,
Portugal

ALBERTO DIAZ DE LEON, MD
Assistant Professor of Radiology, University of
Texas Southwestern Medical Center, Dallas,
Texas, USA

SÉRGIO DUARTE, MD
Department of Radiology, Hospital da Luz,
Setúbal, Portugal

JORGE ELIAS Jr, MD, PhD
Associate Professor of Radiology,
Internal Medicine Department, Imaging and
Physics Science Center, Clinical Hospital of
Ribeirao Preto Medical School, University of
Sao Paulo, Ribeirao Preto, Sao Paulo,
Brazil

JULIA R. FIELDING, MD
Professor of Radiology, Chief,
Abdominal Imaging Division, UT
Southwestern University Hospitals,
Dallas, Texas, USA

FILIPA FIGUEIREDO, MD
Department of Radiology, Hospital Garcia de
Orta, Almada, Portugal

ADALGISA GUERRA, MD
Department of Radiology, Hospital da Luz,
Lisboa, Portugal

NICOLE HINDMAN, MD
Associate Professor, Department of Radiology,
Abdominal Imaging Section, Director of
Female Pelvic Imaging, NYU Langone Health,
New York, New York, USA

BOBBY T. KALB, MD
Associate Professor, Department of Medical
Imaging, Vice Chair, Quality and Safety,
Director of MRI and Chief, Body Section,
University of Arizona College of Medicine,
Tucson, Arizona, USA

PAYAL KAPUR, MD
Professor of Pathology and Urology,
Co-leader, Kidney Cancer Program,
Harold C. Simmons Comprehensive Cancer
Center, University of Texas Southwestern
Medical Center, Dallas, Texas, USA

DIEGO R. MARTIN, MD, PhD, FRCPC
Chairman, Department of Medical Imaging,
The Cosden Professor of Medical Imaging,
Biomedical Engineering and Physiology,
University of Arizona College of Medicine,
Banner University Medical Center, Tucson,
Tucson, Arizona, USA

MELVY SARAH MATHEW, MD
Assistant Professor, Department of Radiology,
University of Chicago, Chicago, Illinois, USA

MAHAN MATHUR, MD
Assistant Professor of Radiology and
Biomedical Imaging, Section of Body Imaging,
Director, Medical Student Education,
Associate Director, Diagnostic Radiology
Residency Program, Yale School of Medicine,
New Haven, Connecticut, USA

ANTÓNIO P. MATOS, MD
Department of Radiology, Hospital Garcia de
Orta, Almada, Portugal

VALDAIR FRANCISCO MUGLIA, MD, PhD
Associate Professor of Radiology,
Internal Medicine Department, Imaging
and Physics Science Center, Clinical
Hospital of Ribeirao Preto Medical School,
University of Sao Paulo, Ribeirao Preto, Sao
Paulo, Brazil

AYTEKIN OTO, MD, MBA
Professor, Department of Radiology, University
of Chicago, Chicago, Illinois, USA

IVAN PEDROSA, MD, PhD
Professor of Radiology, Urology, Advanced
Imaging Research Center, and Biomedical
Engineering, Chief of MRI, Co-leader,
Kidney Cancer Program, Harold C. Simmons
Comprehensive Cancer Center, University of
Texas Southwestern Medical Center, Dallas,
Texas, USA

MIGUEL RAMALHO, MD
Department of Radiology, Hospital Garcia
de Orta, Almada, Portugal; Department
of Radiology, Hospital da Luz, Setúbal,
Portugal

MANOJKUMAR SARANATHAN, PhD
Department of Medical Imaging, University of
Arizona, Tucson, Arizona, USA

MICHAEL SPEKTOR, MD
Assistant Professor of Radiology and
Biomedical Imaging, Section of Body
Imaging, Fellowship Director, Body/MRI,
Director of Teleradiology, Yale School
of Medicine, New Haven, Connecticut,
USA

GIRI SURA, PhD, MD
Fellow, Abdominal Imaging Division, UT
Southwestern University Hospitals, Dallas,
Texas, USA

ERIC ZEIKUS, MD
Assistant Professor of Radiology, Chief
Radiology Officer, UT Southwestern University
Hospitals, Dallas, Texas, USA

Contents

> Renal tumors encompass a heterogeneous disease spectrum, which confounds patient management and treatment. Percutaneous biopsy is limited by an inability to sample every part of the tumor. Radiomics may provide detail beyond what can be achieved from human interpretation. Understanding what new technologies offer will allow radiologists to play a greater role in caring for patients with renal cell carcinoma. In this article, we review the use of radiomics in renal cell carcinoma, in both the pretreatment assessment of renal masses and posttreatment evaluation of renal cell carcinoma, with special emphasis on the use of multiparametric MR imaging datasets.

> Hematuria evaluation remains a common problem, particularly in patients who smoke and are at risk for urothelial tumors. Lifetime surveillance of the urothelium is often required once urothelial cancer is diagnosed. Computed tomography urography (CTU) has exquisite sensitivity and specificity for identification of renal and urothelial lesions. The examination is well accepted by patients and physicians. Possible harms include radiation exposure and contrast-induced nephropathy. MR imaging is also an accurate test, but requires longer exam times, and may not demonstrate stones. We present the technical and interpretation skills required to use MR urography and CTU effectively.

> Superior soft tissue and contrast resolution of MR imaging benefits sensitivity to kidney cyst features and classification, which may have an impact on patient management and outcomes. Contrast-enhanced ultrasound (CEUS) may have nearly similar sensitivity for detection of cyst features yet is dependent on patient body habitus and adequacy of visualization windows for the kidneys, which does not have the same impact on MR imaging results. Both MR imaging and CEUS may provide superior kidney cyst assessment compared with contrast-enhanced CT; however, further research is needed, particularly for the identification of role of CEUS.

used for population-level screening. We can expect standardization of multiparametric MR imaging and increased use of quantitative multiparametric MR imaging, which will lead to more reproducible results and improved interpretation. The development and integration of new acquisition techniques and use of artificial intelligence for image interpretation can lead to implementation of new clinical MR methods. These will lead to increased adoption of multiparametric MR imaging for prostate cancer diagnosis and for guiding intervention and follow-up.

MR Imaging–Guided Focal Therapies of Prostate Cancer   131

Melvy Sarah Mathew and Aytekin Oto

MR imaging-guided focal therapy is a viable treatment option for patients with localized prostate cancer. After the identification of a malignant focus in the prostate gland on multiparametric MR imaging, treatment can be directed in a precise fashion to the area of interest. The goal of focal therapy is to eradicate prostate cancer while minimizing complications that can affect quality of life. Currently, the most commonly used methods of focal treatment of prostate cancer are cryotherapy, high-intensity focused ultrasound, and laser ablation.

MR Imaging of the Penis and Urethra   139

Ersan Altun

MR imaging has been increasingly used as a problem-solving adjunct after an initial ultrasound examination for a variety of penile disorders, and is the best cross-sectional imaging modality for the assessment of urethra and periurethral disease. Critical advantages of MR imaging for penile and urethra imaging include high soft tissue contrast resolution providing detailed anatomic evaluation, which is important for the demonstration and assessment of critical structures such as tunica albuginea or walls of the urethra, larger field of view for better evaluation of extent of disease, and demonstration of proteinaceous material and varying ages of the blood products.

MR Imaging of the Testicular and Extratesticular Tumors: When Do We Need?   151

Mahan Mathur and Michael Spektor

Testicular ultrasound is typically the first-line imaging examination in evaluating scrotal pathology. However, MR imaging can often provide valuable additional information, especially when ultrasound and/or clinical examinations are inconclusive. This is particularly evident when encountering testicular or paratesticular lesions, where accurate localization and characterization are paramount for management and prognosis. After reviewing normal scrotal anatomy as seen on MR imaging and offering a sample imaging protocol, the article describes specific indications for scrotal MR imaging and highlights imaging findings unique to various benign and malignant causes.

MAGNETIC RESONANCE IMAGING CLINICS OF NORTH AMERICA

SERIES OF RELATED INTEREST

Neuroimaging Clinics of North America
Available at: www.Neuroimaging.theclinics.com
PET Clinics
Available at: www.pet.theclinics.com
Radiologic Clinics of North America
Available at: www.Radiologic.theclinics.com

VISIT THE CLINICS ONLINE!
Access your subscription at:
www.theclinics.com

PROGRAM OBJECTIVE

The goal of *Magnetic Resonance Imaging Clinics of North America* is to keep practicing physicians up to date with current clinical practice by providing timely articles reviewing the state of the art in patient care.

TARGET AUDIENCE

All practicing physicians and healthcare professionals who provide patient care utilizing findings from Magnetic Resonance Imaging.

LEARNING OBJECTIVES

Upon completion of this activity, participants will be able to:

1. Review magnetic resonance imaging as a diagnostic technique to assess retroperitoneal diseases
2. Discuss magnetic resonance imaging, non-contrast and contrast enhanced, techniques available for evaluating kidney structure and function in patients with renal impairment
3. Recognize role of magnetic resonance imaging for the evaluation of infectious and inflammatory disease processes of the Urinary Tract

ACCREDITATION

The Elsevier Office of Continuing Medical Education (EOCME) is accredited by the Accreditation Council for Continuing Medical Education (ACCME) to provide continuing medical education for physicians.

The EOCME designates this enduring material for a maximum of 15 *AMA PRA Category 1 Credit*(s)™. Physicians should claim only the credit commensurate with the extent of their participation in the activity.

All other healthcare professionals requesting continuing education credit for this enduring material will be issued a certificate of participation.

DISCLOSURE OF CONFLICTS OF INTEREST

The EOCME assesses conflict of interest with its instructors, faculty, planners, and other individuals who are in a position to control the content of CME activities. All relevant conflicts of interest that are identified are thoroughly vetted by EOCME for fair balance, scientific objectivity, and patient care recommendations. EOCME is committed to providing its learners with CME activities that promote improvements or quality in healthcare and not a specific proprietary business or a commercial interest.

The planning committee, staff, authors and editors listed below have identified no financial relationships or relationships to products or devices they or their spouse/life partner have with commercial interest related to the content of this CME activity:

Ersan Altun, MD; Hina Arif-Tiwari, MD, DNB; Jaspreet K. Bisla, MD; Aritrick Chatterjee, PhD; João Cruz, MD; Alberto Diaz de Leon, MD; Sérgio Duarte, MD; Jorge Elias Jr, MD, PhD; Julia R. Fielding, MD; Filipa Figueiredo, MD; Adalgisa Guerra, MD; Nicole Hindman, MD; Bobby T. Kalb, MD; Payal Kapur, MD; Alison Kemp; Pradeep Kuttysankaran; Diego R. Martin, MD, PhD, FRCPC; Mahan Mathur, MD; António P. Matos, MD; Valdair Francisco Muglia, MD, PhD; Suresh K. Mukherji, MD, MBA, FACR; Ivan Pedrosa, MD, PhD; Miguel Ramalho, MD; Manojkumar Saranathan, PhD; Michael Spektor, MD; Lynne S. Steinbach, MD, FACR; Giri Sura, PhD, MD; John Vassallo; Eric Zeikus, MD.

The planning committee, staff, authors and editors listed below have identified financial relationships or relationships to products or devices they or their spouse/life partner have with commercial interest related to the content of this CME activity:

Melvy Sarah Mathew, MD: receives research support from Guerbet LLC.

Aytekin Oto, MD, MBA: receives research support from Koninklijke Philips NV and Guerbet LLC, is a speaker for Bracco, and is a consultant/advisor and receives research support from Profound Medical Corp.

UNAPPROVED/OFF-LABEL USE DISCLOSURE

The EOCME requires CME faculty to disclose to the participants:

1. When products or procedures being discussed are off-label, unlabelled, experimental, and/or investigational (not US Food and Drug Administration [FDA] approved); and
2. Any limitations on the information presented, such as data that are preliminary or that represent ongoing research, interim analyses, and/or unsupported opinions. Faculty may discuss information about pharmaceutical agents that is outside of FDA-approved labelling. This information is intended solely for CME and is not intended to promote off-label use of these medications. If you have any questions, contact the medical affairs department of the manufacturer for the most recent prescribing information.

TO ENROLL

To enroll in the *Magnetic Resonance Imaging Clinics of North America* Continuing Medical Education program, call customer service at 1-800-654-2452 or sign up online at http://www.theclinics.com/home/cme. The CME program is available to subscribers for an additional annual fee of USD 260.

METHOD OF PARTICIPATION

In order to claim credit, participants must complete the following:

1. Complete enrolment as indicated above.
2. Read the activity.
3. Complete the CME Test and Evaluation. Participants must achieve a score of 70% on the test. All CME Tests and Evaluations must be completed online.

CME INQUIRIES/SPECIAL NEEDS

For all CME inquiries or special needs, please contact elsevierCME@elsevier.com.

Foreword

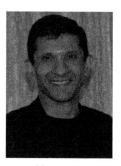

Suresh K. Mukherji, MD, MBA, FACR
Consulting Editor

I would like to thank Dr Ersan Altun for editing this wonderful issue of *Magnetic Resonance Imaging Clinics of North America* entitled, "MR Imaging of the Genitourinary System." This important issue provides the reader with a state-of-the-art update on new imaging techniques and their applications to the various complex pathologies of the genitourinary system. This issue is a collection of eleven review articles covering the entire gamut of genitourinary disorders with a focus on MR imaging technique and diagnosis. The issue is very clinically oriented but also has articles dedicated to novel techniques that include radiomics, multiparametric prostate imaging, and MR-guided focused treatment of prostate.

These articles are written by international leaders in the field of genitourinary imaging, and I personally thank all of the authors for creating such outstanding contributions. The information is timely and relevant, which will add value to our daily clinical practice.

On a personal note, this topic is very poignant for me as my mother had polycystic kidney disease and required a renal transplant. Although I opted to focus on "Neuro"radiology, "Uro"radiology has played an important role in the health and well-being of my family. Thank you again to all who contributed to this wonderful issue of *Magnetic Resonance Imaging Clinics of North America*!

Suresh K. Mukherji, MD, MBA, FACR
Department of Radiology
Michigan State University
Michigan State University Health Team
846 Service Road
East Lansing, MI 48824, USA

E-mail address:
sureshkm@msu.edu

Magn Reson Imaging Clin N Am 27 (2019) xi
https://doi.org/10.1016/j.mric.2018.10.002
1064-9689/19/© 2018 Published by Elsevier Inc.

Preface
Update on Genitourinary MR Imaging

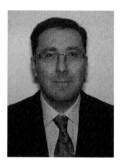

Ersan Altun, MD
Editor

This issue of *Magnetic Resonance Imaging Clinics of North America* is focused on Genitourinary Imaging. Updated clinically relevant information, including state-of-the-art MR imaging techniques, is given in each article in addition to future perspectives and insights on new horizons. Moreover, clinically important questions have been addressed in multiple articles. The main points of the articles are summarized below.

The radiomics of kidney cancer with MR imaging could be critical in the near future, particularly with the clinical use of artificial intelligence (AI). AI could detect qualitative and/or quantitative parameters with the potential to differentiate renal tumors from each other, but cannot be visually detected. The current status of MR imaging in the assessment of tumors of the renal collecting systems and ureters is also discussed and compared with computed tomographic urography illustrating multiple disease entities.

Contrast-enhanced ultrasound could be particularly helpful in the diagnosis of complex cystic renal cystic masses, particularly in patients with renal impairment and patients at risk for further renal damage or nephrogenic systemic fibrosis, if intravenous contrast is used for cross-sectional imaging. However, the accuracy of contrast-enhanced ultrasound in the diagnosis of complex cystic masses has not been well defined yet compared with cross-sectional imaging. The use of noncontrast MR imaging techniques in patients with renal impairment has been getting increasing attention in the medical community due to their critical use, particularly in critically sick in-patients.

The current role of MR imaging in the evaluation of infection and inflammatory disease processes of the urinary tract, perirenal space, and retroperitoneum, illustrating multiple disease entities, is discussed. MR imaging staging of urinary bladder cancer is reviewed due to the recent interest among the medical community with particular emphasis on hybrid imaging (ie, PET-MR imaging), although the role of PET-MR imaging has not been established yet in the staging of bladder cancer.

Future perspectives on multiparametric MR imaging prostate MR are discussed with possible new promising imaging techniques. Techniques of MR imaging–guided focal therapies with postablation MR imaging features, particularly for low-grade prostate cancers, are demonstrated with multiple cases.

The current role of MR imaging in the evaluation of the penis and urethra, and testicular and

Magn Reson Imaging Clin N Am 27 (2019) xiii–xiv
https://doi.org/10.1016/j.mric.2018.10.001
1064-9689/19/© 2018 Published by Elsevier Inc.

extratesticular tumors, is reviewed with various cases. The role of MR imaging compared with ultrasound is also discussed for specific disease entities, when possible.

In conclusion, this issue summarizes the current status of MR imaging in the assessment of various genitourinary disease processes and presents the clinically relevant but still unanswered questions that need to be addressed in the near future regarding the use of MR imaging compared with other imaging modalities, or relatively newer imaging techniques.

Ersan Altun, MD
Department of Radiology
Abdominal Imaging Section
The University of North Carolina
at Chapel Hill
UNC Hospitals
101 Manning Drive
2021 Old Clinic
Chapel Hill, NC 27514, USA

E-mail address:
ersan_altun@med.unc.edu

Radiomics in Kidney Cancer: MR Imaging

Alberto Diaz de Leon, MD[a], Payal Kapur, MD[b,c], Ivan Pedrosa, MD, PhD[a,c],*

KEYWORDS

- Radiomics • Kidney cancer • MR imaging • Quantitative imaging

KEY POINTS

- Radiomics includes various techniques for the extraction of quantitative features from imaging to improve diagnostic, prognostic, and predictive accuracy of image interpretation, but mandates standardization and large and well-designed databases for optimal use.
- Radiomics in the pretreatment assessment of kidney cancer may provide additional insight into the subtyping and tumor biology of renal cell carcinoma.
- In the posttreatment setting, radiomics may assist in predicting a response to systemic therapy, including to antiangiogenic treatment, which may not be adequately assessed with traditional size-based criteria.

INTRODUCTION

Renal tumors encompass a broad disease spectrum, from benign and indolent lesions to aggressive and invasive malignancies. Imaging plays a critical role in the management of patients with renal tumors. Small renal masses (SRMs), defined as those 4 cm or less in size, account for more than 50% of all renal masses with approximately 20% of these demonstrating malignant behavior.[1] The American Urologic Association guidelines for management of renal masses contemplate active surveillance as a valid option for patients with comorbidities and T1a ($\leq$4 cm) or T1b (4–7 cm) tumors. The ability to predict the histology of these renal lesions to distinguish aggressive forms of renal cell carcinoma (RCC) from benign and indolent malignant lesions with imaging has been a primary topic of interest. Furthermore, despite the reported low risk of metastases in larger tumors

(ie, cT1b/T2, >4 cm) followed on active surveillance, the lack of reliable predictors of oncologic behavior and low reliability of biopsies to grade larger, heterogeneous tumors limit the applicability of active surveillance in clinical practice for these tumors. Moreover, there is currently no accepted neoadjuvant therapy regimen in the management of kidney cancer. The inherent heterogeneous nature of renal tumors[2,3] drives the need to better characterize the disease and overcome the sampling variability of percutaneous biopsies. Imaging provides a whole tumor assessment that has the potential to help select effective therapies for specific histologic subtypes. Nevertheless, the known histologic and molecular heterogeneity within the subtypes of RCC, and even within a single tumor, is such that the development of reliable imaging biomarkers to predict the histology and biologic behavior of these lesions is challenging.

This article was supported by NIH Grant U01 CA207091 (I. Pedrosa), P50CA196516 (I. Pedrosa, P. Kapur) and R01CA154475 (I. Pedrosa).

[a] Department of Radiology, University of Texas Southwestern Medical Center, 2201 Inwood Road, 2nd Floor, Suite 202, Dallas, TX 75390, USA; [b] Department of Pathology, University of Texas Southwestern Medical Center, 6201 Harry Hines Boulevard, Room 04.257, Dallas, TX 75390, USA; [c] Kidney Cancer Program, Harold C. Simmons Comprehensive Cancer Center, University of Texas Southwestern Medical Center, 5323 Harry Hines Boulevard, Dallas, TX 75390, USA
* Corresponding author. 2201 Inwood Road. 2nd Floor, Suite 202, Dallas, TX 75390-9085.
E-mail address: ivan.pedrosa@UTSouthwestern.edu

Radiomics is an emerging field that attempts to extract data from imaging to provide information beyond what can be achieved from human imaging interpretation alone. The correlation of these imaging data with genomics (ie, radiogenomics), metabolomics (ie, radiometabolomics), and beyond offers an opportunity to generate objective, quantitative biomarkers of tumor biology that may be used to predict patient's prognosis and likelihood of response to therapy, overcoming some of the challenges associated with disease heterogeneity (**Fig. 1**). Magnetic resonance (MR) imaging provides rich imaging datasets because of the multiple image contrast mechanisms available with this technique (ie, multiparametric MR imaging). These datasets offer a unique opportunity to implement radiomic analysis. In this article, we review the use of radiomics in RCC, in both the pretreatment assessment of renal masses and the posttreatment evaluation of RCC, with a special emphasis on the use of multiparametric MR imaging datasets.

RADIOMICS OVERVIEW

Radiomics is a term that includes various techniques for the extraction of quantitative features from imaging to improve diagnostic, prognostic, and predictive accuracy of image interpretation. Gillies and colleagues[4] define radiomics as "the conversion of images to higher dimensional data

and the subsequent mining of these data for improved decision support." Radiomics approaches provide a mechanism to identify complex patterns in images that are not obvious to the naked eye. The recent breakthroughs in artificial intelligence and computer power have accelerated the application of this type of analysis to medical imaging to guide clinical decisions.[5]

The process begins with the selection and standardization of an imaging protocol. Uniformity in image acquisition is vital in any radiomics assessment to decrease variability and improve the reproducibility and comparability of studies. Mackin and colleagues[6] reported a similar level of variability in the values of radiomics features calculated on computed tomography (CT) images obtained from different CT scanners to that of the variability of these radiomics features found in CT images of patients with non-small cell lung cancers. In MR imaging, standardization of image acquisition may represent a greater challenge owing to the interplay of numerous factors including hardware (ie, magnet strength, coil selection, etc), sequence parameters, and contrast agents. For example, with dynamic contrast-enhanced (DCE) MR imaging, the type and dose contrast agent, software used to extract the pharmacokinetic parameters, and pulse sequence used for image acquisition must be accounted for.[7] Nevertheless, several organizations

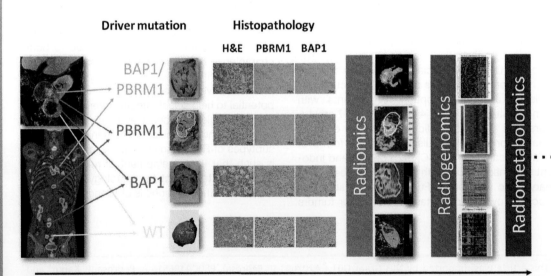

Fig. 1. Schematic representation of the goal of image-based analysis in kidney cancer. Imaging provides analysis of the entire tumor and virtually every metastatic lesion in the patient. The imaging phenotype in the primary tumor and metastatic lesions may correlate to specific underlying molecular alteration (eg, mutation status), which can be confirmed with genomics or immunohistochemistry during histopathologic evaluation. Mining of imaging data (radiomics) offers the opportunity to correlate objective, quantitative in vivo data with datasets generated with tissue-based analyses such as histopathology, genetic data (radiogenomics), metabolomics data (radiometabolomics), and potentially others. The spatial colocalization of imaging data with tissue-based data provides an avenue to address tumor heterogeneity in kidney cancer. BAP1, BRCA1-associated protein 1; H&E, hematoxylin and eosin; PBRM1, polybromo 1; WT, wild-type.

have attempted to introduce standardization of imaging techniques for quantitative analyses, such as the Quantitative Imaging Biomarkers Alliance[8], and the Image Biomarker Standardization Initiative (IBSI).[9]

Once an appropriate imaging protocol is selected, a volume of interest is identified. Depending on the prediction target, analyses can be performed on an entire lesion, metastases, and/or normal tissues. Additionally, analyses may be performed on subvolumes of tumor known as habitats, regions that may exhibit unique physiologic characteristics from the remainder of the tumor.[9] Volume of interests are then segmented, either manually or automatically, to determine which voxels are analyzed.

Segmentation is considered a critical component of radiomics, because the subsequent features data are generated from the segmented volumes. Manual segmentation is considered as ground truth, but it is labor intensive, may not be feasible with large volumes of data, and suffers from inter-operator variability.[10] Semiautomatic segmentation methods, such as region-growing and level set methods, may maximize outputs and provide greater reproducibility, although they still require some level of manual input by the operator. The method of segmentation can also affect the radiomic analysis.[11] Once the volumes are segmented, feature extraction can then be performed.

Feature extraction involves the mining of quantitative attributes from the segmented volumes and encompasses the center of radiomics. The number of radiomic features that can be extracted is essentially limitless and requires careful selection, because the inclusion of too many features could result in overfitting. Predictive and prognostic radiomic features should be extracted from training sets and validated in independent datasets, when possible, to diminish the opportunity of overfitting. Features can be subdivided into 2 broad categories: semantic and agnostic features.[4] Semantic features include descriptors commonly used in image interpretation by the radiologist, such as lesion shape, margin, and location. Agnostic features are those mathematically extracted from the image and can be further subdivided into first-, second-, and higher-order statistical outputs.[12]

First-order statistics are obtained from the histogram of voxel intensities to provide characteristics such as the mean, skewness/asymmetry, kurtosis/sharpness, and measures of randomness, including entropy and uniformity. First-order features describe the distribution of intensities without taking into account the spatial relationship of voxels. Second-order, or texture or grayscale features, are based on matrices depicting spatial intensity distribution and describe the relationship between voxels with similar or different intensity values and can provide a measurement of intratumoral heterogeneity. Examples of these include gray-level cooccurrence matrix (**Fig. 2**) and run-length matrix.[12] Haralick first described a series

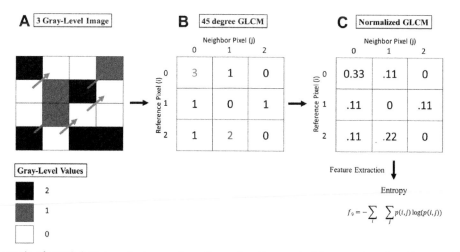

Fig. 2. Example of Haralick texture features using a 3 gray-level image. In this example, a 4 × 4 image with 3 gray levels is assessed (A). The first step in is constructing a gray-level cooccurrence matrix (GLCM) in a specified direction (B). In this example, a 45° (*diagonal*) direction is used. The value of the reference pixel (i) establishes the appropriate row, and the value of the neighbor pixel (j) determines the column. In this example, for the reference value of 0, the cooccurrence of a neighbor pixel of 0 in the 45° is 3 (annotated by the *green arrows*), and for a reference value of 2, the cooccurrence with a neighbor pixel of 1 is 2 (annotated by the *red arrows*). The GLCM can then be normalized by the sum of the elements to generate a probability of each combination to occur in the image (C). Haralick statistical features can then be subsequently extracted from the region of interest.

> **Box 1**
> **List of common Haralick features**
>
> Angular second momentum
>
> Contrast
>
> Correlation
>
> Difference entropy
>
> Difference variance
>
> Energy
>
> Entropy
>
> Homogeneity
>
> Information measure of correlation 1
>
> Information measure of correlation 2
>
> Max correlation coefficient
>
> Sum average
>
> Sum entropy
>
> Sum variance

of texture features commonly applied to medical imaging (**Box 1**).[13] Finally, higher-order statistical outputs use filter grids on the image to identify repetitive or nonrepetitive patterns.

Ultimately, the goal of radiomics is to use imaging features to identify patterns that can be used individually or correlated with patient characteristics beyond imaging (eg, histology, immunohistochemistry, and genomic and proteomic profiles) to generate objective, quantitative biomarkers of disease status that can improve diagnosis, inform patient prognosis, and predict response to therapy. This requirement for expansive datasets mandates the creation of large databases through which data may be mined and patterns may be discovered. An intermediate step toward the described radiomic analysis is the use of quantitative MR imaging techniques for characterization of disease aggressiveness in kidney cancer. Understanding the correlation between these quantitative techniques and histopathologic, metabolic, and genetic conditions will facilitate the implementation of radiomic analyses. Here we discuss some of these techniques for evaluation of patients with renal masses in general, localized kidney cancer, and locally advanced and/or metastatic kidney cancer.

RADIOMICS IN THE PRETREATMENT ASSESSMENT OF RENAL MASSES

Intratumor heterogeneity presents a challenge in the preoperative assessment of renal masses. Percutaneous biopsy is an invasive procedure with excellent accuracy for the diagnosis of kidney cancer. However, biopsies are limited by the inability to sample every part of the tumor or at multiple time points, potentially limiting the accurate characterization of renal masses (ie, subtyping, tumor grading). MR imaging is well-suited for a comprehensive evaluation of renal masses, particularly with its ability to provide quantitative and functional assessments, such as diffusion-weighted imaging (DWI), arterial spin labeling (ASL), and DCE imaging. MR imaging may also be used at multiple time points without the drawback of radiation exposure, allowing renal masses to be followed over time to detect changes in lesion characteristics, which may reflect changes in tumor histology and aggressiveness.

Radiomics for Subtyping of Renal Masses

The noninvasive characterization of renal masses using qualitative features on MR imaging has been well-described.[14–16] The more common subtypes of RCC can be differentiated primarily using a combination of T2-weighted and postcontrast imaging. Clear cell RCC (ccRCC), the most common and aggressive subtype, most often exhibits hyperintense signal on T2-weighted images and avid enhancement, in addition to intravoxel fat. In contrast, papillary RCC tends to show hypointense signal on T2-weighted imaging and show low-level enhancement. Finally, chromophobe RCC can demonstrate variable signal intensity relative to renal parenchyma on T2-weighted images and show moderate enhancement.

Quantitative assessment of renal mass enhancement is not just an academic exercise. Indeed, there are several clinical scenarios where these measures can have substantial impact on patient management.[17] Therefore, attention to the acquisition technique and standardization across patients is important.[18] For example, a high arterial-to-delay enhancement ratio (>1.5) on multiphasic contrast-enhanced MR imaging, combined with homogeneous low signal intensity on T2-weighted images, has a sensitivity of 73% and specificity of 99% in distinguishing an angiomyolipoma without visible fat (ie, fat-poor angiomyolipoma [fpAML]) from RCC.[19] Quantification of contrast enhancement on multiphasic contrast-enhanced MRI can play a complementary role to tissue biopsies in patients presenting with locally advanced and/or synchronous metastatic disease at diagnosis and can assist in the selection of optimal therapy for these patients (**Fig. 3**).

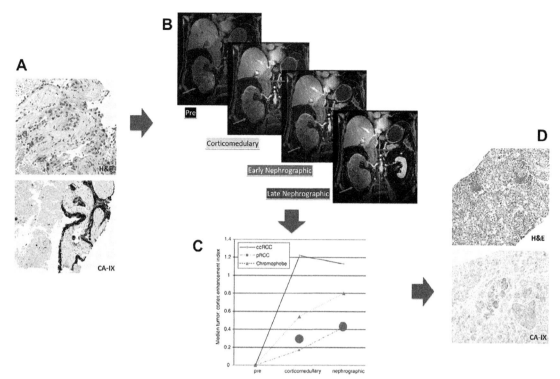

Fig. 3. Use of tumor enhancement characteristics on MR imaging to guide treatment. Biopsy of a renal mass (*A*) in a patient presenting with a large tumor and inferior vena cava (IVC) thrombus and synchronous pulmonary metastasies. The biopsy specimen was largely necrotic with only a small foci of high-grade tumor with some clearing of cytoplasm present on hematoxylin and eosin staining (*top*) exhibiting positive membranous staining with CAIX (*bottom*). The tumor was positive for PAX8 (not shown). The possibility of clear cell renal cell carcinoma (RCC) was considered and antiangiogenic therapy with sunitinib was recommended. MR imaging was performed to assess the possibility of debulking nephrectomy. Multiphasic contrast-enhanced MR imaging (*B*) showed a large right renal mass and IVC thrombus, both exhibiting very low-level progressive enhancement. A quantitative analysis of the renal mass enhancement relative to the renal cortex (*C*) was performed and found to be 35% and 42% during the corticomedullary and nephrographic phases, respectively. These enhancement characteristics would not be typical of clear cell RCC (ccRCC), and more suggestive of a papillary histology. Based on MR imaging findings, a repeat biopsy was performed (*D*) demonstrating tubulo-papillary architecture (*top*) with microcalcifications, negative CAIX stain (*bottom*) and strong CK7 and racemase (not shown). Final diagnosis was high-grade papillary RCC (pRCC) and treatment recommendation was changed to temsirolimus. CAIX, carbonic anhydrase IX protein. ([C] *From* Sun MR, Ngo L, Genega EM, et al. Renal cell carcinoma: dynamic contrast-enhanced MR imaging for differentiation of tumor subtypes–correlation with pathologic findings. Radiology 2009;250(3):800; with permission).

Quantitative assessment with DWI may be useful in assisting with characterizing renal masses as well. Signal on DWI depends on the motion of water molecules in the extracellular space and provides a noninvasive assessment of tissue cellularity, integrity of cell membranes, and microcapillary perfusion. Overall, malignant solid renal masses are reported to demonstrate lower apparent diffusion coefficient (ADC) values than benign lesions.[20] Using qualitative features alone, renal oncocytomas exhibit imaging features that may overlap with subtypes of RCC, particularly ccRCC and chromophobe RCC. A metaanalysis of DWI of renal lesions, however, described ADC

values for renal oncocytomas tend to be higher ($2 \pm 0.08 \times 10^{-3}$ mm^2/s) than RCC ($1.5 \pm 0.08 \times 10^{-3}$ mm^2/s). For example, Taouli and colleagues[21] reported significantly higher ADC values for renal oncocytomas (mean ADC, $1.91 \pm 0.97 \times 10^{-3}$ mm^2/s) than solid RCCs (mean ADC, $1.54 \pm 0.69 \times 10^{-3}$ mm^2/s).

Nevertheless, absolute ADC values are affected by numerous factors and may vary between MR systems and field strengths. Histogram analyses may help to overcome these limitations and provide a more reliable quantitative assessment, because distribution parameters are independent of signal intensity. A histogram analysis of DWI features may be used to differentiate benign from malignant neoplasms, because histogram-based assessment provides the benefit of quantitatively assessing the heterogeneity characteristically exhibited by ccRCC. Gaing and colleagues[22] used whole lesion histogram analysis of intravoxel incoherent motion (IVIM) on renal lesions, and of the distribution parameters, kurtosis (ie, a measure of flatness of the histogram) of the perfusion fraction was the only variable to distinguish renal oncocytomas from ccRCC. These authors also found that the mean and standard deviation of tissue diffusivity and kurtosis of perfusion fraction could distinguish ccRCC from fpAML. Histogram analysis of contrast enhancement patterns has been used to differentiate among different renal masses as well. Chandarana and colleagues[23] found the histogram distribution parameters of kurtosis and skewness on contrast-enhanced MR imaging

acquisitions to be significantly different between ccRCC and papillary RCC.

Textural analyses have also been used on CT to predict histologic subtypes and grade. On portal venous phase images, entropy, a measure of histogram uniformity, and standard deviation correlate positively with ccRCC subtype on whole lesion analyses.[24] In the same study, an association between texture features and survival measures, including overall survival and time to disease recurrence, was seen with the histogram distribution parameters of standard deviation, mean, and entropy on unenhanced CT images. Global heterogeneity features, including run-length nonuniformity and gray-level nonuniformity, were significantly greater for sarcomatoid RCC tumors, an aggressive differentiation of RCC associated with a poor prognosis, when compared with non-sarcomatoid ccRCC.[25]

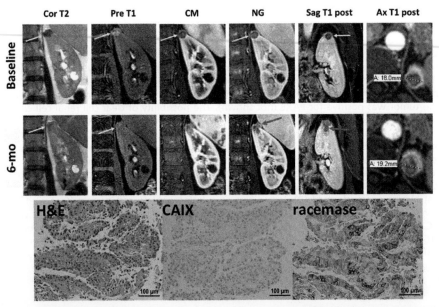

Fig. 4. Aggressive behavior detected by change in the imaging phenotype in small renal mass. A 48-year-old woman with an incidentally detected small renal mass. Baseline MR imaging examination (*top row*) shows a well-encapsulated, round, 1.8-cm renal mass in the upper pole of the left kidney (*yellow arrow*) with homogeneous low signal intensity on coronal T2-weighted single shot fast spin echo image (Cor T2), high signal intensity on coronal precontrast T1-weighted fat-saturated spoiled gradient echo images (Pre T1), and low-level progressive enhancement on same images acquired during the corticomedulary (CM), early nephrographic (NG), and sagittal images during excretory phase after administration of 0.1 mmol/kg body weight of gadobutrol. MR imaging findings are consistent with papillary renal cell carcinoma. The patient remained asymptomatic and follow-up MR imaging examination 6 months later (*middle row*) shows a change in signal intensity on coronal Cor T2 and (Pre T1) images (*yellow arrows*). Importantly, postcontrast images demonstrate an interval change in tumor shape now infiltrating the perirenal fat (NG, *red arrow*) and renal parenchyma (Sag T1 post, *red arrow*) despite minimal change in size (1.9 cm on an axial T1-weighted postcontrast image). Percutaneous biopsy (*bottom row*) obtained before percutaneous ablation confirmed high-grade (International Society of Urological Pathology grade 3 out of 4) papillary renal cell carcinoma, type II. Ax T1 post, axial delayed postcontrast T1-weighted; CAIX, carbonic anhydrase IX protein; H&E, hematoxylin and eosin.

Future Role for Radiomics in Predicting Tumor Biology

Over the past decade, the incidence of incidentally detected renal masses has increased with the majority of those made up of small renal masses ($\leq$4 cm).[1] Approximately 20% of these masses are benign and many others exhibit an indolent growth pattern. In patients with comorbidities and increased surgical risk, active surveillance may be pursued as a management option. In this setting, the prediction of tumor grade within each specific subtype of RCC would be an essential part in the assessment of renal lesions. Furthermore, a non-invasive method to further assess changes in histopathologic and molecular tumor characteristics on subsequent follow-up imaging that predict a change in oncologic behavior would be of great value in managing these patients. As tumors undergo transformation from a low-grade neoplasm to a high-grade and aggressive tumor, detection of these changes would allow for early intervention, before the tumor acquires the ability to metastasize or invade locally (**Fig. 4**). This transformation is likely the result of changes in genetic and metabolic alterations, which are difficult to determine in clinical practice owing to the impracticality of performing multiple serial biopsies, so a method to assess for this change noninvasively, such as liquid biopsies or imaging, would radically transform the management of patients undergoing active surveillance.

Ideally, such imaging methods would rely on robust, reproducible imaging techniques. The described variability of MR imaging protocols, sequences, and hardware challenge this concept. T2-weighted single-shot fast spin echo acquisitions, however, are known to be robust and reliable in most state-of-the-art MR imaging scanners and, therefore, could be an optimal candidate for radiomics. Texture analysis of T2-weighted single-shot fast spin echo images may be helpful in predicting tumor grade in ccRCC (**Fig. 5**). Similarly, texture features on T2-weighted images have been shown to be predictive of molecular alterations in other tumors such as glioblastomas.[26]

Quantitative MR imaging techniques have been explored to evaluate for imaging features that may correlate with histologic and metabolic features. Insight into the von Hippel-Lindau tumor suppressor gene (*VHL*) and its importance in regulation of the hypoxia pathway was revolutionary in understanding the tumor biology of ccRCC. Mutation/inactivation of *VHL* result in the unregulated expression of hypoxia response elements and ultimately angiogenesis, which has been described to be associated with ccRCC prognosis and ability to metastasize.[27,28] An imaging technique that can estimate tumor microvascular density may provide a noninvasive method to assess tumor angiogenesis and perhaps aggressiveness. ASL is one such potential technique, which uses arterial blood protons to assess tissue perfusion without the use of an exogenous contrast agent. Tumor perfusion estimated by ASL imaging has been shown to correlate with microvessel density on histopathology both in human samples and RCC xenografts.[29-31] In human studies of ccRCC, ASL was able to detect intratumoral heterogeneity within a single tumor by showing areas with different degrees of tissue perfusion, which correlate with differences in microvessel density and tumor cellularity on histologic assessment.[30,32]

Multiecho Dixon-based MR imaging, which uses a chemical shift technique to detect and

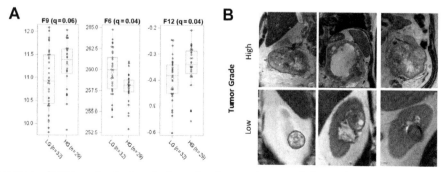

Fig. 5. Extraction of MR imaging texture features for characterization of clear cell renal cell carcinoma. Haralick features extracted from T2-weighted single-shot turbo spin echo (*A*) MR imaging exhibiting a statistically significant correlation with histopathologic tumor grade. Representative examples of tumors with high and low entropy on T2-weighted images (*B*) and high and low tumor grade at histopathology. F6 = sum average. F9, entropy; F12, information measures of correlation; HG, high grade (International Society of Urological Pathology grade 3–4 out of 4); LG, low grade (International Society of Urological Pathology grade 1–2 out of 4); q, false discovery rate.

quantify lipid, has been used as a noninvasive method to assess the metabolic features of ccRCC. Alterations in lipid metabolism result in the storage of lipids in intracytoplasmic vacuoles, characteristically manifested on imaging as decreased signal intensity on T1-weighted opposed-phase images relative to in-phase images. Furthermore, ccRCC expresses high levels of enzymes necessary to produce fatty acids and lipids, and 2 of these, fatty acid synthase and stearoyl-CoA desaturase, are associated with a poor prognosis.[33,34] Multiecho Dixon acquisitions with multipeak fat spectral modeling provide a method to further quantify the presence of fat by providing a fat fraction (FF)—MR imaging signal arising from fat relative to the total MR imaging signal (ie, fat plus water).[35]

Zhang and colleagues[36] reported that FF quantification provided by Dixon MR imaging correlated with intracellular lipid at histopathology. ccRCCs showed heterogeneous accumulation of fat independent of tumor grade, although the most aggressive tumors (International Society of Urological Pathology grade 4/4) exhibited a statistical significant decrease in FF compared with grade 3 tumors. FF measures in ccRCC also correlated positively with triglyceride levels in tumor samples and negatively with phosphoethanolamine, a predominantly membrane-localized lipid; the latter finding is consistent with previous reports suggesting that the downregulation of the phosphoethanolamine pathway is another significant feature promoting growth in ccRCC.[37]

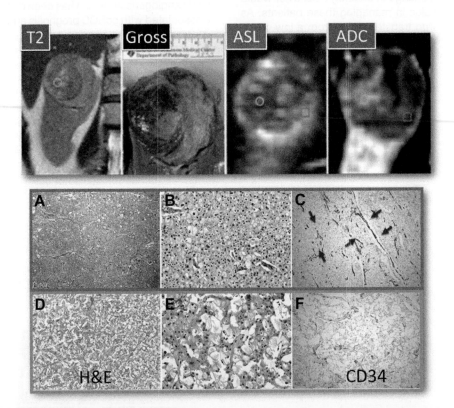

Fig. 6. Quantitative MR imaging techniques for the evaluation of the tumor microenvironment in chromophobe renal cell carcinoma. Coronal T2-weighted single-shot turbo spin echo (T2), gross specimen sectioned in the same anatomic plane after nephrectomy (gross image), and corresponding coronal arterial spin labeling perfusion map (ASL) and apparent diffusion coefficient map (ADC) in the same location of the tumor are shown in the top panel. The bottom panel shows low (A, D; original magnification ×10) and high (B, E; original magnification ×200) magnification hematoxylin and eosin (H&E) stains and CD34 immunohistochemistry (C, F; original magnification ×200) slides corresponding with the tumor areas indicated on the MR imaging by the red square (top row) and green circle (bottom row). Areas with high flow on arterial spin labeling (red square) also have marked restricted diffusion (ie, low apparent diffusion coefficient) and this finding correlates with increased cellularity (B) and microvascular density (blue arrows, C). In contrast, areas with low flow on arterial spin labeling (green circle) have increased diffusion (ie, high apparent diffusion coefficient), indicating increased motion of water, which is likely the result of ischemia-induced damage leading to the presence of cell membrane defects (E, yellow arrows). Decreased vascularity is also noted in the same area of the tumor (F). HG, high grade; LG, low grade.

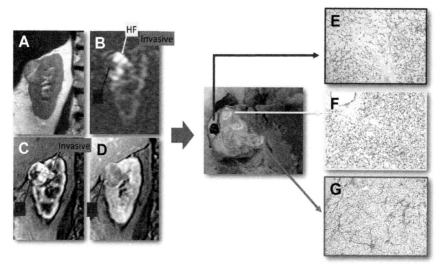

Fig. 7. Multiparametric MR imaging as a platform to detect intratumor histologic heterogeneity in vivo. Coronal T2-weighted single shot fast spin echo (*A*), arterial spin labeled (ASL) difference image (*B*), and T1-weighted gradient echo images acquired during the corticomedullary (*C*) and delayed (*D*) phases of a dynamic contrast-enhanced acquisition. After nephrectomy, tumor specimen (*center*) was sectioned with the help of fiducial markers placed during surgery in a coronal plane matching the anatomic location of the MR imaging images. Tumor samples were obtained in areas colocalized to regions of high flow (HF), low flow (LF), and invasive component on MR imaging. Histopathologic analysis of these samples revealed clear cell renal cell carcinoma (International Society of Urological Pathology grade 3 out of 4). Note the differences in tumor architecture; a small acinar pattern with the more hyalinized stroma in the LF region (*E*), prototypical ("classic") clear cell renal cell carcinoma with a small acinar pattern and thin arborizing vasculature in the high flow region (*F*), and a different trabecular pattern in the invasive area (*G*).

Several studies have also described the use of ADC values to differentiate low-grade from high-grade ccRCC. Using an ADC cut-off of 1.20×10^{-3} mm^2/s, a group reported a sensitivity and specificity of 0.65 and 0.96, respectively.[38] Another report indicated a sensitivity and specificity of 0.90 and 0.71, respectively, when using an ADC cut-off of 1.87×10^{-3} mm^2/s.[39]

These MR imaging techniques may be useful in patients on active surveillance where increases in tumor perfusion, changes in intratumor fat, and/or decrease in ADC may indicate evolution of the tumor toward a more aggressive phenotype. A better understanding of the correlation of MR imaging quantitative measures with histopathologic findings is crucial to adopt these biomarkers in the assessment of patients with renal masses (**Fig. 6**).

Studies have also evaluated the use of quantitative and qualitative imaging features on CT to predict genetic mutations in RCC. Qualitative features of ccRCC including ill-defined tumor margins, calcifications, and renal vein invasion have been reported to correlate with mutations in BRCA1-associated protein 1, which is known to be associated with high-grade ccRCC.[40,41] Jamshidi and colleagues[42] reported the construction of a predictive image phenotype-based system, using 28 imaging features on CT that correlate with a previously reported supervised principal component (SPC) risk score. The SPC risk score is a quantitative multigene assay consisting of 259 genes that predict poor prognosis in ccRCC. They composed a radiogenomic risk score using 4 of the 28 traits, including the pattern of tumor necrosis, tumor transition zone, tumor–parenchyma interactions, and tumor–parenchyma interface, that demonstrated a significant association with the SPC risk score. Importantly, the radiogenomic risk score performed similarly to the SPC score in the differentiation of aggressive from more indolent disease in a training set and a validation cohort,

Quantitative multiparametric MR imaging protocols can be used to create objective composite phenotypes of the tumor. These phenotypes can be used to study histologic heterogeneity (**Fig. 7**). Colocalization of imaging features in vivo with pathology and molecular analysis requires however careful coregistration of patient imaging with tissue specimens. This goal can be achieved with in vivo segmentation of tumors based on imaging datasets and subsequent creation of a physical mold using state-of-the-art 3-dimensional

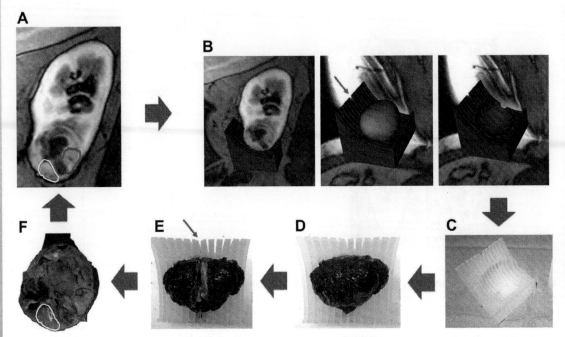

Fig. 8. Registration of imaging and pathology specimens for radiogenomic analysis. (*A*) Coronal contrast-enhanced three-dimensional (3D) gradient echo image of a renal mass in the lower pole of the right kidney. (*B*) After segmentation of the tumor, a virtual 3D mold is created. Note an indentation in the 3D mold (*arrow*), corresponding to the anatomic location of the coronal MRI image displayed in A. (*C*) Creation of the physical mold with 3D printing technology. (*D*) After partial nephrectomy, the specimen is oriented and placed within the 3D mold. (*E*) The surgical specimen is sectioned using the indentation in the 3D mold (*arrow*). (*F*) A near per-fect co-localization of the surgical specimen and MRI imaging is achieved allowing the sampling of specific areas in the tumor and subsequent correlation of tumor features on MRI with histopathology and other tissue based analysis (e.g. radiogenomics, radiometabolomics, etc).

printing technology.[43] The 3-dimensional molds are then used to orient and section the tissue specimen after surgical resection so that samples of the tumor colocalized to imaging findings can be obtained (**Fig. 8**).

MR elastography is a relatively new technology that allows to quantitate the biomechanical prop-erties of tissue (ie, stiffness) and has been vali-dated in the detection and estimation of liver fibrosis.[44] This technique can be also applied to assess the tissue properties in renal tumors. Of special interest is the detection of fibromuscular stroma in ccRCC. The presence of fibromuscular stroma has been reported in both low-grade tu-mors (*TCEB1* mutated) and high-grade tumors (without *TCEB1* mutation)[45] (**Fig. 9**).

RADIOMICS IN THE POSTTREATMENT ASSESSMENT OF RENAL CELL CARCINOMA

In routine clinical practice, imaging is used to monitor for treatment response in patients under-going systemic therapy. Several criteria have been produced to assess for response in the oncologic setting, such as the Response Evaluation Criteria in Solid Tumors (RECIST) criteria. However, traditional size-based response criteria do not incorporate early predictors of response, and size measurements alone may not be sufficient to assess response with antiangio-genic therapies. Additionally, a method to predict response before initiating therapy would be a step toward providing personalized medicine.

Assessment of tissue perfusion via ASL and DCE MR imaging has been evaluated as a method to predict response and outcome in patients with metastatic ccRCC. These quantitative MR imaging sequences depict changes in tissue perfusion/permeability early after the initiation of therapy. Treatment with tyrosine kinase inhibitors de-creases the vessel density of tumors on histologic analysis, and this change correlates with de-creases in vessel permeability on DCE analyses.[46] In patients with metastatic ccRCC receiving sora-fenib, significant decreases in tumor vascular permeability on DCE MR imaging manifest as changes in the transfer constant K_{trans}. Early changes in K_{trans} at 3 to 12 weeks after initiation of therapy and decrease tumor size at 12 weeks correlated with progression-free survival.[47] In a

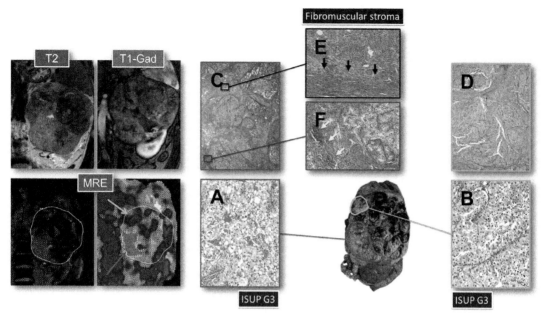

Fig. 9. MR elastography (MRE) for the characterization of tissue properties in renal tumors. Coronal T2-weighted single-shot fast spin echo image (T2) and contrast-enhanced T1-weighted gradient echo image (T1-Gad) acquired during the corticomedulary phase of a dynamic contrast-enhanced acquisition and corresponding magnitude and stiffness map from an MRE acquisition performed at the same anatomic level. Note an area of increased stiffness in the lower medial aspect of the mass (*red arrow*) compared with a relatively softer area in the upper medial aspect of the mass (*light blue arrow*). After nephrectomy, tumor specimen (*right panel*) was sectioned with the help of fiducial markers placed during surgery in a coronal plane matching the anatomic location of the MR images. Histopathologic assessment of both areas indicated by the red and light blue regions of interest (ROIs), which correspond with the *red* and *light blue arrows* on MRE, demonstrated no obvious differences in the International Society of Urological Pathology grade (ISUP grade 3 out of 4) of clear cell carcinoma (*A, B*; original magnification ×200). Histopathologic images at lower magnification; however, show obvious morphologic/architectural differences between both tumor areas (*C, D*; original magnification ×10). Detailed analysis of the tumor region within red ROI (ie, area of increased stiffness) confirms the presence of nodular fibrosis (*black arrows, E*; original magnification ×100) and smooth muscle in the stroma (*yellow arrows, F*; original magnification ×100). The presence of fibromuscular stroma explains the increase stiffness detected by MRE.

mouse model of RCC, after the initiation of sorafenib, changes in tissue perfusion with ASL were detected within 3 days of therapy,[31] and histopathologic findings of decreased microvascular density also correlated with decreased perfusion on ASL. In patients with metastatic RCC receiving antiangiogenic therapy, decreasing tumor blood flow on ASL seen as early as 1 month after the initiation of therapy were shown to be associated with subsequent changes in tumor size.[48] Changes in tumor perfusion can be detected by ASL 2 weeks after initiation of antiangiogenic therapy.[49]

Studies have also evaluated the use of imaging features on CT to predict response to therapeutic agents. Smith and colleagues[50] used a custom postprocessing software and algorithm to develop a novel system to quantify changes in the amount of vascularized tumor within specific attenuation thresholds, termed the vascular tumor burden. This semiautomated biomarker, in addition to other tumor metrics, such as length,

area, and mean attenuation, were used to predict response to antiangiogenic therapy with sunitinib. Changes in the vascular tumor burden metric on initial posttherapy imaging after the initiation of sunitinib showed a better separation of progression free survival between nonresponders and responders compared with other commonly used response criteria changes in tumor metrics, including length, area, mean attenuation, RECIST, CHOI, modified CHOI, MASS, and 10% sum long diameter. Goh and colleagues[51] also used textural analysis on CT imaging to assess for treatment response after 2 cycles of treatment on a tyrosine kinase inhibitor. Using arterial phase images, regions of interest were placed on CT images on all metastases at baseline and after 2 cycles of treatment to calculate absolute and percentage changes in image entropy and uniformity. Both baseline entropy and uniformity were significantly correlated with time to progression. Additionally, the percent change in uniformity was found to be an independent predictor of time to progression.

SUMMARY

Renal cell carcinoma (RCC) exhibits a heterogeneous disease spectrum, which may confound patient management and accurate image interpretation. Semiquantitative and quantitative analyses of MR imaging data can aid in the characterization of this disease. Quantitative MR imaging acquisitions and radiomic analysis provide a method to address heterogeneity for better tumor characterization. Extension of radiomic analysis through radiogenomics, radiometabolomics, and correlation with other epidemiologic, clinical, and tissue-based datasets have the potential to improve patient management in the era of personalized medicine. Understanding what these technologies can offer will allow radiologists to play a larger role in the care of patients with RCC.

REFERENCES

1. Weikert S, Ljungberg B. Contemporary epidemiology of renal cell carcinoma: perspectives of primary prevention. World J Urol 2010;28(3):247–52.
2. Durinck S, Stawiski EW, Pavia-Jimenez A, et al. Spectrum of diverse genomic alterations define non-clear cell renal carcinoma subtypes. Nat Genet 2015;47(1):13–21.
3. Gerlinger M, Rowan AJ, Horswell S, et al. Intratumor heterogeneity and branched evolution revealed by multiregion sequencing. N Engl J Med 2012; 366(10):883–92.
4. Gillies RJ, Kinahan PE, Hricak H. Radiomics: images are more than pictures, they are data. Radiology 2016;278(2):563–77.
5. Aerts H. Data science in radiology: a path forward. Clin Cancer Res 2018;24(3):532–4.
6. Mackin D, Fave X, Zhang L, et al. Measuring computed tomography scanner variability of radiomics features. Invest Radiol 2015;50(11):757–65.
7. Yang X, Knopp MV. Quantifying tumor vascular heterogeneity with dynamic contrast-enhanced magnetic resonance imaging: a review. J Biomed Biotechnol 2011;2011:732848.
8. Buckler AJ, Bresolin L, Dunnick NR, et al. A collaborative enterprise for multi-stakeholder participation in the advancement of quantitative imaging. Radiology 2011;258(3):906–14.
9. Chang YC, Ackerstaff E, Tschudi Y, et al. Delineation of tumor habitats based on dynamic contrast enhanced MRI. Sci Rep 2017;7(1):9746.
10. Rios Velazquez E, Aerts HJ, Gu Y, et al. A semiautomatic CT-based ensemble segmentation of lung tumors: comparison with oncologists' delineations and with the surgical specimen. Radiother Oncol 2012;105(2):167–73.
11. Larue RT, Defraene G, De Ruysscher D, et al. Quantitative radiomics studies for tissue characterization: a review of technology and methodological procedures. Br J Radiol 2017;90(1070):20160665.
12. Lubner MG, Smith AD, Sandrasegaran K, et al. CT texture analysis: definitions, applications, biologic correlates, and challenges. Radiographics 2017; 37(5):1483–503.
13. Haralick RM, Shanmugam K, Dinstein I. Textural features for image classification. IEEE Trans Syst Man Cybern 1973;3(6):610–21.
14. Sun MR, Ngo L, Genega EM, et al. Renal cell carcinoma: dynamic contrast-enhanced MR imaging for differentiation of tumor subtypes–correlation with pathologic findings. Radiology 2009;250(3):793–802.
15. Young JR, Coy H, Kim HJ, et al. Performance of relative enhancement on multiphasic MRI for the differentiation of clear cell renal cell carcinoma (RCC) from papillary and chromophobe RCC subtypes and oncocytoma. AJR Am J Roentgenol 2017; 208(4):812–9.
16. Wang H, Cheng L, Zhang X, et al. Renal cell carcinoma: diffusion-weighted MR imaging for subtype differentiation at 3.0 T. Radiology 2010;257(1):135–43.
17. Campbell N, Rosenkrantz AB, Pedrosa I. MRI phenotype in renal cancer: is it clinically relevant? Top Magn Reson Imaging 2014;23(2):95–115.
18. Zhang J, Pedrosa I, Rofsky NM. MR techniques for renal imaging. Radiol Clin North Am 2003;41(5): 877–907.
19. Sasiwimonphan K, Takahashi N, Leibovich BC, et al. Small (<4 cm) renal mass: differentiation of angiomyolipoma without visible fat from renal cell carcinoma utilizing MR imaging. Radiology 2012;263(1): 160–8.
20. Lassel EA, Rao R, Schwenke C, et al. Diffusion-weighted imaging of focal renal lesions: a meta-analysis. Eur Radiol 2014;24(1):241–9.
21. Taouli B, Thakur RK, Mannelli L, et al. Renal lesions: characterization with diffusion-weighted imaging versus contrast-enhanced MR imaging. Radiology 2009;251(2):398–407.
22. Gaing B, Sigmund EE, Huang WC, et al. Subtype differentiation of renal tumors using voxel-based histogram analysis of intravoxel incoherent motion parameters. Invest Radiol 2015;50(3):144–52.
23. Chandarana H, Rosenkrantz AB, Mussi TC, et al. Histogram analysis of whole-lesion enhancement in differentiating clear cell from papillary subtype of renal cell cancer. Radiology 2012;265(3):790–8.
24. Lubner MG, Stabo N, Abel EJ, et al. CT textural analysis of large primary renal cell carcinomas: pretreatment tumor heterogeneity correlates with histologic findings and clinical outcomes. AJR Am J Roentgenol 2016;207(1):96–105.

25. Schieda N, Thornhill RE, Al-Subhi M, et al. Diagnosis of sarcomatoid renal cell carcinoma with CT: evaluation by qualitative imaging features and texture analysis. AJR Am J Roentgenol 2015;204(5):1013–23.

26. Korfiatis P, Kline TL, Coufalova L, et al. MRI texture features as biomarkers to predict MGMT methylation status in glioblastomas. Med Phys 2016;43(6):2835–44.

27. Mertz KD, Demichelis F, Kim R, et al. Automated immunofluorescence analysis defines microvessel area as a prognostic parameter in clear cell renal cell cancer. Hum Pathol 2007;38(10):1454–62.

28. Iakovlev VV, Gabril M, Dubinski W, et al. Microvascular density as an independent predictor of clinical outcome in renal cell carcinoma: an automated image analysis study. Lab Invest 2012;92(1):46–56.

29. Noguchi T, Yoshiura T, Hiwatashi A, et al. Perfusion imaging of brain tumors using arterial spin-labeling: correlation with histopathologic vascular density. AJNR Am J Neuroradiol 2008;29(4):688–93.

30. Yuan Q, Kapur P, Zhang Y, et al. Intratumor heterogeneity of perfusion and diffusion in clear cell renal cell carcinoma: correlation with tumor cellularity. Clin Genitourin Cancer 2016;14(6):e585–94.

31. Schor-Bardach R, Alsop DC, Pedrosa I, et al. Does arterial spin-labeling MR imaging–measured tumor perfusion correlate with renal cell cancer response to antiangiogenic therapy in a mouse model? Radiology 2009;251(3):731–42.

32. Zhang Y, Kapur P, Yuan Q, et al. Tumor vascularity in renal masses: correlation of arterial spin-labeled and dynamic contrast-enhanced magnetic resonance imaging assessments. Clin Genitourin Cancer 2016;14(1):e25–36.

33. Horiguchi A, Asano T, Asano T, et al. Fatty acid synthase over expression is an indicator of tumor aggressiveness and poor prognosis in renal cell carcinoma. J Urol 2008;180(3):1137–40.

34. von Roemeling CA, Marlow LA, Wei JJ, et al. Stearoyl-CoA desaturase 1 is a novel molecular therapeutic target for clear cell renal cell carcinoma. Clin Cancer Res 2013;19(9):2368–80.

35. Reeder SB, McKenzie CA, Pineda AR, et al. Water-fat separation with IDEAL gradient-echo imaging. J Magn Reson Imaging 2007;25(3):644–52.

36. Zhang Y, Udayakumar D, Cai L, et al. Addressing metabolic heterogeneity in clear cell renal cell carcinoma with quantitative Dixon MRI. JCI Insight 2017; 2(15) [pii:94278].

37. Saito K, Arai E, Maekawa K, et al. Lipidomic signatures and associated transcriptomic profiles of clear cell renal cell carcinoma. Sci Rep 2016;6:28932.

38. Rosenkrantz AB, Niver BE, Fitzgerald EF, et al. Utility of the apparent diffusion coefficient for distinguishing clear cell renal cell carcinoma of low and high nuclear grade. AJR Am J Roentgenol 2010;195(5):W344–51.

39. Sandrasegaran K, Sundaram CP, Ramaswamy R, et al. Usefulness of diffusion-weighted imaging in the evaluation of renal masses. AJR American journal of roentgenology 2010;194(2):438–45.

40. Shinagare AB, Vikram R, Jaffe C, et al. Radiogenomics of clear cell renal cell carcinoma: preliminary findings of the cancer genome atlas-renal cell carcinoma (TCGA-RCC) imaging research group. Abdom Imaging 2015;40(6):1684–92.

41. Karlo CA, Di Paolo PL, Chaim J, et al. Radiogenomics of clear cell renal cell carcinoma: associations between CT imaging features and mutations. Radiology 2014;270(2):464–71.

42. Jamshidi N, Jonasch E, Zapala M, et al. The radiogenomic risk score: construction of a prognostic quantitative, noninvasive image-based molecular assay for renal cell carcinoma. Radiology 2015;277(1):114–23.

43. Dwivedi DK, Chatzinoff Y, Zhang Y, et al. Development of a patient-specific tumor mold using magnetic resonance imaging and 3-dimensional printing technology for targeted tissue procurement and radiomics analysis of renal masses. Urology 2018;112:209–14.

44. Venkatesh SK, Yin M, Ehman RL. Magnetic resonance elastography of liver: technique, analysis, and clinical applications. J Magn Reson Imaging 2013;37(3):544–55.

45. Favazza L, Chitale DA, Barod R, et al. Renal cell tumors with clear cell histology and intact VHL and chromosome 3p: a histological review of tumors from the Cancer Genome Atlas database. Mod Pathol 2017;30(11):1603–12.

46. Drevs J, Muller-Driver R, Wittig C, et al. PTK787/ZK 222584, a specific vascular endothelial growth factor-receptor tyrosine kinase inhibitor, affects the anatomy of the tumor vascular bed and the functional vascular properties as detected by dynamic enhanced magnetic resonance imaging. Cancer Res 2002;62(14):4015–22.

47. Flaherty KT, Rosen MA, Heitjan DF, et al. Pilot study of DCE-MRI to predict progression-free survival with sorafenib therapy in renal cell carcinoma. Cancer Biol Ther 2008;7(4):496–501.

48. de Bazelaire C, Alsop DC, George D, et al. Magnetic resonance imaging-measured blood flow change after antiangiogenic therapy with PTK787/ZK 222584 correlates with clinical outcome in metastatic renal cell carcinoma. Clin Cancer Res 2008;14(17):5540–54.

49. Pedrosa I, Alsop DC, Rofsky NM. Magnetic resonance imaging as a biomarker in renal cell carcinoma. Cancer 2009;115(10 Suppl):2334–45.

50. Smith AD, Zhang X, Bryan J, et al. Vascular tumor burden as a new quantitative CT biomarker for predicting metastatic RCC response to antiangiogenic therapy. Radiology 2016;281(2):484–98.

51. Goh V, Ganeshan B, Nathan P, et al. Assessment of response to tyrosine kinase inhibitors in metastatic renal cell cancer: CT texture as a predictive biomarker. Radiology 2011;261(1):165–71.

Tumors of Renal Collecting Systems, Renal Pelvis, and Ureters

Role of MR Imaging and MR Urography Versus Computed Tomography Urography

Eric Zeikus, MD[a],*, Giri Sura, PhD, MD[b],
Nicole Hindman, MD[c], Julia R. Fielding, MD[b]

KEYWORDS

- MR urography • CT urography • Urothelial carcinoma kidney • Urothelial carcinoma ureter

KEY POINTS

- Computed tomography (CT) urography is the single best examination for comprehensive evaluation of the upper urinary tract.
- MR urography is an appropriate substitute for CT urography when there are contraindications to CT, including both ionizing radiation (young patients, pregnancy, serial examinations) and iodinated contrast (renal insufficiency, allergic reaction).
- Because transitional cell carcinoma is so uncommon in young, nonsmoking patients, MR urography or ultrasound may serve as an appropriate screening study following a negative renal colic CT examination.

INTRODUCTION

Magnetic resonance urography (MRU) and computed tomography urography (CTU) are useful tools that provide a comprehensive assessment of the renal parenchyma, renal collecting systems, and ureters.[1] Cystoscopy remains the reference standard for bladder evaluation, which is not discussed here.[2,3] This article reviews the indications and optimal technique for MRU and CTU. The appearance of benign and malignant disease is also reviewed.

BACKGROUND

CTU has become the most frequently used screening test for upper urinary tract tumors because of its widespread availability, short imaging time, and high spatial resolution. It is the reference standard for evaluation of the upper urinary tract.[3,4] Drawbacks include use of iodinated contrast, which can exacerbate renal insufficiency and cause allergic-type reactions. CTU also imparts a relatively high level of ionizing radiation exposure, which is undesirable in the setting of pregnancy, pediatric patients, and frequent imaging.

MRU has the benefits of improved soft tissue resolution, absence of ionizing radiation, and a greater safety profile for intravenous contrast agents due in part to lower doses relative to CTU.[5–7] Disadvantages include long scan times, more limited availability, and difficulties due to

The authors have nothing to disclose.
[a] UT Southwestern University Hospitals, 5323 Harry Hines Boulevard, Dallas, TX 75390-8827, USA; [b] Abdominal Imaging Division, UT Southwestern University Hospitals, 5323 Harry Hines Boulevard, Dallas, TX 75390-8827, USA; [c] Department of Radiology, Abdominal Imaging Section, NYU Langone Health, 660 First Avenue, Third Floor, New York, NY 10016, USA
* Corresponding author.
E-mail address: eric.zeikus@utsouthwestern.edu

Magn Reson Imaging Clin N Am 27 (2019) 15–32
https://doi.org/10.1016/j.mric.2018.09.002
1064-9689/19/© 2018 Elsevier Inc. All rights reserved.

imaging artifacts and respiratory motion. Diuretics are important adjuncts for the examination. Rarely, these may be associated with allergic reactions. The American College of Radiology (ACR) Contrast Manual version 10.3 reports screening for renal impairment is now optional when using a macrocyclic agent such as Gadavist (gadobutrol; Bayer, Leverkusen, Germany) or Dotarem (gadoterate meglumine; Guerbet, Villepinte, France).

IMAGING TECHNIQUES
Magnetic Resonance Urography

MRU can be performed on 1.5-T or 3.0-T systems using an identical protocol with similar results. The patient is placed in supine position with arms raised above the head if possible. External torso phased array coils are placed over the patient to cover the kidneys and bladder in a single field of view.

Adequate distention of the urinary tract is essential for evaluation of nonobstructed collecting systems. If contrast is to be administered, gadolinium chelates can cause paradoxic low signal intensity due to the T2* effect overcoming the effect of T1 shortening. This can be minimized by administration of diuretics, normal saline, or both. At our institution, 10 mg furosemide is administered intravenously 5 minutes before administration of contrast agent; 250 mL intravenous (IV) saline can be used in the setting of diuretic allergy or dehydration. If a bladder catheter is present, it is clamped before diuretic or fluid administration.

Sample protocols from our institution, including both contrast-enhanced and noncontrast MRU, are given in **Tables 1** and **2**. Both protocols include axial and coronal single-shot fast spin-echo (SSFSE) images and axial T1 in-phase and opposed-phase T1-weighted images of the abdomen, and an axial T2-weighted fast spin-echo sequence of the bladder. In noncontrast technique, additional thick slab and 3-dimensional (3D) or thin-section highly T2-sensitive MR cholangiopancreatography (MRCP)-like sequences are acquired (**Fig. 1**). If contrast is used, 0.1 mmol/kg is administered at 2 mL/s and 3D fat-saturated T1-weighted spoiled gradient echo (SPGR) images are obtained at 40 seconds, 90 seconds, and 10 minutes, usually in the coronal projection. Fat saturation can be achieved with spectral fat suppression, or Dixon technique, the latter using the water-only reconstructed images. From the delayed sequence, an MIP (maximum intensity projection) is obtained, generating an IV pyelogram (IVP)-like image (**Fig. 2**). Subtraction images also can be obtained. If the technologist notices a region with suboptimal imaging, additional images can be obtained. This is an advantage compared with CTU, in which each acquisition results in additional radiation exposure.

Computed Tomography Urography

Most CTU protocols consist of 3 phases (unenhanced, nephrographic, and excretory). Unenhanced images are obtained of the kidneys, ureters, and bladder (3-mm slice thickness, 3-mm gap); 100 mL iodinated contrast (Omnipaque 350 [iohexol], GE Healthcare Inc, Marlborough, MA or Isovue 370 [iopamidol], Bracco, Monroe Township, NJ) is then administered at 3 mL/s followed by 150 mL of 0.9 normal saline at the same rate via power injector. Nephrographic-phase images of the entire abdomen and pelvis are obtained at 100-second delay. Slice thickness is typically 3 mm, but the gap can be variable. Ten-minute delayed-phase images are obtained in the axial plane (3-mm slice thickness, 3-mm gap) of the kidneys, ureters, and bladder. Coronal and sagittal multiplanar reconstruction (MPR) images (2-mm thick, 2-mm gap) of all phases are obtained. Review of all planes is essential for detection of small urothelial lesions, particularly on the delayed-phase images. Furthermore, the delayed-phase images must be evaluated with appropriate window and level settings to detect subtle abnormalities that can be obscured by dense contrast. To reduce radiation dose, the split bolus technique optimizes contrast timing to obtain both nephrographic and excretory phases simultaneously in a single acquisition. Iterative reconstruction, low dose unenhanced scans, and dual energy strategies are other useful or promising techniques for dose reduction.

Indications

Indications for MRU and CTU include hematuria (both microscopic and macroscopic), urinary obstruction, evaluation for renal and urothelial neoplasms, and characterization of congenital abnormalities. As renal stones are the most common cause of hematuria, ultrasound or noncontrast CT are often the first tests obtained.

Both the ACR[8] and the American Urologic Association (AUA)[9] have generated recommendations for the evaluation of hematuria in adults, albeit with several important differences. Specifically, the AUA guidelines do not address radiation dose in young patients without significant risk factors or the cumulative radiation exposure of serial examinations. Summaries of the ACR and AUA recommendations are given in **Boxes 1** and **2**.

Two retrospective observational studies of large numbers of at-risk patients with hematuria reported upper tract urothelial malignancy rate

Table 1
Contrast-enhanced MR Urogram protocol

Coil: External Phased Array Torso

Plane	Sequence	Size/Gap (2D) or Slice/Interval (3D) in mm	Region/Comment	Matrix	FOV cm	TR ms	TE ms
COR	2D T2 SSFSE	6/1	Abdomen and Pelvis (K, U, B)	288 × 248	40 × 40	507	80
AX	2D T2 FSE	6/1	Pelvis	265 × 217	21 × 21	4819	120
AX	2D T1 IP/OP	6/1	Abdomen	220 × 217	33 × 40	91	2.3/4.6
AX	2D T2 SSFSE	6/1	Abdomen	236 × 239	26 × 26	1299	80
SAG	3D T1 mDIXON Pre	3/1.5	Left Kidney Single Phase	200 × 210	30 × 31	5.9	1.8/4.0
SAG	3D T1 mDIXON Pre	3/1.5	Right Kidney Single Phase	200 × 210	30 × 31	5.9	1.8/4
CLAMP BLADDER CATHETER IF PRESENT 10 mg IV furosemide given slowly over 1 min prior to dynamic contrast enhanced sequences							
COR	3D T1 mDIXON Dynamic	3/1.5	Abdomen and Pelvis Pre 40 sec 90 sec 10 min	176 × 173	35 × 35	5.8	1.80/4
SAG	3D T1 mDIXON Post	3/1.5	Left Kidney Single phase	200 × 210	30 × 31	5.9	1.8/4
SAG	3D T1 mDIXON Post	3/1.5	Right Kidney Single phase	200 × 210	30 × 31	5.9	1.8/4
AX	3D T1 mDIXON Top	3/1.5	Single Phase Abdomen	176 × 160	35 × 31	5.9	1.8/4
AX	3D T1 mDIXON Bottom	3/1.5	Single Phase Pelvis	176 × 160	35 × 31	5.9	1.8/4
COR	3D T1 SPGR	3/1.5	Flip Angle = 40° 10 min delay	176 × 160	35 × 35	20	4.6

Scan time: 13 min
Total table time: 45 min
Abbreviations: AX, Axial; COR, Coronal; DYN, dynamic; LSAG, Left sagittal; mDIXON, T1 spoiled gradient recalled echo with 2 point Dixon technique; Pre, pre-contrast; Post, post-contrast; RSAG, Right sagittal; XL, extra large.

Table 2
Non-contrast MR Urogram protocol

Coil: External Phased Array Torso

Plane	Sequence	Size/Gap (2D) or Slice/Interval (3D) in mm	Region/Comment	Matrix	FOV cm	TR ms	TE ms
CLAMP BLADDER CATHETER IF PRESENT							
10 mg IV furosemide given slowly over 1 min at beginning of examination							
COR	2D T2 SSFSE	6/1	Abdomen and Pelvis (K, U, B)	288 × 248	40 × 40	507	80
SAG	3D T2 FSE	4/2	Pelvis	200 × 145	20 × 20	2000	200
AX	2D T2 SSFSE	5/1	Abdomen	236 × 239	26 × 26	1299	80
AX	2D T2 SSFSE	5/1	Pelvis	265 × 217	21 × 21	4819	120
AX	3D T1 mDIXON Top	3/1.5	Abdomen	176 × 160	35 × 31	5.9	1.8/4
AX	3D T1 mDIXON Bottom	2/1	Pelvis	176 × 160	35 × 31	5.9	1.8/4
SAG	2D T2 fs SSFSE	4/0.4	Left Kidney	200 × 210	30 × 31	5.9	1.8/4
SAG	2D T2 fs SSFSE	4/0.4	Right Kidney	200 × 210	30 × 31	5.9	1.8/4.0
AX	DWI	5/0.5	Abdomen and Pelvis	104 × 121	31 × 37	1411	61
COR	3D T1 mDIXON	3/1.5	Abdomen and Pelvis	176 × 173	35 × 35	5.8	1.80/4
RAD	2D T2 SSFSE Thick Slab	40/0	MRCP-like	320 × 256	30 × 30	8000	800
COR	3D T2 SSFSE Thin	2/1	MRCP-like	260 × 260	26 × 26	1024	600

Scan time: 11 min
Total table time: 30 min
Abbreviations: 2D, 2 Dimensional; 3D, 3 Dimensional; AX, Axial; COR, Coronal; DWI, Diffusion Weighted Images; FOV, Field of View; fs, Fat Suppressed; FSE, Fast Spin Echo; K, U, B, Kidneys, Ureters, Bladder; mDIXON, T1 spoiled gradient recalled echo with 2 point Dixon technique; MRCP, Magnetic Resonance Cholangiopancreatography; RAD, Radial; SAG, Sagittal; SSFSE, Single Shot Fast Spin Echo; TE, Echo Time; TR, Repetition time.

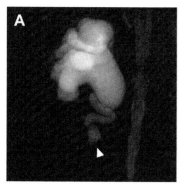
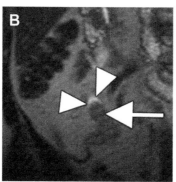
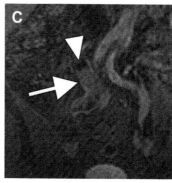

Fig. 1. A 56-year-old female smoker with gross hematuria. (*A*) Slab T2-weighted image showing severe hydro-nephrosis and ureteral tortuosity. There is a rounded filling defect (*white arrowhead*) causing obstruction. At this point, the etiology of the filling defect is uncertain. (*B, C*) Coronal SSFSE (*B*) and postcontrast T1-weighted (*C*) images demonstrate an intermediate signal intensity enhancing right ureteral mass (*white arrows*). A stone would demonstrate low signal intensity on all pulse sequences. Note the crescentic areas of high signal intensity urine at the periphery of the lesion (*white arrowheads*). This is the MR imaging equivalent of the classic "goblet" sign from IVP. Pathology revealed papillary urothelial carcinoma.

of less than 3%.[10] An older study with similar methodology reported malignancy in 10.7%.[11] Review of these studies suggests that CTU alone has a positive predictive value of approximately 50%, increased to 92% when associated with positive urine cytology. Lesions <5 mm are rarely detected.

When avoidance of ionizing radiation is paramount or there are contraindications to iodinated contrast, MRU is a reasonable alternative to CT for detection of urothelial tumors.[2,4,12–14]

Summary

- Given the low yield of CTU screening for asymptomatic hematuria in patients younger than 30 years, or without risk factors for urinary tract malignancy, ultrasound or noncontrast CT may be appropriate first-line examinations.
- When there are risk factors present for urinary tract malignancy and the patient is older than 50 years, CTU is the examination of choice.

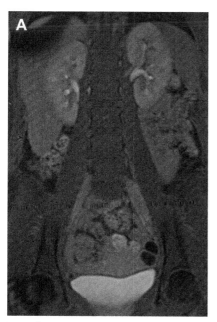
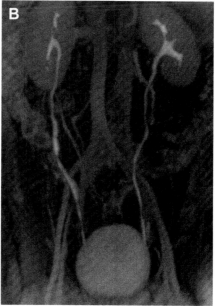

Fig. 2. (*A*) Coronal postcontrast T1-weighted image including the kidneys and bladder. The excreted contrast is uniform, without areas of T2* artifact. There is coverage of both kidneys, ureters, and bladder in the field of view. (*B*) Coronal MIP image demonstrates excellent visualization of the ureters.

MRU is a substitute for patients with contraindications to iodinated contrast, but a noncontrast CT also may be warranted to exclude calculi.

- In young patients for characterization of complex congenital abnormalities or warranting multiple serial follow-up examinations, and pregnant patients, MRU is the first-line examination.

- The combination of suspicious findings on CTU and positive urine cytology should prompt detailed urologic evaluation given the high positive predictive value of this combination.

DISEASE PROCESSES
Demographics

In 2018, there will be an estimated 81,000 new carcinoma cases in the bladder, 65,000 new cases of carcinoma of the kidney and renal pelvis, and 4000 new cases of carcinoma of the ureter and other urinary organs, resulting in approximately 17,000, 15,000, and 1000 deaths, respectively.[15] Estimates suggest that urothelial cancers account for approximately 10% to 15% of all renal tumors.[16–18] Urothelial carcinoma incidence is greatest in the sixth and seventh decades of life; the mean age at presentation is approximately 64 years. The male-to-female ratio is approximately 3:1.[19]

Risk factors for urothelial carcinoma include tobacco use, exposures to urinary carcinogens (aniline, aromatic amine, azo dyes, benzidine), cyclophosphamide therapy, and Balkan nephropathy.

Location

The vast majority of urothelial neoplasms occur in the bladder, followed by the renal pelvis, and a small minority in the ureter.[20] Based on 2018 data, and assuming 12.5% of the kidney and renal pelvis carcinomas were urothelial carcinoma, approximately 87% of urothelial carcinomas occur in the bladder, 9% occur in the renal pelvis, and approximately 4% occur in the ureter.[15] When urothelial carcinomas occur in the kidney, the most

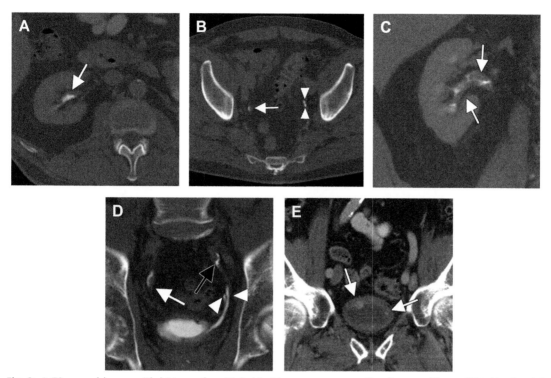

Fig. 3. A 70-year-old man with history of multiple bladder cancers presenting for surveillance CTU. (*A, B*) Axial delay-phase CT images of the right renal pelvis (*A*) and right ureter (*B*). Numerous filling defects are present (*white arrows*). Duplex left renal collecting system (*white arrowheads*). (*C, D*) Coronal MPR images through the right renal pelvis (*C*) and distal ureter (*D*) better depict the multiplicity of lesions (*white arrows*). Note the 2 ureters (*white arrowheads* in [*D*]). Atheromatous calcification mimics the left ureter (*black arrow*). (*E*) Coronal MPR image depicts 2 additional bladder lesions (*white arrows*). Pathology revealed multifocal noninvasive papillary urothelial carcinoma.

frequent site is the extrarenal portion of the pelvis, followed by the infundibulum/calyces.[21] Urothelial carcinoma of the ureter most frequently arises in the distal third (60%–75% of cases).[22]

Tumor Subtypes

Most urothelial tumors of the renal pelvis and collecting system are urothelial (transitional cell) carcinoma (85%–90%). The remaining 10% to 15% are composed of squamous cell carcinoma (9%), mucinous adenocarcinoma (1%); the remainder are extremely rare entities, including small cell undifferentiated carcinoma and carcinosarcoma. Metastatic disease is also possible.[17,18,20]

Hallmarks of urothelial carcinoma include multifocality (**Fig. 3**), and metachronous and recurrent tumors. Multicentric urothelial carcinoma is relatively common, and is associated with a worse prognosis.[23] The presence of urothelial carcinoma at one site increases risk for development at subsequent sites. The relative risk, however, is unequal. Renal pelvis or ureter urothelial carcinoma will occur in approximately 2% to 4% of patients

with bladder cancer, whereas approximately 40% (range 20%–70%) of patients with an upper tract lesion will develop a urothelial carcinoma of the bladder.[24] This higher incidence of metachronous lesions when the incident lesion is in the ureter or renal pelvis is most likely due to the far more common appearance of urothelial carcinomas in the bladder, rather than inherent differences in upper tract lesions. The metachronous tumors may develop years after the primary lesion, so regular surveillance imaging is necessary. Note that many of the series from which these data are obtained are before multidetector row CTU.

Urothelial carcinomas have papillary, invasive papillary, invasive, and carcinoma-in-situ morphologic variants. The papillary variant, accounting for more than 85% of tumors, demonstrates multiple frondlike projections and tends to be low grade; invasion beyond the mucosa is a late feature. As the lesions grow, they project into the collecting system (**Fig. 4**). The invasive lesions are sessile or nodular and tend to be of higher grade, with invasion beyond the mucosa. Invasive tumors of the renal pelvis will often invade the renal medulla.[19]

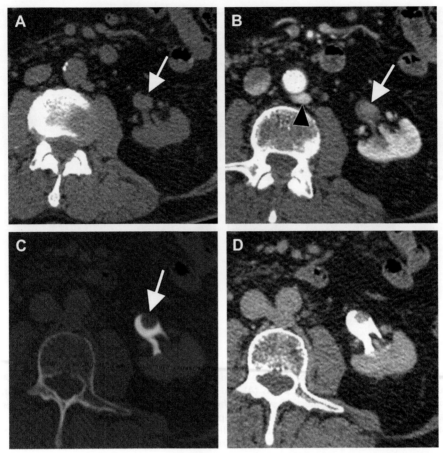

Fig. 4. An 81-year-old man with painless gross hematuria. (*A–C*) Noncontrast (*A*), nephrographic (*B*), and delay (*C*) CT images showing a smoothly marginated enhancing mass in the renal pelvis (*white arrows*). The mass is best visualized in bone window setting on delayed images. Appropriate window/level settings allow the observer to "see through" the excreted contrast. Incidental note is made of a retroaortic left renal vein (*black arrowhead* in [*B*]). (*D*) Image (*C*) in standard abdominal window/level settings. The mass is visible, but is more difficult to discern given the high attenuation of the surrounding contrast. Smaller lesions may be completely obscured. Pathology revealed noninvasive papillary urothelial carcinoma.

RADIOGRAPHIC FEATURES

All currently available imaging modalities for tumors of the renal collecting systems and ureters using excreted contrast (IVP, CT, MR imaging) rely on the same principles: visualization of filling defects, obstruction, and distortion, obliteration, and/or amputation of calyces on excretory phase imaging. MRU can also depict masses and filling defects on unenhanced images.

Renal Pelvis

Papillary urothelial tumors are visualized as filling defects, both on T2-weighted images and excretory postcontrast images, in the renal pelvis or calyces (**Fig. 5**). The masses tend to be of intermediate signal intensity on T2-weighted images and are isointense to renal parenchyma on

T1-weighted images. The presence of enhancement can be confirmed either by region of interest signal intensity comparison or subtraction sequences. It may be difficult to obtain accurate subtraction sequences in the setting of respiratory motion and other causes of misregistration. Urothelial tumors are also usually bright on diffusion-weighted images (DWI), with relatively low apparent diffusion coefficient (ADC) values.

On CTU, papillary urothelial tumors are best depicted on the delayed-phase images as filling defects within the excreted contrast column (see **Figs. 3** and **4**; **Fig. 6**). Larger lesions may visibly enhance (see **Fig. 4**), but enhancement may be difficult to detect in smaller lesions. Urothelial carcinomas frequently cause hydronephrosis. Careful windowing must be done to mitigate the extremely high density of excreted contrast on standard

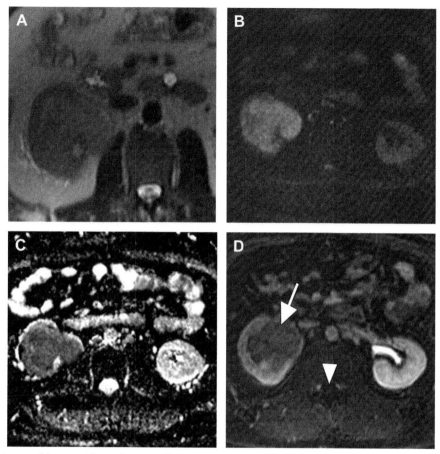

Fig. 5. A 44-year-old man with painless gross hematuria. Axial T2-weighted SSFSE (*A*), DWI (*B*), ADC (*C*), and post-contrast subtraction (*D*) images demonstrate loss of corticomedullary differentiation of the right kidney, the "faceless" appearance. The mass demonstrates restricted diffusion (*B*) and low signal intensity on ADC (*C*). The signal intensity within the mass on the subtraction sequence (*white arrow* on [*D*]) is higher than cerebrospinal fluid (*white arrowhead*), confirming low-level enhancement. Pathology revealed high-grade noninvasive papillary urothelial carcinoma.

abdominal soft tissue window settings. "Bone window" settings are a good starting point, but the window width and level may need to be adjusted further to allow visualization through the excreted contrast (see **Fig. 4**D). In addition, close evaluation of the coronal and sagittal MPR images is essential, as many filling defects may be better depicted in the coronal plane. Special care must be given to the papillae, as often prominent or compound papillae may simulate a small filling defect.

Renal stones also may present as filling defects, but are always low in signal intensity on all MR imaging pulse sequences, and do not demonstrate enhancement (**Fig. 7**). On CTU, stones are readily apparent, but may be extremely difficult to visualize if surrounded by excreted contrast on delayed-phase images.

Nonpapillary tumors present as areas of abnormal urothelial thickening, nodular thickening, or as infiltrative masses (**Fig. 8**). Diffuse urothelial thickening, however, is nonspecific, and can be seen in the setting of renal stones, indwelling nephrostomy catheters, or nephroureteral stents.

Urothelial carcinoma versus renal cell carcinoma

Urothelial carcinoma is centered in the renal collecting system or renal pelvis, and usually fills the collecting system. The mass may extend to or beyond the ureteropelvic junction. The calyces peripheral to the mass are frequently dilated, causing hydronephrosis or potentially cystic areas within the mass. Papillary variants may form a cast within the involved collecting system, and preserve medullary fat. There is usually preservation of normal reniform shape. Tumor thrombus is uncommon.

Renal cell carcinoma (RCC) is centered in the renal cortex, although large or infiltrative lesions

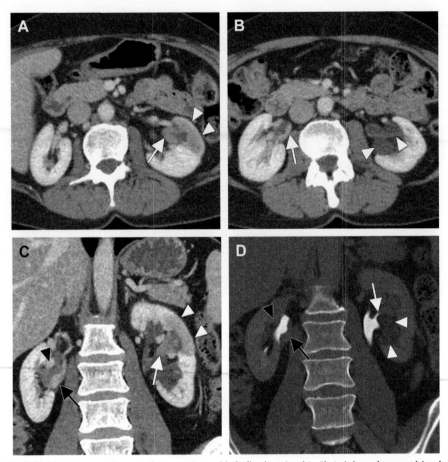

Fig. 6. A 61-year-old woman with gross hematuria and left flank pain. (*A, B*) Axial nephrographic-phase CT images show enhancing lesions (*white arrows*) in the renal pelvis bilaterally. There is focal decreased left cortical enhancement (*white arrowheads* in [*A*]) due to obstruction by the mass. (*C, D*) Coronal MPR images in nephrographic (*C*) and delay (*D*) phases. The left mass is centered on the infundibulum (*white arrow* in [*C*]), causing the amputated calyx sign (*white arrow* in [*D*]). The postobstructive hypoenhancement (*white arrowheads* in [*C*]) is also shown. Left renal sinus cysts are noted (*white arrowheads* in [*B, D*]). The right renal pelvis mass (*black arrows*) is medially located, and an additional potential lesion is visualized laterally (*black arrowhead*). This area was shown to be tubular on adjacent images (not shown), connecting to the renal vein, and represents a vein. Careful scrutiny regarding the location (inside or outside the collecting system) of a potential lesion is essential. Pathology on the right kidney revealed invasive high-grade urothelial carcinoma, on the left revealed noninvasive high-grade papillary urothelial carcinoma.

may be difficult to differentiate from urothelial carcinoma. RCC frequently contains areas of fatty metamorphosis. This can be seen as areas of lower signal intensity on opposed-phase T1-weighted imaging. Renal vein thrombus indicates advanced RCC and is rare otherwise.

Differential diagnosis

In the renal pelvis and calyces, other processes can present as filling defects, including hemorrhagic products, fungus ball, sloughed papillae, and stones. Not all infiltrative appearing lesions are urothelial carcinomas, or necessarily malignant. Multiple neoplastic processes may mimic a urothelial carcinoma including squamous cell

carcinoma, and rare entities such as medullary carcinoma, collecting duct carcinoma (**Fig. 9**), and metastatic disease (**Fig. 10**). Non-neoplastic entities such as xanthogranulomatous pyelonephritis, malakoplakia, focal pyelonephritis, mycobacterial infection[25] (**Fig. 11**) and parenchymal contusions secondary to trauma may all simulate mass lesions. Clinical history, laboratory evaluation, and previous imaging all help direct the radiologist to the appropriate conclusion.

Ureter

Ureter lesions can present areas of abnormal thickening (**Fig. 12**), strictures, or focal masses

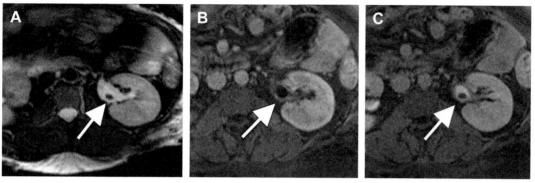

Fig. 7. (A) Axial T2 fat-suppressed image demonstrates a low signal intensity filling defect in the left renal pelvis (*white arrow*) surrounded by high signal intensity urine. (B, C) Axial nephrographic-phase (B) and delayed-phase (C) T1-weighted images. The filling defect remains very low in signal intensity, lower than fat and similar to bowel gas. The low signal intensity on all pulse sequences is indicative of a stone (*white arrows* [B, C]), which can be confirmed with radiographs or CT.

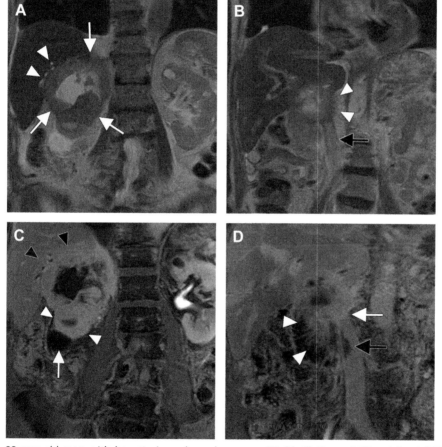

Fig. 8. An 88-year-old man with hematuria and renal mass on CT. (A, B) Coronal T2-weighted SSFSE images through a large right renal mass with central necrosis (*white arrows* in [A]). (B) is posterior to (A). The mass invades the liver with adjacent biliary dilatation (*white arrowheads* in [A]). There is loss of the normal inferior vena cava flow void (*black arrow* in [B]). Note the heterogeneity in the fat along the medial margin of the mass (*white arrowheads* in [B]) representing local fat infiltration. (C, D) Coronal postcontrast T1-weighted images at the same level as (A) and (B). The mass enhances with central necrosis. There is uninvolved renal cortex below the mass (*white arrowheads* in [C]), and a right lower pole cyst (*white arrow*). Note the subtle enhancement in the infiltrated liver (*black arrowheads*). In (D), there is local infiltration of the IVC (*white arrow*) and adjacent duodenum (*white arrowheads*). There is a low signal intensity filling defect in the IVC (*black arrow* in [D]) indicating bland thrombus. The IVC enhances homogeneously. The loss of the IVC flow void was due to slow flow, a known pitfall on the SSFSE images. Biopsy revealed invasive high-grade urothelial carcinoma.

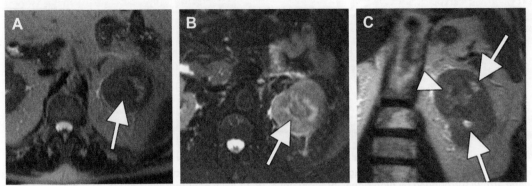

Fig. 9. A 75-year-old man with painless gross hematuria. (*A, B*) Axial T2-weighted SSFSE image (*A*) and axial fat-suppressed T2-weighted image (*B*) of the kidneys demonstrating an intermediate signal intensity mass centered on the left renal collecting system (*white arrow*). (*C*) Coronal T2-weighted SSFSE image shows that the mass (*white arrowhead*) is infiltrative, the upper pole is slightly expanded, and the reniform shape is maintained. There is focal upper and lower pole caliectasis (*white arrows*). Initial radiographic interpretation favored urothelial carcinoma. Pathology revealed carcinoma of the collecting ducts of Bellini.

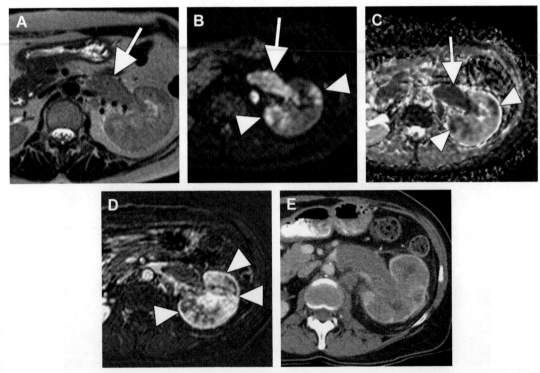

Fig. 10. A 58-year-old female smoker with history of non–small-cell lung cancer. (*A–D*) Axial T2-weighted SSFSE (*A*), DWI (*B*), ADC (*C*), and postcontrast subtraction (*D*) images demonstrate a large infiltrative left renal mass with expansion of the left renal vein (*white arrows*). The venous filling defect demonstrates similar signal intensity to the renal mass, and demonstrates elevated signal on DWI and low signal on ADC (*B, C*), all suggestive of tumor thrombus. The signal in the venous filling defect on the subtraction image (*D*) is higher than cerebrospinal fluid, indicating enhancement, which confirms tumor thrombus. Note the thin band of preserved renal cortical enhancement. The mass has similar areas of elevated DWI signal and low ADC correlating with areas of enhancing infiltrative tumor (*white arrowheads*). (*E*) Axial nephrographic-phase CT image demonstrates similar findings. The differential diagnosis offered for this mass was primary RCC due to the presence of tumor thrombus. An infiltrative urothelial carcinoma was also considered. Biopsy revealed metastatic poorly differentiated carcinoma, consistent with lung primary.

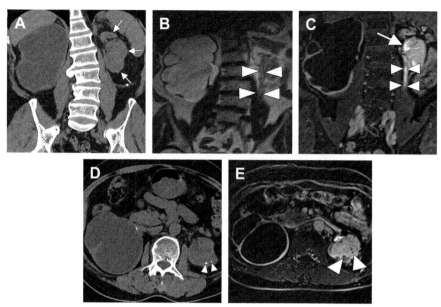

Fig. 11. A 55-year-old Asian man with history of renal failure, initial evaluation by noncontrast CT, and subsequent MRU. (A–C) Coronal noncontrast CT (A), T2-weighted SSFSE (B), and postcontrast T1-weighted (C) images. There is severe right hydronephrosis with cortical thinning. The left kidney (*white arrows*) is small and faceless, concerning for infiltrative mass. There is diffuse thickening and enhancement of the left ureter (*white arrowheads* in [B, C]). (D, E) Axial noncontrast CT (D), and postcontrast T1-weighted images (E) showing similar findings. Note the foci of calcification in the left kidney (*white arrowheads*), which are foci of signal void on MR. Pathology revealed chronic granulomatous inflammation with central caseous necrosis. The abnormalities in both kidneys were due to renal tuberculosis. In most cases, infiltrative neoplastic masses result in renal enlargement. The spectrum of radiographic findings in tuberculosis is broad, and often nonspecific. Urine cultures or histologic proof are required for definitive diagnosis.

(**Fig. 13**). The lesions are isointense to renal parenchyma on T1-weighted images, intermediate signal intensity on T2-weighted images, and show enhancement with contrast. The lesions are usually bright on DWI and show lower signal intensity on ADC images. Noncontrast MRU is an effective examination in the setting of obstruction (see **Fig. 13**), as the site can be well depicted, and usually mass lesions can be differentiated from blood clot or other causes. At the minimum,

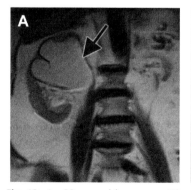 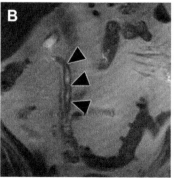 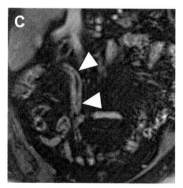

Fig. 12. An 82-year-old woman with painless hematuria. (A, B) Coronal T2-weighted SSFSE images through the right kidney (A) and right ureter (B). There is a duplex collecting system with hydronephrosis and cortical thinning of the upper pole moiety (*black arrow*). Note irregular nodular thickening of the right upper moiety ureter (*black arrowheads*). (C) Coronal delayed-phase T1-weighted image at the same level as (B). The thickened upper pole moiety ureter (*white arrowheads*) diffusely enhances. Diffuse urothelial thickening is nonspecific and can be seen in the setting of indwelling stents. No nephroureteral stent was present. Pathology revealed multifocal urothelial carcinoma.

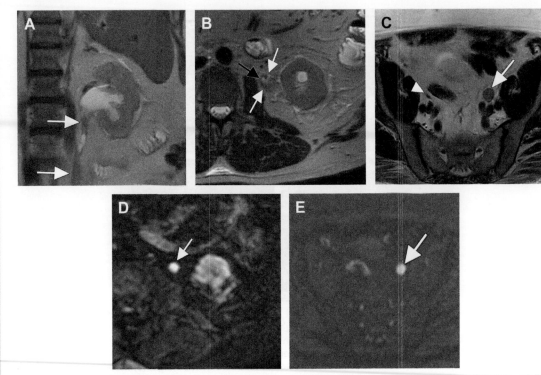

Fig. 13. A 70-year-old man with history of bladder cancer undergoing surveillance imaging. (*A*) Coronal T2-weighted SSFSE image demonstrates multiple obstructing masses (*white arrows*) at the left ureteropelvic junction and in the left ureter. The mass extended farther inferiorly into the pelvis (not shown). (*B, C*) Axial T2-weighted SSFSE images through the upper (*B*) and lower (*C*) ureteral masses (*white arrows*, [*B* and *C*]). There is minimal or no bright signal from urine (*black arrow* in [*B*], *white arrow* in [*C*]) within the upper lesion or distal lesion. Normal right ureter (*white arrowhead*, [*C*]). (*D, E*) Axial DWI of the upper (*D*) and lower (*E*) ureteral masses showing abnormally restricted diffusion (*white arrows*). Despite noncontrast technique, the cause of obstruction was identified, and a neoplastic etiology was favored. Pathology revealed high-grade noninvasive papillary urothelial carcinoma involving the entire ureter.

it can direct further evaluation with retrograde pyelogram, ureteroscopy, and/or biopsy.

Ureteral masses are usually associated with hydronephrosis. Focal masses may demonstrate the classic "goblet" sign equivalent on MRU as seen on IVP and CTU (see **Fig. 1**). There is dilation of the ureter proximal to the soft tissue mass that is displaced inferiorly during peristalsis. Strictures may occur.

In cases of focal or diffuse thickening, the images should be carefully evaluated for the presence of a stent, which can be difficult to visualize on MR imaging, and may require review of a radiograph. Stents are best visualized on T2-weighted images, where the stent walls are low in signal intensity with central high signal intensity of urine. They are most easily identified on T2-weighted images, by visualization of the retaining loops in the renal pelvis or bladder. Urothelial thickening and enhancement may be diffuse in the setting of a stent, but special attention should be paid to areas in which there is asymmetrical or irregular

thickening, or masslike areas. DWIs are also helpful in evaluating focal areas of abnormal thickening.

On CTU, ureteral tumors are depicted as areas of intraluminal masses (**Fig. 14**) or as areas of focal or diffuse thickening. Masses of significant size usually obstruct, but not all lesions cause ureteral obstruction, particularly when small. Careful ureteral evaluation using appropriate window/level setting, and in multiple planes, particularly coronal, is essential. As on MRU, diffuse thickening is nonspecific, particularly in the setting of indwelling stents. Ureteral stents, when present, may also present a challenge on CT, as the high density of the stent may obscure the underlying obstructing mass that warranted its placement.

Differential diagnosis

Ureteral stones may also present as filling defects, but are low in signal intensity on all pulse sequences and do not enhance, although ureteral thickening and enhancement may be present at

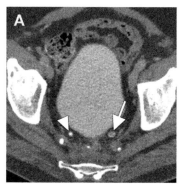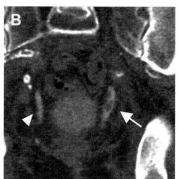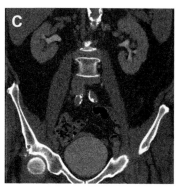

Fig. 14. A 75-year-old man with painless gross hematuria. (*A, B*) Axial (*A*) and magnified coronal MPR (*B*) delay-phase CT images through the distal ureters showing enlargement of the left ureter (*white arrow*) compared with the right ureter (*white arrowheads*), with an internal filling defect. (*C*) Coronal delayed-phase MPR image through the kidneys demonstrates no hydronephrosis. Not all ureteral masses cause obstruction. Urine cytology positive for high-grade urothelial carcinoma. Biopsy revealed fragments of urothelial carcinoma.

the site of an impacted ureteral calculus. Clot or other debris may also present as a filling defect.

Ureteritis cystica may also present as multiple filling defects in the ureter on CTU or IVP, but details regarding the MR imaging appearance are limited. Fibroepithelial polyp is an additional differential consideration for a filling defect. Extramedullary hematopoiesis has been reported but is uncommon.

Differential considerations for focal and diffuse ureteral thickening are more numerous, including indwelling stents, ureteritis, tuberculosis (see **Fig. 11**), metastases, and amyloidosis. Other processes may displace the ureter, including retroperitoneal fibrosis, lymphoma, and nodal metastases.[26]

Pitfalls in Technique and Interpretation

Interpretation of MRU cases can be clinically challenging, as a multitude of artifacts may simulate disease.[27] Some are due to physiologic phenomena, others related to MR imaging physics.

Inadequate distention or peristalsis of the ureter may mimic strictures. These are usually transient. A fixed stricture is present throughout the examination. Patient motion can cause blurring of the images as well as misregistration. Motion can often be mitigated by coaching the patient and using motion insensitive sequences. Unfortunately, 3D T1-weighted images are most susceptible to artifact (**Fig. 15**).

Other disease processes may cause filling defects in the renal collecting systems that can be mistaken for masses. The most common causes include blood products (**Fig. 16**), stones/debris, fungus balls, and sloughed papillae. Blood products typically demonstrate higher signal intensity

than the renal parenchyma on precontrast T1-weighted images. Care must be given if precontrast images are obtained after a test bolus of gadolinium-based contrast agent. The signal intensity of blood products can be variable over time, so images also should be analyzed on the

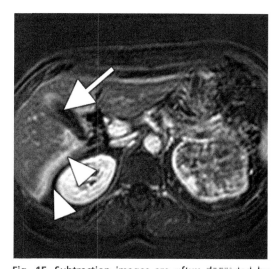

Fig. 15. Subtraction images are often degraded by respiratory motion and misregistration. The band of increased signal along the posterior liver surface (*white arrowheads*) is due to misregistration. In the authors' experience, the liver is more susceptible to this type of artifact. Renal position is less affected by inspiration, and the kidneys are often spared, as in this case. The gallbladder lumen (*arrow*) should be devoid of signal, and can be used as an internal control for low-level enhancement. Despite the reduced image quality, enhancement is clearly discerned in the infiltrative left renal mass compared with the gallbladder lumen.

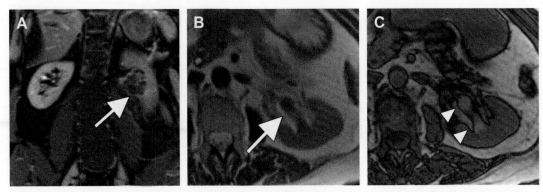

Fig. 16. (*A*) Coronal postcontrast T1-weighted image shows expansion of the left renal collecting system with low signal intensity material, concerning for a solid lesion (*white arrow*). (*B, C*) Axial SSFSE (*B*) and OP T1-weighted (*C*) images demonstrate loss of normal bright T2 signal in the left renal pelvis (*B*). On the OP T1-weighted image, however, the filling defect (*white arrowheads*) has intrinsically high signal intensity before contrast administration, suggesting blood products. Region of interest signal intensity evaluation (not shown) revealed no enhancement.

precontrast and postcontrast images for the presence of enhancement. Blood products should not enhance. Subtraction sequences, if successful, also will demonstrate the area to be void of signal. Stones should maintain low signal intensity on all pulse sequences, and associated hallmarks might include ureteral thickening or surrounding inflammation, and hydronephrosis. Clinical history will usually aid in the diagnosis of fungus ball, and other signs of papillary necrosis should point to the diagnosis of a sloughed papilla.

Flowing urine may produce an artifactual low signal intensity filling defect on spin-echo or turbo spin-echo sequences that can mimic a stone or other filling defect (**Fig. 17**). This artifact can be overcome by imaging in multiple planes and varying the slice-select and phase encode

gradients. Flow-related artifacts should be absent on excretory postcontrast images.

Similarly, the normal low signal intensity flow void in major vessels can also demonstrate areas of artifactually high signal intensity due to flowing blood on SSFSE images (see **Fig. 8B**). The artifact can be confirmed by review of other sequences (T1 in-phase [IP]/opposed-phase [OP]) and most convincingly on postcontrast images (see **Fig. 8D**).

At high concentrations, the T2* (magnetic susceptibility) effect of gadolinium can overwhelm the T1 shortening effect, resulting in areas of paradoxically very low signal intensity on T1-weighted images (**Fig. 18**). When this occurs in a small amount, it may simulate a filling defect. In a large area, pathology could be potentially obscured. Although less commonly visualized,

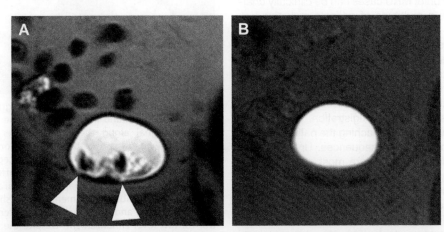

Fig. 17. Coronal T2-weighted SSFSE (*A*) and postcontrast T1 (*B*) image showing several irregular filling defects in the bladder (*white arrowheads* in [*A*]). On the postcontrast image, there is no filling defect. The low signal intensity areas in (*A*) are artifactual due to ureteral jets. The same artifact can occur in the renal pelvis.

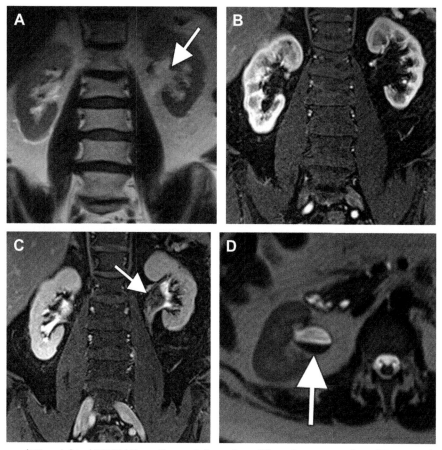

Fig. 18. Coronal T2-weighted SSFSE (*A*), corticomedullary phase (*B*), and excretory phase (*C*) T1-weighted images. There is normal high signal intensity of urine in the left renal pelvis (*white arrow* in [*A*]), and no abnormality on the corticomedullary image (*B*). (*C*) demonstrates a low signal intensity filling defect in the left renal pelvis (*white arrow*). As no abnormality was seen on other sequences, the finding in (*C*) is artifactual, due to the T2* effect of concentrated gadolinium. The same principle is demonstrated on an axial T2-weighted image from a different patient (*D*).

the effect also can be seen on T2-weighted images, if they are obtained after contrast administration. Adequate distention of the collecting systems and diuretic administration, both of which dilute the excreted gadolinium, minimizing the T2* effect, mitigate this artifact.

SUMMARY

CTU remains the modality of choice for comprehensive radiographic evaluation of the upper urinary tract. However, there are clinical settings in which MRU may be a preferable alternative, including in patients with renal insufficiency or allergy to iodinated contrast, during pregnancy, and in the pediatric population. MRU also should be considered in young patients requiring serial imaging.

Both CTU and MRU demonstrate tumors of the renal collecting system as enhancing filling defects

or infiltrative masses. To optimize MRU, steps must be taken to ensure adequate distention of the collecting system and dilution of excreted gadolinium. It is important to recognize normal physiologic characteristics and expected findings on various pulse sequences to avoid misinterpretation of physiologic and/or artifactual findings. Adequate visualization and evaluation of the entire urinary tract is critical due to the small risk of synchronous and metachronous lesions.

The sensitivity of MRU is likely comparable to CT for urothelial lesions in the renal pelvis, but the accuracy of MRU in the ureter remains debatable. In screening for hematuria, MRU can be paired with a noncontrast CT examination to exclude nephrolithiasis.

The diagnostic yield of screening CTU and by extrapolation for microscopic and/or asymptomatic hematuria has been the subject of multiple recent studies, demonstrating the incidence of urothelial cancers in this isolated setting is extremely rare. The prevalence of synchronous lesions has also been shown to be less than previously estimated. In addition, although sensitivity of CTU is not in doubt, its positive predictive value warrants further evaluation, particularly in the ureter, and in the setting of small lesions. The combination of positive urine cytology and findings on CTU and MRU increases the positive predictive value. Additional studies are needed to establish optimal utilization of MRU in the clinical armamentarium, particularly in younger patients and patients without known risk factors for urothelial carcinoma.

REFERENCES

1. Takahashi N, Kawashima A, Glockner JF, et al. MR urography for suspected upper tract urothelial carcinoma. Eur Radiol 2009;19(4):912–23.

2. Sudah M, Masarwah A, Kainulainen S, et al. Comprehensive MR urography protocol: equally good diagnostic performance and enhanced visibility of the upper urinary tract compared to triple-phase CT urography. PLoS One 2016;11(7): e0158673.

3. Shinagare AB, Sadow CA, Sahni VA, et al. Urinary bladder: normal appearance and mimics of malignancy at CT urography. Cancer Imaging 2011;11: 100–8.

4. Jinzaki M, Kikuchi E, Akita H, et al. Role of computed tomography urography in the clinical evaluation of upper tract urothelial carcinoma. Int J Urol 2016; 23(4):284–98.

5. Leyendecker JR, Barnes CE, Zagoria RJ. MR urography: techniques and clinical applications. Radiographics 2008;28(1):23–46 [discussion: 46–7].

6. Leyendecker JR, Gianini JW. Magnetic resonance urography. Abdom Imaging 2009;34(4):527–40.

7. Takahashi N, Glockner JF, Hartman RP, et al. Gadolinium enhanced magnetic resonance urography for upper urinary tract malignancy. J Urol 2010;183(4): 1330–65.

8. ACR. ACR Appropriateness Criteria for Hematuria. 2014. Available at: https://acsearch.acr.org/docs/69490/Narrative/. Accessed April 2018.

9. AUA. Diagnosis, evaluation and follow-up of asymptomatic microhematuria (AMH) in adults. 2016. Available at: http://www.auanet.org/guidelines/asymptomatic-microhematuria-(2012-reviewed-and-validity-confirmed-2016). Accessed April 2018.

10. Commander CW, Johnson DC, Raynor MC, et al. Detection of upper tract urothelial malignancies by computed tomography urography in patients referred for hematuria at a large tertiary referral center. Urology 2017;102:31–7.

11. Sudakoff GS, Dunn DP, Guralnick ML, et al. Multidetector computerized tomography urography as the primary imaging modality for detecting urinary tract neoplasms in patients with asymptomatic hematuria. J Urol 2008;179(3):862–7 [discussion: 867].

12. Lee KS, Zeikus E, DeWolf WC, et al. MR urography versus retrograde pyelography/ureteroscopy for the exclusion of upper urinary tract malignancy. Clin Radiol 2010;65(3):185–92.

13. Razavi SA, Sadigh G, Kelly AM, et al. Comparative effectiveness of imaging modalities for the diagnosis of upper and lower urinary tract malignancy: a critically appraised topic. Acad Radiol 2012;19(9):1134–40.

14. Krishnan V, Chawla A, Sharbidre KG, et al. Current techniques and clinical applications of computed tomography urography. Curr Probl Diagn Radiol 2018; 47(4):245–56.

15. Siegel RL, Miller KD, Jemal A. Cancer statistics, 2018. CA Cancer J Clin 2018;68(1):7–30.

16. Prando A, Prando P, Prando D. Urothelial cancer of the renal pelvicaliceal system: unusual imaging manifestations. Radiographics 2010;30(6):1553–66.

17. Guinan P, Vogelzang NJ, Randazzo R, et al. Renal pelvic cancer: a review of 611 patients treated in Illinois 1975-1985. Cancer Incidence and End Results Committee. Urology 1992;40(5):393–9.

18. Bree RL, Schultz SR, Hayes R. Large infiltrating renal transitional cell carcinomas: CT and ultrasound features. J Comput Assist Tomogr 1990;14(3):381–5.

19. Wong-You-Cheong JJ, Wagner BJ, Davis CJ Jr. Transitional cell carcinoma of the urinary tract: radiologic-pathologic correlation. Radiographics 1998;18(1):123–42 [quiz: 148].

20. Ramchandani P, Pollack HM. Tumors of the urothelium. Semin Roentgenol 1995;30(2):149–67.

21. Nocks BN, Heney NM, Daly JJ, et al. Transitional cell carcinoma of renal pelvis. Urology 1982;19(5): 472–7.

22. Kirkali Z, Tuzel E. Transitional cell carcinoma of the ureter and renal pelvis. Crit Rev Oncol Hematol 2003;47(2):155–69.

23. Chan V, Pantanowitz L, Vrachliotis TG, et al. CT demonstration of a rapidly growing transitional cell carcinoma of the ureter and renal pelvis. Abdom Imaging 2002;27(2):222–3.

24. Vikram R, Sandler CM, Ng CS. Imaging and staging of transitional cell carcinoma: part 2, upper urinary tract. AJR Am J Roentgenol 2009;192(6):1488–93.

25. Gibson MS, Puckett ML, Shelly ME. Renal tuberculosis. Radiographics 2004;24(1):251–6.

26. Wasnik AP, Elsayes KM, Kaza RK, et al. Multimodality imaging in ureteric and periureteric pathologic abnormalities. AJR Am J Roentgenol 2011;197(6): W1083–92.

27. Chung AD, Schieda N, Shanbhogue AK, et al. MRI evaluation of the urothelial tract: pitfalls and solutions. AJR Am J Roentgenol 2016;207(6):W108–16.

Classification and Diagnosis of Cystic Renal Tumors
Role of MR Imaging Versus Contrast-Enhanced Ultrasound

Hina Arif-Tiwari, MD, DNB[a],*, Bobby T. Kalb, MD[b],
Jaspreet K. Bisla, MD[c], Diego R. Martin, MD, PhD, FRCPC[d]

KEYWORDS

- Contrast-enhanced ultrasound • Magnetic resonance imaging • Cystic renal tumors

KEY POINTS

- Superior soft tissue and contrast resolution of MR imaging benefits sensitivity to kidney cyst features and classification, which may have an impact on patient management and outcomes.
- Contrast-enhanced ultrasound evaluation is a safe alternative imaging modality for the assessment of complex cystic renal masses in patients with renal impairment.
- Further research is needed to identify the role of contrast-enhanced ultrasound in the differentiation of benign complex cystic lesions from malignant complex cystic lesions and to determine its accuracy compared with MR imaging.
- Determination of subtypes of cystic renal cell carcinomas by imaging is still challenging due to overlap of common imaging features.

INTRODUCTION

Renal cysts are common incidental findings on imaging studies performed for nonurologic indications. Autopsy series report 50% incidence of at least 1 renal cyst in adults. Commonly encountered cysts on ultrasound (US) and cross-sectional imaging (CT and MR imaging) mostly are benign simple cortical renal cysts. Complex cysts, on imaging, may be seen as part of benign cysts, renal infection, and cystic neoplasms, including cystic renal cell carcinoma (RCC), which can be distinctly identified due to characteristic imaging features.

Cystic renal tumors, overall, have excellent prognosis and less aggressive metastatic behavior compared with solid renal tumors.[1,2] Imaging plays a critical role in management, differentiating benign cysts, which do not require treatment, from cystic neoplasms, which may benefit from partial or radical nephrectomy, or percutaneous ablation under imaging guidance. Neoplastic cysts show complex features that include wall thickening, intracystic lobulated soft

The authors have nothing to disclose.

[a] Department of Medical Imaging, South Campus Hospital, University of Arizona, College of Medicine, 1501 North Campbell Avenue, PO Box 245067, Tucson, AZ 85724, USA; [b] Quality and Safety, Body Section, University of Arizona, College of Medicine, 1501 North Campbell Avenue, PO Box 245067, Tucson, AZ 85724, USA; [c] Department of Medical Imaging, University of Arizona, College of Medicine, 1501 North Campbell Avenue, PO Box 245067, Tucson, AZ 85724, USA; [d] Department of Medical Imaging, College of Medicine, University of Arizona, Banner University Medical Center, Tucson, 1501 North Campbell Avenue, PO Box 245067, Tucson, AZ 85724, USA
* Corresponding author.
E-mail address: hinaarif@radiology.arizona.edu

tissue, irregular thick cyst walls with thickened septations, and with these soft tissue components demonstrating enhancing elements on contrast-enhanced imaging.

BOSNIAK CLASSIFICATION OF RENAL CYSTS

Since its introduction in 1986, Bosniak classification for renal cysts has been used by radiologists and urologists as a method to stratify patients to plan treatment. Bosniak classification is based on findings on contrast-enhanced CT scans, dividing renal cysts into 4 broad categories (I–IV) proposed to distinguish malignant from benign cystic lesions. In 2005,[3] a new II-F category was added to classification to the Bosniak classification system.[4]

Bosniak category I represent cysts are simple and outlined by a thin wall, without internal septa or contrast enhancement (**Fig. 1**). Category II corresponds to cysts with thin septations, minimally smooth thick walls but without contrast enhancement or nodularity (**Fig. 2**). Category III includes complex cysts with irregular and/or thick septa, coarse calcifications, and presence of enhancement after injection of iodinated contrast (**Fig. 3**). Enhancing well-defined solid components and thickened septations with irregular cyst walls comprise category IV (**Fig. 4**). Category II-F is assigned to indeterminate lesions, between category II and III, which are clearly not benign, and warrant follow-up imaging ("F" refers to follow-up). These patients require several follow-up examinations for longitudinal evaluation, allowing the natural course of growth to reveal a neoplasm warranting intervention. These multiple CT studies expose patients to a cumulative x-ray dosing and risks related to iodinated contrast. The Bosniak classification system has been extended to apply to contrast-enhanced ultrasound (CEUS) and gadolinium contrast-enhanced MR imaging.

MR imaging has excellent intrinsic soft tissue and contrast resolution, which makes the appearance of septa more conspicuous and enhancement of the solid components, septa, and cystic walls more evident. This may yield higher Bosniak classification grading compared with CT.[5–7] Graumann and colleagues[8] report MR imaging both upgraded and downgraded 22% of the cases in their series, because of better contrast resolution, which aided distinction of solid and cystic elements within cysts. Higher-contrast resolution of CEUS, coupled with microbubble postcontrast imaging, helps identify details within a cyst (solid nodules, septa, cystic walls, and enhancement of soft tissue). Compared with the same CT study cohort, CEUS also both upgraded and downgraded 21% of the lesions, suggesting superior results to CT and similar results to MR imaging, when comparing delineation of solid and cystic components.

CONTRAST-ENHANCED ULTRASOUND

US is easily available and frequently used for imaging kidneys. Complex cysts may show internal septations, solid components, or thickened walls, with vascularity of these soft tissue elements assessable with duplex Doppler technique. US contrast agents have been recently used in assessing blood flow with solid renal masses and soft tissue components of complex cysts masses. Vascularity in fine septations and small mural nodules may be challenging to elicit on conventional US using duplex Doppler. Enhancement can be improved, however, after contrast administration with use of tissue harmonic imaging in real time, differentiating benign complicated cysts from cystic tumors.

US contrast comprises synthetic microbubbles with diameters in the range of 1 μm to 10 μm, up to the size of red blood cells. These microbubbles are small enough to flow through capillaries but too large extravasate into the interstitium. The distribution volume represents the intravascular compartment. Thus, microbubbles are useful for determining vascularity, perfusion, and angiogenesis. Microbubbles are typically composed of a

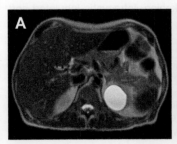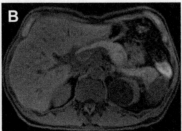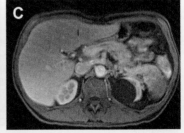

Fig. 1. Bosniak category I simple cyst. Axial T2WI (*A*), precontrast (*B*), and postcontrast (*C*) gadolinium-enhanced T1W FS GRE images. There is high signal on T2W images (*A*) and low signal on T1WI (*B*) with imperceptible wall and no septations in the cyst, characteristic of a simple cyst. No enhancement is seen after gadolinium contrast administration (*C*).

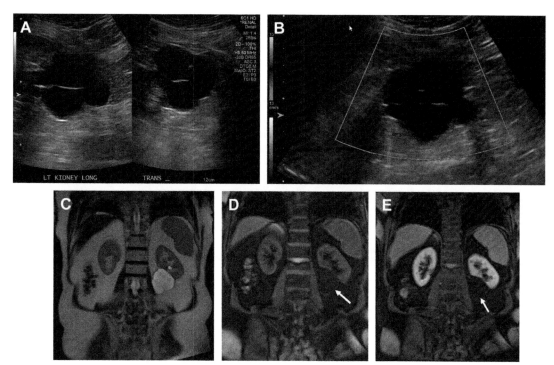

Fig. 2. Bosniak category II simple cyst. Sagittal and transverse B-mode US images show left renal cyst with thin smooth internal septations (*A*), which does not show internal vascularity on color doppler image (*B*). Coronal T2W images (*C*) show left renal cyst with smooth thin wall and septations. Precontrast (*D*) and postcontrast (*E*) gadolinium-enhanced coronal T1W FS GRE images show no enhancement within the septations (*arrows* [*D* and *E*]) in keeping with Bosniak category II simple cyst.

phospholipid shell containing low solubility complex gas, such as a perfluoro gas.[9–12] Conventional B-mode sonographic frequencies can burst the microbubbles. Therefore, it is essential to use low mechanical index US waves to capture postcontrast sonographic imaging. Both linear and nonlinear oscillations occur in the microbubbles after exposure to low mechanical index US, which leads to generation of harmonics overtone signals from the blood due to increased backscatter. Generation of signal from microbubbles is independent of blood flow or vessel diameter

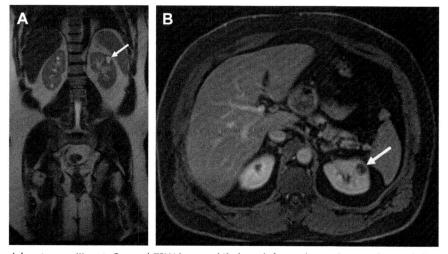

Fig. 3. Bosniak category III cyst. Coronal T2W images (*A*) show left renal complex cyst (*arrow* [*A*]) with smooth thin wall and septations with mildly irregular and thickened septae (*arrow* [*B*]), which show nodular enhancement (*B*) on axial postcontrast gadolinium-enhanced coronal T1W FS GRE images.

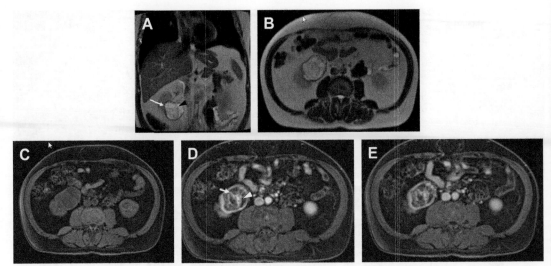

Fig. 4. Bosniak category IV cyst. Coronal (*A*) and axial T2W (*B*) images, precontrast (*C*), early (*D, arrowheads*), and delayed postcontrast (*E*) gadolinium-enhanced axial T1W FS GRE images show complex right cyst (*arrows*) with intracystic irregular septations and nodular solid components, which show irregularity on (*A*) coronal T2W image and enhancement on postcontrast gadolinium-enhanced axial T1W FS GRE images (*arrowheads*). Hypervascularity and early enhancement in solid nodular component favor CC-RCC.

and is based on US imaging with optimized spatial resolution. These characteristics of CEUS differentiate from duplex Doppler US for the evaluation of smaller vascularized soft tissue structures, which may not be resolved by Doppler due to lower intrinsic spatial resolution.

Microbubbles have a short half-life (approximately 5 min) after intravenous injection. Usual doses are 1 mL to 2.4 mL of microbubble preparation, suspended in saline, followed by a saline bolus. The microbubbles are disintegrated into its constituting parts; phospholipid shells are metabolized by the liver and the gas exhaled by the lungs.

CEUS gives an opportunity to image tissue vascularity (including arterial) in real-time, rapid, and continuous fashion over several minutes. More than 1 injection may be administered safely to evaluate both kidneys. US contrast agents have the benefit of being safe and with less severe adverse effects, compared with CT or MR contrast agents. Microbubbles are not hepatotoxic or nephrotoxic and can be given to patients with renal insufficiency and has a very good safety profile in terms of adverse reactions.

CEUS can reveal details of cyst wall, including nodularity and thickness, accurate number and thickness of septations, and the presence of enhancing solid components[13] (**Fig. 5**). Wash-in times and peak-to-enhancement values can used to assess enhancement patterns. An

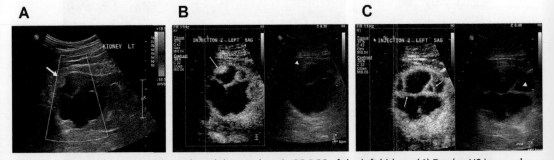

Fig. 5. A 47-year-old woman with incidental detected cystic CC-RCC of the left kidney. (*A*) Duplex US image shows complex left renal cyst with internal septations with a mural nodule along the wall of the cyst. No vascularity is seen on duplex doppler with in the septations or nodular component. (*B*) CEUS image obtained 36 seconds after contrast injection shows contrast enhancement in the soft tissue nodule (*arrow*) along the wall of the cyst (*arrowhead*) as seen on grayscale image. (*C*) After 46 seconds following contrast injection, striking enhancement of the intracyst septations is seen (*arrows*), which appear more conspicuous on CEUS image compared with B-mode.

increasing body of literature supports that CEUS is as good or better in showing enhancing fine septa in cystic renal masses than CECT.[14-18] Xu and colleagues[14] were able to differentially characterize benign and malignant cystic renal masses based on CEUS appearances. The presence of enhancing nodules was the most common feature leading to Bosniak category IV classification and subsequent correlation with histologic subtypes of malignant cystic tumors (cystic clear cell RCC [cystic CC-RCC] and cystic papillary RCC [cystic P-RCC]). A multilocular cystic nephroma (MLCN) was classified as Bosniak category III, based on the multiloculated appearance and the lack of solid components in this particular study.

MAGNETIC RESONANCE IMAGING

MR imaging in recent years has established a valuable role in the evaluation of cystic renal lesions due to its superior contrast resolution. Fluid-sensitive T2-weighted (T2W) sequences provide exquisite details of contents within renal cysts, including nodularity, septation, and solid components. Precontrast and dynamic postcontrast fat-saturated (FS) T1-weighted (T1W) 3-D gradient-echo (GRE) sequences are valuable in identifying enhancement of septation and/or solid nodules, which indicate malignancy.

Diffusion-weighted imaging (DWI) relies on the random motion of free water molecules and it has been widely used for the characterization of benign versus malignant processes in the abdomen. DWI and apparent diffusion coefficient are now increasingly used for the evaluation of kidney tumors, including categorization and staging of solid renal tumors. Solid components of cystic tumors show restriction on DWI, aiding accurate identification of malignant cystic tumors.[19,20]

Rosenkrantz and colleagues[20] report increased demonstration of septations, septal and/or mural thickening and irregularity, and mural nodules in cystic renal tumors using 3T MR imaging, compared with 1.5T and suggested more accurate cyst classification on 3T MR imaging. If 1.5T MR imaging is used, these investigators have recommended longitudinal evaluation of a patient should be performed at a consistent field strength, thereby leading to consistent evaluation.

CYSTIC RENAL TUMORS

Imaging plays a crucial role in stratifying renal cystic lesions, into benign simple cysts, mildly complex benign cysts (blood-protein cysts), or complicated cysts representing low malignant-potential tumors (MLCN or multilocular cystic RCC) and malignant cystic renal tumors (CC-RCC and P-RCC) with internal necrosis, cystic change, or focal hemorrhage. Identification of lesion complexity has a critical impact on patient management. Although nephron-sparing surgery is offered to low malignant-potential tumors (MLCN or multilocular cystic RCC), nephrectomy/radical nephrectomy may be considered in larger malignant tumors.

Renal Cell Carcinoma

A rising incidence of RCC has been observed in recent years, which may be attributed to both increasing exposure to risk factors and increasing use of imaging technologies.[21,22] RCC represents a spectrum of disease, encompassing a family of differing neoplasms with different cytogenetic and molecular defects and varying prognoses and potential morbidities. The World Health Organization (WHO) classification divides these tumors into different classes based on histologic, immunohistochemical, and genetic differences as follows[23,24]:

1. CC-RCCs (65%)
2. P-RCCs (15%; 90% 5-year survival in sporadic cases)
3. Chromophobe RCCs (5% overall best prognosis)
4. Collecting duct carcinomas (1%; very poor prognosis)
5. Renal oncocytomas (5%; benign tumors, similar pathology to chromophobe tumors except by immunohistochemistry)
6. Unclassified tumors (5%)

Cystic clear cell carcinoma

CC-RCC is the most common subtype of RCC. A majority of CC-RCC are solid masses; only approximately 15% may have cystic change.[25] Hartman and colleagues[25] characterize 4 basic pathologic mechanisms resulting in cystic RCC: intrinsic multiloculated growth, intrinsic unilocular growth (cystadenocarcinoma), cystic necrosis (pseudocyst), and origin from the epithelial lining of a preexisting simple cyst. Based on these histologic appearances, CC-RCCs can be classified into 4 morphologic subtypes, seen on imaging:

1. Multilocular cystic RCC
2. Unilocular cystic RCC
3. Cystic RCC with 1 or more mural tumor nodules
4. RCC with extensive necrosis

Multilocular cystic renal cell carcinoma, also known as multilocular cystic renal neoplasm of low malignant potential Multilocular cystic RCC is a rare subtype, first described in 1982, and comprising up to 6% of RCCs and 15% to 40% of all CC-RCCs. These asymptomatic tumors are incidentally discovered in adults (20–76 years of age) with a favorable prognosis, without local recurrence or metastatic disease after resection.[26]

Multilocular cystic RCC is a low-grade tumor comprising cysts of varying sizes that are separated from the renal cortex by a fibrous capsule, which contains serous or hemorrhagic cyst fluid. The cyst wall is lined by a monolayer of epithelial cells with clear cytoplasm.

On MR imaging, these tumors show a T2-hyperintense, well-defined, multilocular cystic structures. FS T1W 3-D GRE postcontrast images reveal enhancement of the cyst wall and septa, without any internal mural enhancing nodules (**Fig. 6**). Aubert and colleagues,[27] in their investigation of preoperatively diagnosed cystic clear cell carcinomas, were able to distinguish cystic CC-RCC from multilocular cystic RCC by the presence of fewer loculations, thicker and more nodular septa, and enhancing mural nodules. Hindman and colleagues,[28] however, report overlapping imaging appearances of multilocular cystic RCC to cystic neoplasms, including cystic nephroma, mixed epithelial and stromal tumor (MEST), extensively cystic RCC, tubulocystic carcinoma, and P-RCC. Most of the peer-reviewed literature lacks validation of MR imaging appearance of cysts by correlative histopathology.

Unilocular cystic renal cell carcinoma and cystic renal cell carcinoma with 1 or more mural tumor nodules Unilocular cystic RCC comprise 10% to 33% of cystic RCCs. Histologically, a solitary cyst with irregular excrescence along its wall can be identified. Tumor mural nodule in the wall of the cyst protruding into the lumen can be seen in cystic RCC variant with 1 or more mural nodules observed in up to 18% of cases.

On fluid-sensitive T2W MR imaging, a well-circumscribed, hyperintense, unilocular cystic mass with an irregularly thickened wall is commonly identified, which may be associated with an enhancing mural nodule on T1W 3-D GRE postcontrast venous or delayed-phase sequences. Septations traversing the lumen of the cysts, however, are usually absent in these 2 variants.[29]

Renal cell carcinoma with extensive necrosis In approximately 20% to 36% of CC-RCCs, cystic change within the mass can be due to extensive tumor necrosis, which is histologically seen as interspersed islands of tumor and cystic spaces filled with necrotic and hemorrhagic material. Cysts maybe of varying sizes and contain irregular walls containing variable amounts of fibrous tissue and epithelial cells.[30,31]

CC-RCC with necrosis, on T2W images, appears as a large, heterogeneous, complex and multilocular mass with intracyst septations, irregularly thickened wall, and intermediate signal

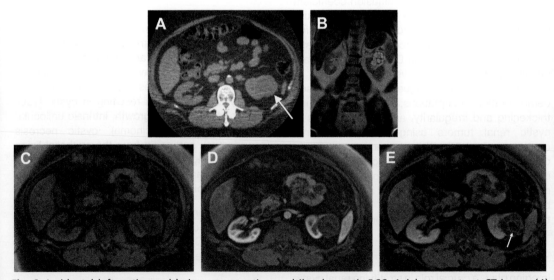

Fig. 6. Incidental left cystic renal lesion, representing multilocular cystic RCC. Axial noncontrast CT image (*A*) through the kidneys show a lobulated indeterminate cystic lesion arising from the left kidney (*arrow*). Coronal T2W image (*B*) and axial precontrast (*C*), arterial (*D*), and delayed postcontrast (*E*) gadolinium-enhanced T1W FS GRE images show internal complexity within the cysts, which comprise multiple thickened but smooth septation without solid components (*arrow* [*E*]).

scattered solid areas.[29] FS GRE T1W postcontrast images are key to demonstrate the solid component of the tumor, which show postgadolinium enhancement. CC-RCCs are vascularized tumors, often showing early avid enhancement when small (**Fig. 7**).

NATURAL HISTORY AND PROGNOSIS

Varying prognoses result from different types of RCCs, relating to different histologies. Worst prognosis is seen with RCC showing extensive necrosis and resultant cystic changes, which may metastasize or even result in death in up to 40% of cases. Multilocular cystic clear cell carcinomas, unilocular cystic RCC, and cystic RCC with mural nodules are rare subtypes, with no reported cases of metastases in the literature. Therefore, it is crucial to differentiate indolent cystic RCC from RCC with necrosis, which is an aggressive neoplasm.

Renal Epithelial and Stromal Tumors

Benign cystic renal tumors, including MLCN and MESTs, are biphasic tumors, comprise both epithelial and stromal components, and represent opposite ends of the same spectrum. Although MLCN is entirely cystic without solid nodules, complex epithelial and stromal components are seen in MEST. Common histogenesis is also proved by similar ultrastructural features, and immunohistochemistry pattern (ovarian-like stroma) in these lesions.[32] Therefore, the WHO classification of renal neoplasms has grouped them together under a unifying term, renal epithelial and stromal tumors,[33,34] to encompass both entities.

MULTILOCULAR CYSTIC NEPHROMA

MLCN is a rare, benign, slow-growing renal tumor, containing mixed mesenchymal and epithelial cells with approximately 200 reported cases, since it was first described in 1892. Estimated prevalence of MLCN is 2.4% in a single-institute experience shared by Gallo and Penchansky.[35]

Bimodal age of presentation is seen in children younger than 2 years and in middle age adults (40–69 years old). Incidence is higher in male children (male-to-female ratio, 3:1) and in postmenopausal women (female-to-male ratio, 9:1).[36–38] Oral estrogen use is a proposed etiology for development of acquired MLCN in women; however, not all women in reported cases had a history of estrogen use or were analyzed for hormone receptors.[39,40]

MLCN is usually detected incidentally in adults. Patients may have nonspecific symptoms, or loin pain (due to mass effect), hematuria (extension into renal pelvis), and urinary tract infection.[39]

Although MLCN is a mixed mesenchymal and epithelial neoplasm, it presents as an entirely cystic mass without associated solid components. Cysts of varying sizes are lined with flat, low cuboidal, or hobnail epithelial cells, and septa are thin with variable cellularity including characteristic ovarian-type stroma.[32]

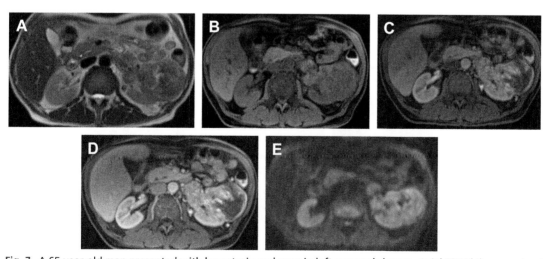

Fig. 7. A 65-year-old man presented with hematuria and mass in left upper abdomen. Axial T2W (*A*), precontrast (*B*), arterial (*C*), and delayed postcontrast (*D*) gadolinium-enhanced axial T1W FS GRE images show heterogenous, partially exophytic left renal tumor with central necrosis. Tumor shows avid early arterial enhancement suggestive of CC-RCC (*C*). Solid components of the tumor show remarkable restriction on DWI (*E*) depicting its malignant nature.

Imaging studies of MLCN usually appear as unilateral mass with irregular cysts and septa of variable thicknesses (Bosniak category III; 60% potential malignant risk).[41,42] On MR imaging, well-circumscribed cystic mass with internal septations and resultant multilocular appearance is seen, which may extend centrally to impinge on the renal pelvis. Solid components are classically absent suggestive of a benign cystic renal mass.[42,43] On T2W images, outer capsule and septa have low signal intensity, and the cysts are hyperintense. T1W 3-D GRE images demonstrate septal enhancement after IV gadolinium administration[44] (Fig. 8).

MIXED EPITHELIAL AND STROMAL TUMOR

MEST is a newly recognized, benign, rare, histologically biphasic renal tumor consisting of epithelial and complex stromal components, which was first reported by Michal and Syrucek in 1998.[45] Only 100 cases of MEST have been reported in the world literature until now, with the tumor occurring almost exclusively in perimenopausal women, many of them on long-term oral estrogen therapy. Only 7 male patients with MEST have been described, of whom 1 had a history of prostatic adenocarcinoma and had been treated with both diethylstilbestrol and Leuprolide for several years, which may have played a role in etiopathogenesis of the tumor.[32,45–47]

Approximately a quarter of these masses are incidentally identified on imaging studies performed for other reasons. Clinical presentation includes hematuria, loin pain and mass, or urinary tract infection.[32,46]

Unlike MLCN, MEST is a complex, mixed, solid cystic mass with biphasic components, including epithelial and stromal cells. Small and large cysts

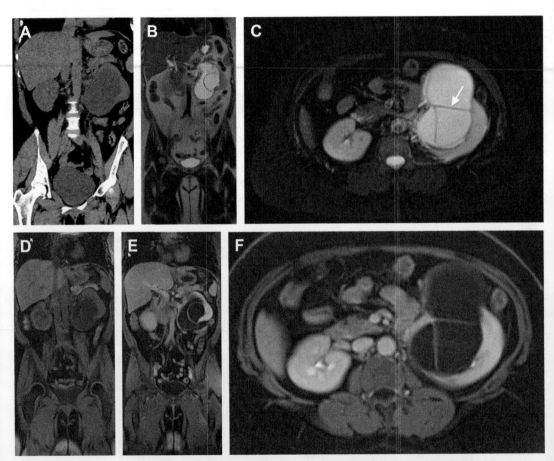

Fig. 8. A 52-year-old woman presented with abdominal pain and palpable mass in left upper quadrant. Unenhanced coronal CT image (A) shows an exophytic complex cystic renal mass in middle third of anterior portion of left kidney extending medially. Coronal (B) and axial (C) T2W images without and with fat saturation show multiple thick but smooth septations (arrow [C]). Coronal precontrast (D) and postcontrast arterial-phase (E) and axial delayed-phase (F) FS GRE T1W images show enhancement in the septations without solid components. Nephrectomy was performed, which confirmed diagnosis of MLCN.

with epithelial lining are seen. Solid stromal elements contain spindle cells mimicking ovarian stroma and express estrogen and progesterone receptors.[48] After resection of MEST, good prognosis with a benign course is usually seen; however, association of MEST with sarcoma is reported in few reports in literature.[18,49–53]

On MR imaging, MEST exhibits features of a well-circumscribed, complex, multiseptate cystic and solid mass with delayed contrast enhancement (Bosniak category III or IV lesions).[32,47,54] On T2W images, the cysts appear hyperintense with low signal intensity related to the septa and solid elements. FS T1W GRE delayed images reveal gadolinium enhancement in solid parts, histologically correlating with regions of spindle cells with densely cellular areas. The relatively less enhancing regions correspond to fibrotic areas. Sahni and colleagues[47] report a well-marginated, partially cystic mass with a central nodule. The cystic part showed T2 hyperintensity, while central nodular component demonstrated T1 hyperintensity, T2 hypointensity, and contrast enhancement on postgadolinium fat-suppressed T1W images.[47] Chu and colleagues[18] in their series report herniation of MEST into the renal pelvis mimicking transitional cell carcinoma, fat containing MEST, which was preoperatively diagnosed as angiomyolipoma and MEST containing hemorrhage.

MEST may show overlapping imaging features with MLCN and cystic RCC. Involvement of the renal pelvis may mimic multicystic dysplastic kidney or obstructed duplicated renal collecting system. Most studies reporting MEST have non–MR imaging modalities, which have limited soft tissue resolution.[18]

Both MLCN and MEST are benign cystic renal masses, which are pathologically related and often treated by surgical excision. Distinction of MLCN and MEST from multilocular cystic RCC and RCC with extensive cystic changes[42] may be challenging in some or many of these rare cases.

Unlike MEST, however, cystic RCCs exhibit thicker, irregularly enhancing septa and enhancing nodular or solid components. Benign complex renal cysts contain thin, nonenhancing internal septa without nodularity.

NEWLY DESCRIBED CYSTIC RENAL TUMORS:

1. Tubulocystic RCC (TC-RCC)
2. Cystic P-RCC

Tubulocystic Renal Cell Carcinoma

TC-RCC is a recently identified renal cystic renal tumor with only approximately 100 reported cases in the pathology literature.[55,56] Most lesions are identified incidentally on imaging for studies performed for other indications; however, patients may complain of hematuria or abdominal discomfort.[57]

Common presenting age is between 50 years and 70 years with strong male predominance and a male-to-female ratio of 7:1,[58–62] in contrast to female predominance seen with multicystic nephroma and MEST.

TC-RCCs are well-defined cysts that lack an outer capsule,[63] describe as a bubble wrap or spongy appearance because tumor contains small cystic spaces with intervening thin septae. On histology, TC-RCC can be differentiated from MLCN and MEST by lack of cellular ovarian-like stroma. Typically, histology shows small cysts with tightly packed tubular and intervening fibrous stroma, filled with serous fluid. Attenuated cuboidal to columnar epithelial cells are seen lining the cysts with hobnail appearance.[55,56]

Conflicting reports on immunohistochemical characteristics of TC-RCC have been published by researchers, which open the scope for further interrogation on their lineage of histogenesis of these cystic tumors. Honda and colleagues[64] reported distinct gene expression for TC-RCC and P-RCC without any overlapping features, although other investigators report similar cytologic, chromosomal, and immunohistochemical profiles closely linked to papillary carcinomas.[61] Various investigators report coexistence of TC-RCC and P-RCC in the same kidney or/and within the same tumor nodule in a cystic mass.[55,56] For instance, Cornelis and colleagues,[58] Yang and colleagues,[62] and Zhou and colleagues[61] report 22.2% (4/18), 38.4% (5/13), and 50% (10/20) association of TCC-RCC and P-RCC in their respective case series.

Multimodality approach is proposed by Cornelis and colleagues[58] to improve identification of TC-RCC. US shows characteristic features of hyperechoic mass with posterior acoustic enhancement, depicting tiny cystic spaces separated by multiple thin septa, resulting in increased acoustic reflections.

Few reports of MR imaging of TC-RCC exist and these describe small cysts with thin septa on T2W images. Enhancing septa or mural nodules can be identified on FS postcontrast T1W 3-D GRE.

TC-RCC currently shows overlapping imaging features to other cystic renal lesions including other cystic RCC, MEST, and multilocular cystic RCC. At this time, differentiation on imaging may be challenging.

Cystic Papillary Renal Cell Carcinoma

P-RCC is the second most frequently encountered RCC after clear cell subtype, which on MR imaging is characteristically seen as homogenous and hypo-intense mass on T2W images, which show mild delayed enhancement on FS T1 GRE sequences.[65]

In recent years, however, increasing reports have identified cystic P-RCC (up to 24%–26%) within series of malignant cystic renal lesions and RCC.[2,30] Although TC-RCCs commonly appeas as a multilocular cystic mass with or without solid components, atypical P-RCCs with dominant cystic change rarely have a multilocular cystic appearance, and the cystic components are commonly secondary to extensive necrosis or hemorrhage within the solid tumor.[30,64,65]

Cystic P-RCCs containing hemorrhage and ne-crosis show heterogeneous high signal intensity on T2W images and DWIs.[66] Bright signal precon-trast T1W images is displayed, which can interfere with identification of enhancing components on postcontrast images; in this scenario, subtraction imaging has been claimed to be useful.[67] Blood products from hemorrhagic changes can be shown on susceptibility-weighted images with high diagnostic accuracy.[68]

MR imaging has been found superior to CT for differentiating cystic P-RCC from hemorrhagic/pro-teinaceous cysts because of better contrast resolu-tion depicting internal tumor details.[69] It is also well established that superior contrast resolution of MR imaging improves identification of internal complexity and septations within the cyst tumor and, therefore, accurately assigns a higher Bosniak classification compared with CT examinations.[7]

The 2016 WHO classification favors overlapping molecular and immunohistochemical profiles of TC- RCC and P-RCC, identifying the fact that TC-RCC can contain components of P-RCC.[61,62] Thus, overlapping imaging features of TC-RCC and cystic P-RCC may be seen. Conversely, distinct chromosomal profiles of TC-RCC and P-RCC have been reported[60,70]; henceforth, more studies are required to improve better under-standing of imaging spectrum of these 2 newly described entities.

SUMMARY

Superior soft tissue and contrast resolution of MR imaging benefits sensitivity to kidney cyst features and classification, which may have an impact on patient management and outcomes. CEUS may have nearly similar sensitivity for detection of cyst features yet is dependent on patient body habitus and adequacy of visualization windows for the kidneys, which does not have the same impact on MR imaging results. Both MR imaging and CEUS may provide superior kidney cyst assessment compared with CECT; however, further research is needed, particularly for the identification of role of CEUS.

ACKNOWLEDGMENTS

The authors would like to acknowledge CEUS image contribution by Dr Alison Harris, Clinical Associate Professor and Abdominal Fellowship Di-rector, Medical Head-Abdominal Division, Depart-ment of Radiology, University of British Columbia, Vancouver, BC, Canada.

REFERENCES

1. Berland LL, Silverman SG, Gore RM, et al. Managing incidental findings on abdominal CT: white paper of the ACR incidental findings committee. J Am Coll Radiol 2010;7(10):754–73.
2. Smith AD, Remer EM, Cox KL, et al. Bosniak cate-gory IIF and III cystic renal lesions: outcomes and associations. Radiology 2012;262(1):152–60.
3. Israel GM, Bosniak MA. An update of the Bosniak renal cyst classification system. Urology 2005;66: 484–8.
4. Israel GM, Bosniak MA. How I do it: evaluating renal masses. Radiology 2005;236:441–50.
5. Bosniak MA. The bosniak renal cyst classification: 25 years later. Radiology 2012;262:781–5.
6. Balci CN, Semelka RC, Patt RH, et al. Complex renal cysts: findings on MR imaging. Am J Roentgenol 1999;172:1495–500.
7. Israel GM, Hindman N, Bosniak MA. Evaluation of cystic renal masses: comparison of CT and MR im-aging by using the Bosniak classification system. Radiology 2004;231(2):365–71.
8. Graumann O, Osther SS, Karstoft J, et al. Bosniak classification system: a prospective comparison of CT, contrast-enhanced US, and MR for categorizing complex renal cystic masses. Acta Radiol 2016; 57(11):1409–17.
9. Quaia E. Microbubble ultrasound contrast agents: an update. Eur Radiol 2007;17(8):1995–2008.
10. Harvey CJ, Blomley MJ, Eckersley RJ, et al. Devel-opments in ultrasound contrast media. Eur Radiol 2001;11(4):675–89.
11. Cosgrove D, Harvey C. Clinical uses of microbub-bles in diagnosis and treatment. Med Biol Eng Com-put 2009;47(8):813–26.
12. Wilson SR, Burns PN. Microbubble-enhanced US in body imaging: what role? Radiology 2010;257(1): 24–39.
13. Park BK, Kim B, Kim SH, et al. Assessment of cystic renal masses based on Bosniak

classification: comparison of CT and contrast-enhanced US. Eur J Radiol 2007;61(2):310–4.

14. Xu Y, Zhang S, Wei X, et al. Contrast enhanced ultrasonography prediction of cystic renal mass in comparison to histopathology. Clin Hemorheol Microcirc 2014;58(3):429–38.

15. Ascenti G, Mazziotti S, Zimbaro G, et al. Complex cystic renal masses: characterization with contrast-enhanced US. Radiology 2007;243:158–65.

16. Clevert DA, Minaifar N, Weckbach S, et al. Multislice computed tomography versus contrast-enhanced ultrasound in evaluation of complex cystic renal masses using the Bosniak classification system. Clin Hemorheol Microcirc 2008;39:171–8.

17. Quaia E, Bertolotto M, Cioffi V, et al. Comparison of contrast-enhanced sonography with unenhanced sonography and contrast-enhanced CT in the diagnosis of malignancy in complex cystic renal masses. AJR Am J Roentgenol 2008;191:1239–49.

18. Chu LC, Hruban RH, Horton KM, et al. Mixed epithelial and stromal tumor of the kidney: radiologic-pathologic correlation. Radiographics 2010;30(6): 1541–51.

19. Taouli B, Thakur RK, Mannelli L, et al. Renal lesions: characterization with diffusion-weighted imaging versus contrast-enhanced MR imaging. Radiology 2009;251(2):398–407.

20. Rosenkrantz AB, Wehrli NE, Mussi TC, et al. Complex cystic renal masses: comparison of cyst complexity and Bosniak classification between 1.5 T and 3.0 T. Eur J Radiol 2014;83:503–8.

21. Ward RD, Remer EM. Cystic renal masses: an imaging update. Eur J Radiol 2018;99:103–10.

22. Chow W-H, Dong LM, Devesa SS. Epidemiology and risk factors for kidney cancer. Nat Rev Urol 2010;7:245–57.

23. Dunnick R, Sandler C, Newhouse J. Renal cystic disease. In: Pine J, editor. Textbook of uroradiology. 5th edition. Philadelphia: Wolters Kluwer Health; 2012. ProQuest Ebook Central, Available at: http://ebookcentral.proquest.com/lib/uaz/detail.action?docID=3418261. Accessed April 20, 2018.

24. Moch H, Cubilla AL, Humphrey PA, et al. The 2016 WHO classification of tumours of the urinary system and male genital organs-part A: renal, penile, and testicular tumours. Eur Urol 2016;70(1):93–105.

25. Hartman DS, Davio CJ, Johns T, et al. Cystic renal cell carcinoma. Urology 1986;28:145–53.

26. Freire M, Remer EM. Clinical and radiologic features of cystic renal masses. AJR Am J Roentgenol 2009; 192(5):1367–72.

27. Aubert S, Zini L, Delomez J, et al. Cystic renal cell carcinomas in adults: is preoperative recognition of multilocular cystic renal cell carcinoma possible? J Urol 2005;174:2115–9.

28. Hindman NM, Bosniak MA, Rosenkrantz AB, et al. Multilocular cystic renal cell carcinoma: comparison of imaging and pathologic findings. AJR Am J Roentgenol 2012;198:W20–6.

29. Yamashita Y, Watanabe O, Miyazaki T, et al. Cystic renal cell carcinoma. Imaging findings with pathologic correlation. Acta Radiol 1994;35:19Y24.

30. Brinker DA, Amin MB, de Peralta-Venturina M, et al. Extensively necrotic cystic renal cell carcinoma: a clinicopathologic study with comparison to other cystic and necrotic renal cancers. Am J Surg Pathol 2000;24(7):988–95.

31. Onishi T, Oishi Y, Goto H, et al. Cyst-associated renal cell carcinoma: clinicopathologic characteristics and evaluation of prognosis in 27 cases. Int J Urol 2001;8:268Y274.

32. Lane BR, Campbell SC, Remer EM, et al. Adult cystic nephroma and mixed epithelial and stromal tumor of the kidney: clinical, radiographic, and pathologic characteristics. Urology 2008;71(6):1142–8.

33. Bonsib SM. Cystic nephroma. Mixed epithelial and stromal tumor. In: Eble JN, Sauter G, Epstein JI, et al, editors. World Health Organization classification of tumours. Pathology and genetics of tumors of the urinary system and male genital organs. Lyon (France): IARC Press; 2004. p. 76.

34. Turbiner J, Amin MB, Humphrey PA, et al. Cystic nephroma and mixed epithelial and stromal tumor of kidney: a detailed clinicopathologic analysis of 34 cases and proposal for renal epithelial and stromal tumor (REST) as a unifying term. Am J Surg Pathol 2007;31:489–500.

35. Gallo GE, Penchansky L. Cystic nephroma. Cancer 1977;39:1322–7.

36. Charles AK, Vujanic GM, Berry PJ. Renal tumours of childhood. Histopathology 1998;32:293–309.

37. Silver IM, Boag AH, Soboleski DA. Best cases from the AFIP: multilocular cystic renal tumor—cystic nephroma. RadioGraphics 2008;28:1221–5 [discussion: 1225–6].

38. Mukhopadhyay S, Valente AL, de la Roza G. Cystic nephroma: a histologic and immunohistochemical study of 10 cases. Arch Pathol Lab Med 2004;128: 1404–11.

39. Stamatiou K, Polizois K, Kollaitis G, et al. Cystic nephroma: a case report and review of the literature. Cases J 2008;1:267.

40. Antic T, Perry KT, Harrison K, et al. Mixed epithelial and stromal tumor of the kidney and cystic nephroma share overlapping features: reappraisal of 15 lesions. Arch Pathol Lab Med 2006;130:80–5.

41. Castillo OA, Boyle ET Jr, Kramer SA. Multilocular cysts of kidney. A study of 29 patients and review of literature. Urology 1991;37:156–62.

42. Eble JN, Bonsib SM. Extensively cystic renal neoplasms: cystic nephroma, cystic partially differentiated nephroblastoma, multilocular cystic renal cell carcinoma, and cystic hamartoma of renal pelvis. Semin Diagn Pathol 1998;15:2–20.

43. Bisceglia M, Galliani CA, Senger C, et al. Renal cystic diseases: a review. Adv Anat Pathol 2006; 13:26–56.

44. Wilkinson C, Palit V, Bardapure M, et al. Adult multilocular cystic nephroma: report of six cases with clinical, radio-pathologic correlation and review of literature. Urol Ann 2013;5(1):13–7.

45. Michal M, Syrucek M. Benign mixed epithelial and stromal tumor of the kidney. Pathol Res Pract 1998; 194(6):445–8.

46. Adsay NV, Eble JN, Srigley JR, et al. Mixed epithelial and stromal tumor of the kidney. Am J Surg Pathol 2000;24(7):958–70.

47. Sahni VA, Mortele KJ, Glickman J, et al. Mixed epithelial and stromal tumour of the kidney: imaging features. BJU Int 2010;105(7):932–9.

48. Zhou M, Kort E, Hoekstra P, et al. Adult cystic nephroma and mixed epithelial and stromal tumor of the kidney are the same disease entity: molecular and histologic evidence. Am J Surg Pathol 2009;33(1): 72–80.

49. Jung SJ, Shen SS, Tran T, et al. Mixed epithelial and stromal tumor of kidney with malignant transformation: report of two cases and review of literature. Hum Pathol 2008;39(3):463–8.

50. Kuroda N, Sakaida N, Kinoshita H, et al. Carcinosarcoma arising in mixed epithelial and stromal tumor of the kidney. APMIS 2008;116(11):1013–5.

51. Nakagawa T, Kanai Y, Fujimoto H, et al. Malignant mixed epithelial and stromal tumours of the kidney: a report of the first two cases with a fatal clinical outcome. Histopathology 2004;44(3):302–4.

52. Sukov WR, Cheville JC, Lager DJ, et al. Malignant mixed epithelial and stromal tumor of the kidney with rhabdoid features: report of a case including immunohistochemical, molecular genetic studies and comparison to morphologically similar renal tumors. Hum Pathol 2007;38(9):1432–7.

53. Svec A, Hes O, Michal M, et al. Malignant mixed epithelial and stromal tumor of the kidney. Virchows Arch 2001;439(5):700–2.

54. Park HS, Kim SH, Kim SH, et al. Benign mixed epithelial and stromal tumor of the kidney: imaging findings. J Comput Assist Tomogr 2005;29(6):786–9.

55. Kuroda N, Matsumoto H, Ohe C, et al. Review of tubulocystic carcinoma of the kidney with focus on clinical and pathobiological aspects. Pol J Pathol 2013;64:233–7.

56. Bhullar JS, Varshney N, Bhullar AK, et al. A new type of renal cancer-tubulocystic carcinoma of the kidney: a review of the literature. Int J Surg Pathol 2013;22:297–302.

57. Srigley JR, Delahunt B. Uncommon and recently described renal carcinomas. Mod Pathol 2009;22: S2–23.

58. Cornelis F, Hélénon O, Correas JM, et al. Tubulocystic renal cell carcinoma: a new radiological entity. Eur Radiol 2016;26(4):1108–15.

59. MacLennan GT, Bostwick DG. Tubulocystic carcinoma, mucinous tubular and spindle cell carcinoma, and other recently described rare renal tumors. Clin Lab Med 2005;25:393–416.

60. Amin MB, MacLennan GT, Gupta R, et al. Tubulocystic carcinoma of the kidney: clinicopathologic analysis of 31 cases of a distinctive rare subtype of renal cell carcinoma. Am J Surg Pathol 2009;33(3): 384–92.

61. Zhou M, Yang XJ, Lopez JI, et al. Renal tubulocystic carcinoma is closely related to papillary renal cell carcinoma: implications for pathologic classification. Am J Surg Pathol 2009;33(12):1840–9.

62. Yang XJ, Zhou M, Hes O, et al. Tubulocystic carcinoma of the kidney: clinicopathologic and molecular characterization. Am J Surg Pathol 2008;32(2): 177–87.

63. MacLennan GT, Cheng L. Tubulocystic carcinoma of the kidney. J Urol 2011;185:2348–9.

64. Honda Y, Goto K, Nakamura Y, et al. Imaging features of papillary renal cell carcinoma with cystic change-dominant appearance in the era of the 2016 WHO classification. Abdom Radiol (NY) 2017;42(7):1850–6.

65. Egbert ND, Caoili EM, Cohan RH, et al. Differentiation of papillary renal cell carcinoma subtypes on CT and MRI. AJR Am J Roentgenol 2013;201(2): 347–55.

66. Akita H, Jinzaki M, Akita A, et al. Renal cell carcinoma in patients with acquired cystic disease of the kidney: assessment using a combination of T2-weighted, diffusion-weighted, and chemical-shift MRI without the use of contrast material. J Magn Reson Imaging 2014;39(4):924–30.

67. Kim S, Jain M, Harris AB, et al. T1 hyperintense renal lesions: characterization with diffusion-weighted MR imaging versus contrast-enhanced MR imaging. Radiology 2009;251(3):796–807.

68. Xing W, He X, Kassir MA, et al. Evaluating hemorrhage in renal cell carcinoma using susceptibility weighted imaging. PLoS One 2013;8(2):e57691.

69. Dilauro M, Quon M, McInnes MD, et al. Comparison of contrast-enhanced multiphase renal protocol CT versus MRI for diagnosis of papillary renal cell carcinoma. AJR Am J Roentgenol 2016;206(2):319–25.

70. Tran T, Jones CL, Williamson SR, et al. Tubulocystic renal cell carcinoma is an entity that is immunohistochemically and genetically distinct from papillary renal cell carcinoma. Histopathology 2016;68(6): 850–7.

MR Imaging Evaluation of the Kidneys in Patients with Reduced Kidney Function
Noncontrast Techniques Versus Contrast-Enhanced Techniques

Jaspreet K. Bisla, MD, Manojkumar Saranathan, PhD,
Diego R. Martin, MD, PhD, FRCPC, Hina Arif-Tiwari, MD, DNB,
Bobby T. Kalb, MD*

KEYWORDS

- Kidneys • Renal impairment • Magnetic resonance imaging techniques
- Contrast-enhanced MR imaging • Noncontrast MR imaging • Functional imaging

KEY POINTS

- MR imaging is a widely used noninvasive method that has intrinsic strengths for evaluating a wide range of renal pathology and has the ability to provide functional analysis of the kidney (eg, renal blood flow, oxygenation and glomerular filtration rate), that is not practically available with any other imaging technology.
- There are a wide variety of noncontrast MR imaging techniques available for evaluating both kidney structure and function, which are especially useful in patients with reduced kidney function and obviate the use of intravenous contrast.
- Contrast-enhanced techniques improve diagnostic accuracy for a wide range of clinical indications, including tumor evaluation, and are used increasingly for functional analysis of quantitative biometrics, such as glomerular filtration rate and kidney blood flow.

INTRODUCTION

MR imaging is a widely used noninvasive imaging method that has intrinsic strengths for evaluating a wide range of renal pathology. Advantages of MR imaging include excellent soft tissue contrast and no ionizing radiation exposure. In addition, MR imaging has the ability to provide functional analysis of the kidney (eg, renal blood flow, oxygenation, and glomerular filtration rate), that is not practically available with any other imaging technology. Contrast-enhanced imaging is an important component of MR imaging examinations of the kidney. Although there are potential safety concerns with gadolinium-based chelate agent (GBCA) administration, the overall safety profile is excellent and, by comparison, favorable to iodinated contrast agents. In addition, there is a growing array of diagnostically useful noncontrast MR imaging techniques available. This review highlights the various noncontrast and contrast enhanced MR techniques available for kidney imaging, and highlights their utility in clinical practice.

The authors have nothing to disclose.
Department of Medical Imaging, University of Arizona, 1501 North Campbell Avenue, PO Box 245067, Tucson, AZ 85724-5067, USA
* Corresponding author.
E-mail address: bkalb@radiology.arizona.edu

Magn Reson Imaging Clin N Am 27 (2019) 45 57
https://doi.org/10.1016/j.mric.2018.09.004

NONCONTRAST TECHNIQUES
T2-Weighted Imaging

T2-weighted (T2W) imaging is a fundamental component of any abdomen-pelvis MR Exam, and for body imaging. Acquisition with a single-shot technique provides the most robust, high-quality fluid-sensitive imaging for renal pathology. Single-shot T2W sequences (ssT2) are truly the workhorse of noncontrast body MR imaging, and provide excellent structural and morphologic evaluation of the kidneys and collecting system. Compared with standard, multi-shot turbo spin-echo T2 images, ssT2 images can suffer from some image blurring due toT2 decay along the long readout as well as the use of partial Fourier acquisition to reduce specific absorption rate (SAR). Multi-breath-hold T2 fast spin-echo (T2 FSE) sequences are another option, which have the advantage of increased image sharpness and some improvements in T2 contrast between lesions and normal tissues. However, the need for multiple breath holds increases the time and complexity of the examination, and is not possible in patients who have difficulty in breath-holding. By using the single-shot technique, robust image quality can be performed even in free-breathing patients, ideal for patients of varying levels of cognition and health status. Recently, the image quality of ssT2 sequences has been significantly improved by using a variable refocusing flip angle methodology, which has the combined benefit of increasing image sharpness and also decreasing SAR and scan times (**Fig. 1**).[1,2]

T2W imaging is key for differentiation of the normal renal cortex and medulla (**Fig. 2**), a differentiation that is lost in both acute and chronic kidney disorders (**Fig. 3**). The bright signal intensity of fluid in T2W MR imaging is excellent for depiction of the renal collecting system, and provides a highly sensitive method for evaluating hydronephrosis. Although MR imaging is not sensitive for the detection of calcified urologic stones, it is highly sensitive for the secondary changes of obstruction and perinephric fluid that occurs with obstructing urolithiasis (**Fig. 4**), correctly identifying the source of pain in patients who may want to avoid exposure to ionizing radiation, such as pregnant and pediatric patients.

Diffusion-Weighted Imaging

Diffusion-weighted imaging (DWI) is based on the Brownian motion of water molecules and used to distinguish between the rapid, unrestricted diffusion of protons versus impeded or slow diffusion of protons (restricted diffusion). The impendence of water molecules is related to high tissue cellularity and the presence of intact cell membranes, whereas unrestricted diffusion is associated with low tissue cellularity that permits rapid diffusion of protons. Therefore, restricted diffusion is most often identified in highly cellular tumors, cytotoxic edema, abscesses, and fibrosis. Apparent diffusion coefficient (ADC) maps are generated from diffusion images obtained at different b values and provides a quantitative metric of differences in tissue diffusivity.[3]

The addition of DWI in abdominal imaging protocols has become standard over the past decade, with an oncologic emphasis based on a high sensitivity for the detection of early metastatic disease in a variety of tumor subtypes.[4–9] DWI is relatively less useful for the primary diagnosis of renal cell carcinoma (RCC), due to a lower contrast differentiation between RCC and normal renal parenchyma (compared with hepatic tumor demonstration, for example). However, there has been extensive work investigating the diffusion characteristics of benign versus malignant renal masses, subtyping RCCs, and tumor grading. Multiple studies have suggested that malignant renal tumors may demonstrate statistically significant lower ADC values as compared with benign lesions (**Figs. 5** and **6**).[10–13] A meta-analysis based on 17 studies with 764 patients showed that

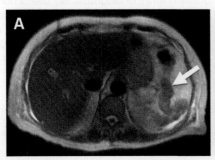
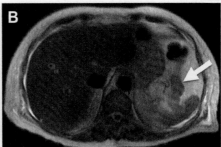

Fig. 1. Standard ssT2 image (*A*) and ssT2 image with a variable flip angle acquisition (*B*). Note the edge blurring seen along the colonic margin with standard single-shot images (*A, arrow*), versus the variable flip angle single-shot sequence (*B, arrow*).

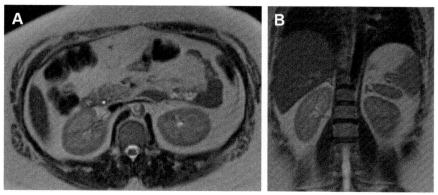

Fig. 2. A 42-year-old woman with acute appendicitis, but no history of renal disease, diabetes, or hypertension. Axial (*A*) and coronal (*B*) ssT2 images show the higher signal renal medulla that contrasts well against the renal cortex in this patient without known renal dysfunction.

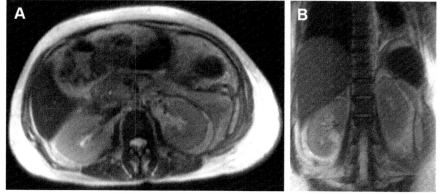

Fig. 3. A 50-year-old woman with acute pancreatitis, acute kidney injury. Axial (*A*) and coronal (*B*) ssT2 images show the kidneys are diffusely increased in signal and do not show the normal differentiation between the renal cortex and medulla.

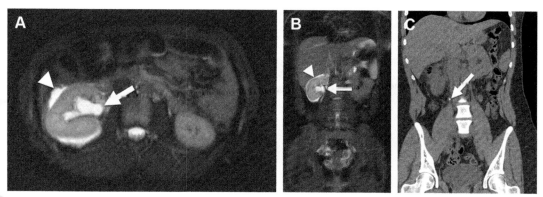

Fig. 4. A 25-year-old woman with right upper quadrant pain. Fat-saturated axial (*A*) and coronal (*B*) ssT2 images demonstrate moderate right-sided hydronephrosis (*A and B, arrow*) and prominent perinephric fluid (*A and B, arrowhead*). Subsequent noncontrast CT (*C*) demonstrated a small, obstructing stone in the mid right ureter (*C, arrow*).

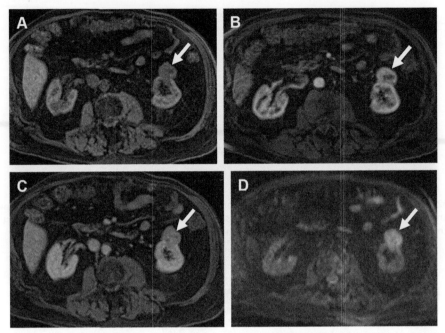

Fig. 5. An 81-year-old man with clear cell RCC. Axial precontrast (*A*), arterial (*B*), and delayed (*C*) phase fat-saturated 3D T1W GRE postcontrast images demonstrate a solid, arterial enhancing left renal mass (*arrows, A–C*), shown to be a clear cell RCC on surgical resection. Note the diffusion-weighted sequence with moderate restricted diffusion (*D, arrow*).

RCCs have significantly lower ADC values than benign tissue ($1.61 \pm 0.08 \times 10^{-3}$ mm^2/s versus $2.10 \pm 0.09 \times 10^{-3}$ mm^2/s; $P<.0001$).[14] Sandrasegaran and colleagues[15] determined that ADC measurements may aid in differentiating benign cystic lesions from cystic renal cell cancers. They found that ADC values of the benign lesions were significantly higher than those of the malignant

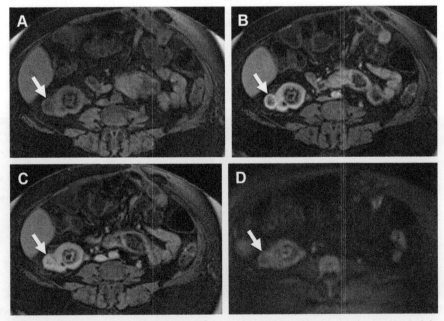

Fig. 6. A 54-year-old woman with oncocytoma, confirmed on surgical resection. Axial precontrast (*A*), arterial (*B*), and delayed (*C*) phase fat-saturated 3D T1W GRE postcontrast images demonstrate a solid, arterial enhancing right renal mass (*arrows, A–C*), shown to be an oncocytoma on surgical resection. Note the diffusion-weighted sequence with relatively low level of restricted diffusion (*D, arrow*).

lesions (mean, 2.72 vs 1.88 × 10^{-3} mm²/s; $P<.0001$); the ADCs of the 31 benign cysts were significantly higher than those of the 7 cystic renal cancers (2.77 vs 2.02 × 10^{-3} mm²/s; $P<.001$).

The diagnosis of lymphoma is a clinical scenario in which DWI has significant added benefit, as lymphomatous tissue demonstrates markedly restricted diffusion (especially compared with background renal parenchyma), providing some added diagnostic specificity for this tumor type (**Fig. 7**).

In addition, DWI is very useful in the assessment of pyelonephritis and abscess. In pyelonephritis, DWI demonstrates a striated pattern of restricted diffusion (**Fig. 8**) that may demonstrate abnormality even before contrast-enhanced images. Abscesses form as a later sequelae of severe pyelonephritis, and manifest as a fluid-filled cavity in the renal parenchyma that demonstrates marked restricted diffusion (**Fig. 9**), which allows for ready differentiation from renal cysts. Rathod and colleagues[16] examined the role of DWI in diagnosing infection and found that areas of nephritis had significantly lower ADC values than the normal renal cortical parenchyma. Also, renal abscesses had significantly lower ADC values than areas of nephritis. In a retrospective study of 88 patients, Goyal and colleagues[17] found that abscesses and RCC both show statistically significant restricted diffusion as compared with the renal parenchyma (1.12 and 1.56, respectively, vs 2.34 ×10^{-3} mm²/s for normal kidney; $P<.0001$ for both), and abscesses restricted to a greater extent than RCCs, which was also statistically significant.

Angiography

Several noncontrast MR angiography techniques have been developed in the past decade, which use either flow-related enhancement, phase-dependent enhancement, or flow-independent enhancement. The most common noncontrast MR techniques to image the renal vasculature include time of flight (TOF), inflow-balanced steady-state free precession (SSFP), and phase contrast.

In conventional TOF angiography, the background stationary volume in an imaging slab is saturated, whereas the inflowing fresh blood appears bright.[18] Although this technique is prevalent for evaluation of the intracranial vasculature, TOF is challenging in renal imaging due to of the limited saturation of vessels with in-plane flowing blood, respiratory motion artifacts, arterial pulsation artifacts, and signal loss at severe stenoses.[19,20]

SSFP angiography is a flow-independent bright blood technique deriving image contrast from the

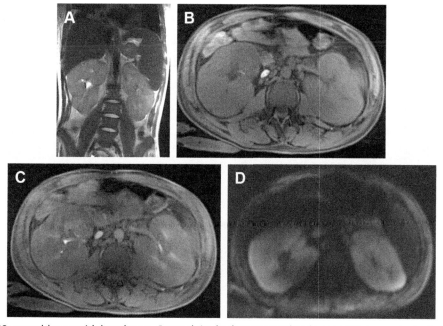

Fig. 7. A 20-year-old man with lymphoma. Coronal single-shot T2-weighted image (*A*) demonstrates both kidneys to be markedly enlarged, showing abnormal signal. Axial precontrast (*B*) and delayed (*C*) phase fat-saturated 3D T1W GRE postcontrast images demonstrate diffuse infiltration of both kidneys by homogeneous, hypovascular soft tissue. DWI (*D*) demonstrates markedly abnormal restricted diffusion throughout both kidneys, in keeping with the diagnosis of lymphoma.

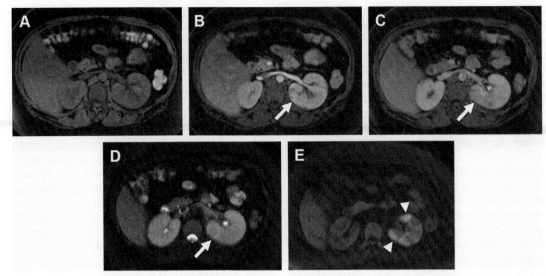

Fig. 8. A 35-year-old woman with pyelonephritis. Axial precontrast (*A*), arterial (*B*), and delayed (*C*) phase fat-saturated 3D T1W GRE postcontrast images demonstrate heterogeneous enhancement of the left kidney with striated areas of hypoperfusion (*B and C, arrows*). Fat-saturated ssT2 image shows abnormal T2 signal (*D, arrow*) in this area of striated enhancement, with some mild perinephric fluid. DWI (*E*) shows multiple wedge-shaped areas of restricted diffusion (*arrowheads*).

T1 and T2 properties of blood pool. SSFP is based on a gradient-echo (GRE) sequence in which steady-state longitudinal and transverse magnetizations are maintained. This technique uses a slab selective adiabatic inversion pulse to suppress the stationary background tissue. The long inflow time of several hundred milliseconds ensures adequate inflow of fresh arterial blood into the imaging slab,

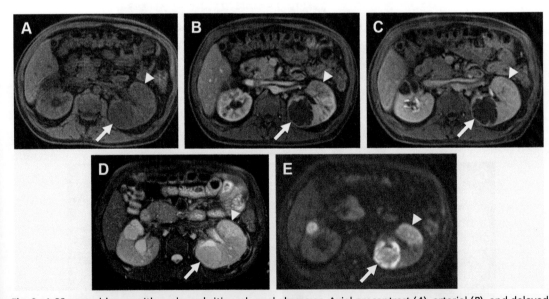

Fig. 9. A 32-year-old man with pyelonephritis and renal abscesses. Axial precontrast (*A*), arterial (*B*), and delayed (*C*) phase fat-saturated 3D T1W GRE postcontrast images demonstrate heterogeneous enhancement of the left kidney with striated areas of hypoperfusion (*A–C, arrowheads*). A large cystic lesion is also present medially in the left kidney without internal enhancement (*A–C, arrows*). Fat-saturated ssT2 image (*D*) shows abnormal T2 signal (*arrowhead*) in the areas of striated enhancement, with complex T2 signal in the cystic lesion (*arrow*). DWI (*E*) shows multiple wedge-shaped areas of restricted diffusion (*arrowhead*) in the area of pyelonephritis, whereas the cystic lesion also shows marked restricted diffusion (*arrow*), in keeping with a parenchymal abscess.

which imparts a high signal-to-noise ratio (SNR). Given that this method relies on brisk arterial inflow, it is suboptimal in individuals with slow flow or poor cardiac output.[20] Advantages of this SSFP are high SNR, shorter acquisition times, and widespread availability; this technique has been used for the preoperative evaluation of renal donors to depict renal vascular anatomy (**Fig. 10**). Limitations of the technique are susceptibility to field heterogeneity and interference from background signals requiring additional preparatory pulses.

Phase-contrast MR angiography uses bipolar or flow-compensated pulses to detect a phase shift caused by blood flowing through a magnetic field.[21–24] Bipolar magnetic field gradients are added to a GRE pulse sequence so that the phase of the MR imaging signal is proportional to the velocity of the flowing blood.[20] Angiographic images are produced by subtracting the 2-dimensional (2D) or 3D flow-compensated acquisition from the uncompensated acquisition. Flow-encoded data must be acquired in 3 orthogonal planes.[20,25] The advantages of this technique are ability to quantify arterial flow velocity, good suppression of background signal, and it is independent of flow direction. A significant limitation of phase-contrast angiography is long acquisition times. Also, there is signal loss in turbulent flow and this technique is motion sensitive and parameter dependent.[25]

Other noncontrast methods of angiography have been developed, such as quiescent-interval single-shot (QISS) angiography, which uses an in-plane radiofrequency saturation pulse to saturate the static tissue, which is followed by a tracking venous saturation pulse to suppress the venous inflow signal. Subsequently, there is a quiescent interval of approximately 230 ms during which time there is rapid systolic arterial inflow of unsaturated blood, after which a chemical shift-selective fat saturation is performed to destroy any fat signal that has recovered followed by a readout.[26] However, this technique has primarily been used for evaluation of the lower extremity peripheral vasculature (primarily in patients unable to receive gadolinium contrast), with limited experience involving the renal vasculature.[27]

Functional Imaging

MR imaging has the advantage of being able to provide functional information in addition to structural information. Many of the noncontrast MR imaging techniques for renal functional imaging remain developmental in nature, and are the focus of current research, but with the potential to provide a noninvasive assessment of a variety of renal functional parameters.

Blood oxygenation level (BOLD) imaging is a technique for assessing renal hypoxia and providing information regarding metabolic status of the kidney. Imaging sensitive to the local tissue oxygen concentration is acquired by using the paramagnetic properties of deoxyhemoglobin, which at higher concentrations results in increased T2* relaxation time and accelerated dephasing, with subsequent signal loss in the surrounding tissues.[28,29] The renal medulla typically functions in a hypoxic environment and is susceptible to small changes in blood oxygenation. This technique has been applied in renal perfusion for the evaluation of renal artery stenosis, transplant allograft dysfunction, and diabetic nephropathy.[29] However, because it is based on an echo-planar imaging technique (which is very sensitive to B0 inhomogeneity), it is relatively limited in spatial resolution and suffers marked image distortion in the presence of metal.

MR elastography (MRE) is an imaging method that uses mechanical waves to quantitatively

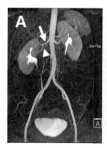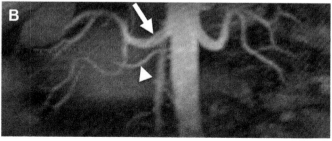

Fig. 10. A 56-year-old woman undergoing preoperative evaluation for possible kidney donation. Contrast-enhanced 3D GRE MR angiography (*A*) demonstrates 2 right renal arteries, a dominant superior artery (*arrow*) and a smaller inferior artery (*arrowhead*). A noncontrast, 3D balanced SSFP technique (*B*) also clearly demonstrates both the dominant superior artery (*arrow*) and also the inferior accessory artery (*arrowhead*), although with a more limited anatomic coverage.

assess the shear modulus of tissues. Shear waves with frequencies ranging from 50 to 500 Hz are induced in tissues using an external driver, and are then propagated into the imaged tissue. The degree of displacement of the imaged tissue is dependent on the viscoelastic properties of that tissue, and these displacements can be visualized and directly quantified in MRE.[29,30] Assessment of renal fibrosis, particularly in renal allografts, is an actively researched topic using MRE, among other developmental techniques. It should be noted that a study of kidney stiffness in using ultrasound elastography showed that other factors contributing to kidney stiffness are filling pressure of the renal collecting system, arterial and venous blood flow, and direction of sound wave relative to the kidney.[31]

Arterial spin labeling is a technique in which the inflowing arterial blood supplying a tissue of interest is labeled by alteration of its longitudinal magnetization. The signal differences in the images between the applied labeled arterial blood and nonlabeled images is a measure of perfusion. Clinical applications of this technique include evaluation of renal artery stenosis and allograft dysfunction. Although this is a powerful technique with the potential to assess tissue perfusion without the use of intravenous contrast, it remains subject to artifacts from insufficient suppression of background tissue and poor SNR.

MR IMAGING CONTRAST MEDIA

The administration of intravenous contrast for MR imaging improves diagnostic accuracy for a wide range of clinical indications, including tumor characterization and staging, assessment of vascular disease, and evaluation of infectious processes and abscess. In addition to the most commonly used GBCAs, there are several other contrast agents available for MR imaging, including manganese agents and superparamagnetic iron oxide agents.[32] As with any drug administered to patients, the risks of drug administration must be weighed against the benefits.

Gadolinium-Based Chelate Agents

Since the US Food and Drug Administration (FDA) approval for intravenous administration in 1988, GBCAs have been the most widely used contrast agents for MR imaging. GBCAs have an excellent safety profile, with an exceedingly low rate of severe contrast reactions and immediate adverse events, especially when compared with iodinated contrasts.[33–38] In addition, GBCAs do not negatively affect renal function in the standard doses administered for clinical imaging,[38–42] another advantage when compared with iodinated contrast agents.

Nephrogenic systemic fibrosis (NSF) is a rare fibrosing disorder primarily affecting the skin and subcutaneous tissues but known to involve organs such as heart, lungs, esophagus, and skeletal muscle. In 2006, a strong association between NSF and patients with impaired renal function,[43] usually undergoing dialysis, was identified. GBCAs are excreted primarily by the kidneys, and it is hypothesized that delayed excretion and prolonged exposure in patients with severe renal disease results in increased the amount of gadolinium agent released from the chelating agent.[32,44]

Since the discovery of NSF, extensive research has shown that the risk of developing the disease is highly dependent on the stability of the gadolinium chelate, with lower stability agents showing higher rates of tissue deposition. In addition, the lowest stability (typically linear and nonionic) agents were responsible for the vast majority of NSF cases across the world. In contrast, the more stable linear ionic and macrocyclic agents were associated with very few cases of NSF. Because of this, the American College of Radiology (ACR) Committee on Drugs and Contrast Media, the European Medicines Agency, and the FDA have classified GBCAs into different groups based on reported NSF associations. Per ACR Manual on contrast media, group I agents are associated with the greatest number of NSF cases and include gadodiamide (Omniscan), gadopentetate dimeglumine (Magnevist), and gadoversetamide (OptiMark). Group II agents including, gadobenate dimeglumine (Multihance), gadobutrol (Gadavist), gadoteridol (Prohance), and gadoterate meglumine (Dotarem), are associated with few, if any, unconfounded cases of NSF. Finally, there are limited data regarding NSF risk for group III agents including gadoxetic acid (Eovist), but few or if any unconfounded cases have been reported.[45] Multiple studies have demonstrated 0% incidence of NSF after switching contrast agents,[44,46–48] and there have been no new cases of NSF in the past 9 years. However, the recently discovered deposition of gadolinium in the brain in even patients with normal renal function again necessitates careful assessment of the need to use GBCAs since the mechanisms and clinical effects of deposition are still not known.[45]

Ferumoxytol

Ferumoxytol (Feraheme) is an ultrasmall superparamagnetic iron oxide agent that was developed as an MR imaging contrast agent in the early 2000s. In 2009, it received FDA approval as an intravenous treatment for iron deficiency anemia in adults with chronic kidney disease. However, Feraheme has been increasingly used as an MR imaging contrast agent by researchers and clinicians, especially since concerns regarding NSF became known. In contrast to GBCAs, Feraheme poses no risk for NSF. Ferumoxytol is a relatively large molecular compound (approximately 750 kDa) made of iron oxide particles and a carbohydrate coating that acts as a blood pool agent with relatively little leakage of the agent into the extravascular/interstitial clearance with a circulating half-life of 14 to 21 hours.[49–51] Advantages of the longer temporal window of increased vascular signal are possibilities of repeat imaging without the requirement for additional contrast material for up to 72 hours, longer imaging acquisitions as compared with GBCAs, and excellent venous imaging. However, the iron agent does accumulate in the reticuloendothelial system, and the long-term effects of increased iron uptake are not well known at this time.

CONTRAST-ENHANCED TECHNIQUES
Three-Dimensional Gradient Echo

Fat-saturated, T1-weighted (T1W) 3D spoiled GRE sequences are the mainstay of contrast-enhanced MR renal imaging. Precontrast T1W 3D GRE images are excellent for demonstrating hemorrhage and proteinaceous material, especially important for the assessment of cystic renal lesions (Fig. 11). The dynamic contrast-enhanced images provide essential information for tumor analysis, depicting both the presence of vascularized soft tissue elements and the pattern of contrast enhancement. Assessing the patterns of dynamic contrast enhancement (in combination with assessment of T2 signal) allows for accurate assessment of tumor histology for the most common subtypes of RCC,[52] in addition to the differentiation of RCC from urothelial carcinoma.

Functional Imaging

Obtaining an accurate measure of renal function remains a challenging clinical problem. Laboratory measurements, such as creatinine, are helpful to provide an estimated glomerular filtration rate (GFR), which can be used as a surrogate measure of global renal function; however, laboratory measures of estimated GFR cannot differentiate single kidney GFR, and are often insensitive for early changes of chronic kidney disease. Imaging-based methods of renal functional analysis can provide a more comprehensive examination by coupling both structural and functional information of the kidneys.

Dynamic contrast-enhanced MR imaging can provide accurate GFR values for each kidney,

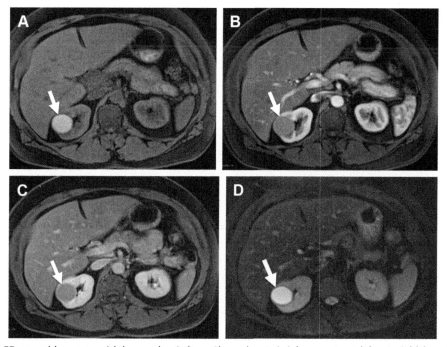

Fig. 11. A 55-year-old woman with hemorrhagic (type 2) renal cyst. Axial precontrast (A), arterial (B), and delayed (C) phase fat-saturated 3D T1-weighted GRE postcontrast images demonstrate uniform, elevated intrinsic T1 signal on the precontrast image (A, arrow), with no enhancement on subsequent postcontrast images (B and C, arrows). Fat-saturated ssT2 image (D) shows a homogeneous cystic lesion in the right kidney (arrow).

enabling the calculation of split renal function; this (coupled with anatomic data) provides essential clinical information for a variety of indications, including preoperative planning (**Fig. 12**). The most commonly used method for quantifying GFR in vivo has been with the injection of a GBCA, and subsequently acquiring a dynamic multiphasic MR imaging examination. However, assessment of GFR with dynamic MR imaging has been challenging due to the competing requirements of high spatial and temporal resolution. Recent breakthroughs in parallel imaging and methods that optimize the trade-off between spatial and temporal resolution have made it feasible to acquire whole coverage of the kidneys with 3-s to 5-s temporal resolution and adequate spatial resolution for characterization of structural features.[53,54] The dynamic data are then post processed using manual or semi-automated image processing to segment different elements like the cortex, medulla, and the aorta. Signal enhancement curves for these elements are then calculated, which are converted to concentration curves using the T1 values of blood and kidney.

These curves are then fed to a pharmacokinetic model that models the renal filtration system to obtain pharmacokinetic parameters that are converted to GFR values.

The simplest model is the Patlak model, which models a nephron space and vascular space. More sophisticated models[55] incorporating finer element of the renal filtration including cortex/medulla/loop of Henle have been developed but require sophisticated fitting algorithms for model fitting. The modified Tofts[56] model seems to be a good compromise between the simplistic Patlak model, which depends on manual identification of enhancement slopes and is hence error prone, and the more sophisticated models that suffer from overfitting poor-quality data. Motion compensation is the most challenging technical issue to overcome to date, because data acquisition typically extends over a 2-minute imaging window, preventing breath-holding. This has been addressed using respiratory gating[57] (which compromises temporal resolution); however, more recent radial imaging[53] methods have shown themselves to be highly robust to patient motion.

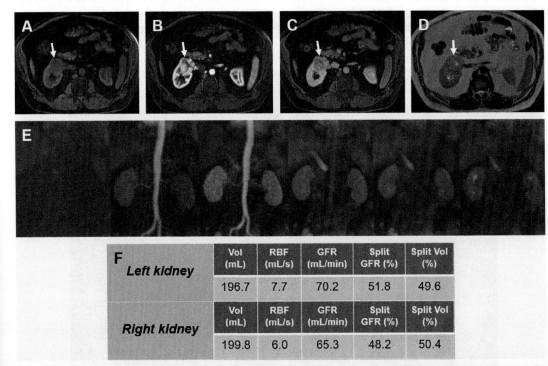

	Vol (mL)	RBF (mL/s)	GFR (mL/min)	Split GFR (%)	Split Vol (%)
F Left kidney					
	196.7	7.7	70.2	51.8	49.6
Right kidney	Vol (mL)	RBF (mL/s)	GFR (mL/min)	Split GFR (%)	Split Vol (%)
	199.8	6.0	65.3	48.2	50.4

Fig. 12. A 67-year-old man with solid renal mass. Axial precontrast (*A*), arterial (*B*), and delayed (*C*) phase fat-saturated 3D T1W GRE postcontrast images demonstrate an arterial enhancing mass in the right kidney (*arrows*). The ssT2 image (*D*) shows mildly elevated, heterogeneous T2 signal (*arrow*). This mass was biopsied as oncocytoma; however, the patient and surgeon decided on surgical resection, with consideration for partial nephrectomy. A functional MR nephrourogram (*E*) was obtained to assess the differential function of each kidney to better aid preoperative planning, demonstrating relatively symmetric function of both kidneys (*F*).

SUMMARY

MR imaging has been optimized for the evaluation of a multitude of disease processes affecting the kidneys. A wide variety of noncontrast methods are available for the evaluation of both kidney structure and function, which are especially useful in clinical scenarios that obviate the use of intravenous contrast. Contrast-enhanced methods remain important, especially for tumor evaluation, and are used increasingly for functional analysis of quantitative biometrics, such as GFR and kidney blood flow.

REFERENCES

1. Loening AM, Saranathan M, Ruangwattanapaisarn N, et al. Increased speed and image quality in single-shot fast spin echo imaging via variable refocusing flip angles. J Magn Reson Imaging 2015;42(6): 1747–58.

2. Loening AM, Litwiller DV, Saranathan M, et al. Increased speed and image quality for pelvic single-shot fast spin-echo imaging with variable refocusing flip angles and full-fourier acquisition. Radiology 2017;282(2):561–8.

3. Qayyum A. Diffusion-weighted imaging in the abdomen and pelvis: concepts and applications. Radiographics 2009;29(6):1797–810.

4. d'Assignies G, Fina P, Bruno O, et al. High sensitivity of diffusion-weighted MR imaging for the detection of liver metastases from neuroendocrine tumors: comparison with T2-weighted and dynamic gadolinium-enhanced MR imaging. Radiology 2013;268(2):390–9.

5. Colagrande S, Castellani A, Nardi C, et al. The role of diffusion-weighted imaging in the detection of hepatic metastases from colorectal cancer: a comparison with unenhanced and Gd-EOB-DTPA enhanced MRI. Eur J Radiol 2016;85(5):1027–34.

6. Taouli B, Beer AJ, Chenevert T, et al. Diffusion-weighted imaging outside the brain: consensus statement from an ISMRM-sponsored workshop. J Magn Reson Imaging 2016;44(3):521–40.

7. Paruthikunnan SM, Kadavigere R, Karegowda LH. Accuracy of whole-body DWI for metastases screening in a diverse group of malignancies: comparison with conventional cross-sectional imaging and nuclear scintigraphy. AJR Am J Roentgenol 2017;209(3):477–90.

8. Jeon SK, Lee JM, Joo I, et al. Magnetic resonance with diffusion-weighted imaging improves assessment of focal liver lesions in patients with potentially resectable pancreatic cancer on CT. Eur Radiol 2018;28(8):3484–93.

9. Liu B, Gao S, Li S. A comprehensive comparison of CT, MRI, positron emission tomography or positron emission tomography/CT, and diffusion weighted imaging-MRI for detecting the lymph nodes metastases in patients with cervical cancer: a meta-analysis based on 67 studies. Gynecol Obstet Invest 2017;82(3):209–22.

10. Taouli B, Thakur RK, Mannelli L, et al. Renal lesions: characterization with diffusion-weighted imaging versus contrast-enhanced MR imaging. Radiology 2009;251(2):398–407.

11. Erbay G, Koc Z, Karadeli E, et al. Evaluation of malignant and benign renal lesions using diffusion-weighted MRI with multiple b values. Acta Radiol 2012;53(3):359–65.

12. Razek AA, Farouk A, Mousa A, et al. Role of diffusion-weighted magnetic resonance imaging in characterization of renal tumors. J Comput Assist Tomogr 2011;35(3):332–6.

13. Kilickesmez O, Inci E, Atilla S, et al. Diffusion-weighted imaging of the renal and adrenal lesions. J Comput Assist Tomogr 2009;33(6):828–33.

14. Lassel EA, Rao R, Schwenke C, et al. Diffusion-weighted imaging of focal renal lesions: a meta-analysis. Eur Radiol 2014;24(1):241–9.

15. Sandrasegaran K, Sundaram CP, Ramaswamy R, et al. Usefulness of diffusion-weighted imaging in the evaluation of renal masses. AJR Am J Roentgenol 2010;194(2):438–45.

16. Rathod SB, Kumbhar SS, Nanivadekar A, et al. Role of diffusion-weighted MRI in acute pyelonephritis: a prospective study. Acta Radiol 2015;56(2):244–9.

17. Goyal A, Sharma R, Bhalla AS, et al. Diffusion-weighted MRI in inflammatory renal lesions: all that glitters is not RCC! Eur Radiol 2013;23(1):272–9.

18. Dumoulin CL, Cline HE, Souza SP, et al. Three-dimensional time-of-flight magnetic resonance angiography using spin saturation. Magn Reson Med 1989;11(1):35–46.

19. Wilson GJ, Maki JH. Non-contrast-enhanced MR imaging of renal artery stenosis at 1.5 tesla. Magn Reson Imaging Clin N Am 2009;17(1):13–27.

20. Lim RP, Koktzoglou I. Noncontrast magnetic resonance angiography: concepts and clinical applications. Radiol Clin North Am 2015;53(3):457–76.

21. Miyazaki M, Lee VS. Nonenhanced MR angiography. Radiology 2008;248(1):20–43.

22. Tatli S, Lipton MJ, Davison BD, et al. From the RSNA refresher courses: MR imaging of aortic and peripheral vascular disease. Radiographics 2003;23 Spec No:S59–78.

23. Ozsarlak O, Van Goethem JW, Maes M, et al. MR angiography of the intracranial vessels: technical aspects and clinical applications. Neuroradiology 2004;46(12):955–72.

24. Pui MH. Cerebral MR venography. Clin Imaging 2004;28(2):85–9.

25. Morita S, Masukawa A, Suzuki K, et al. Unenhanced MR angiography: techniques and clinical applications

in patients with chronic kidney disease. Radiographics 2011;31(2):E13–33.

26. Edelman RR, Sheehan JJ, Dunkle E, et al. Quiescent-interval single-shot unenhanced magnetic resonance angiography of peripheral vascular disease: technical considerations and clinical feasibility. Magn Reson Med 2010;63(4):951–8.

27. Edelman RR, Carr M, Koktzoglou I. Advances in non-contrast quiescent-interval slice-selective (QISS) magnetic resonance angiography. Clin Radiol 2018. [Epub ahead of print].

28. Li LP, Halter S, Prasad PV. Blood oxygen level-dependent MR imaging of the kidneys. Magn Reson Imaging Clin N Am 2008;16(4):613–25, viii.

29. Mannelli L, Maki JH, Osman SF, et al. Noncontrast functional MRI of the kidneys. Curr Urol Rep 2012; 13(1):99–107.

30. Mariappan YK, Glaser KJ, Ehman RL. Magnetic resonance elastography: a review. Clin Anat 2010; 23(5):497–511.

31. Gennisson JL, Grenier N, Combe C, et al. Supersonic shear wave elastography of in vivo pig kidney: influence of blood pressure, urinary pressure and tissue anisotropy. Ultrasound Med Biol 2012;38(9): 1559–67.

32. Czeyda-Pommersheim F, Martin DR, Costello JR, et al. Contrast agents for MR imaging. Magn Reson Imaging Clin N Am 2017;25(4):705–11.

33. Thomsen HS. Contrast media safety—an update. Eur J Radiol 2011;80(1):77–82.

34. Prince MR, Zhang H, Zou Z, et al. Incidence of immediate gadolinium contrast media reactions. AJR Am J Roentgenol 2011;196(2):W138–43.

35. Murphy KJ, Brunberg JA, Cohan RH. Adverse reactions to gadolinium contrast media: a review of 36 cases. AJR Am J Roentgenol 1996;167(4):847–9.

36. Dillman JR, Ellis JH, Cohan RH, et al. Frequency and severity of acute allergic-like reactions to gadolinium-containing i.v. contrast media in children and adults. AJR Am J Roentgenol 2007;189(6): 1533–8.

37. Bleicher AG, Kanal E. Assessment of adverse reaction rates to a newly approved MRI contrast agent: review of 23,553 administrations of gadobenate dimeglumine. AJR Am J Roentgenol 2008;191(6): W307–11.

38. Costello JR, Kalb B, Martin DR. Incidence and risk factors for gadolinium-based contrast agent immediate reactions. Top Magn Reson Imaging 2016; 25(6):257–63.

39. Niendorf HP, Haustein J, Cornelius I, et al. Safety of gadolinium-DTPA: extended clinical experience. Magn Reson Med 1991;22(2):222–8 [discussion: 229–32].

40. Li A, Wong CS, Wong MK, et al. Acute adverse reactions to magnetic resonance contrast media—gadolinium chelates. Br J Radiol 2006;79(941):368–71.

41. Hoffmann U, Fischereder M, Reil A, et al. Renal effects of gadopentetate dimeglumine in patients with normal and impaired renal function. Eur J Med Res 2005;10(4):149–54.

42. Zhang HL, Ersoy H, Prince MR. Effects of gadopentetate dimeglumine and gadodiamide on serum calcium, magnesium, and creatinine measurements. J Magn Reson Imaging 2006;23(3):383–7.

43. Grobner T. Gadolinium—a specific trigger for the development of nephrogenic fibrosing dermopathy and nephrogenic systemic fibrosis? Nephrol Dial Transplant 2006;21(4):1104–8.

44. Martin DR, Krishnamoorthy SK, Kalb B, et al. Decreased incidence of NSF in patients on dialysis after changing gadolinium contrast-enhanced MRI protocols. J Magn Reson Imaging 2010;31(2): 440–6.

45. ACR Committee on Drugs and Contrast Media. ACR-ASNR position statement on the use of gadolinium contrast agents, adverse reaction to gadolinium based contrast agents, nephrogenic systemic fibrosis. ACR Manual on Contrast Media; 2018. p. 76–89. Available at: https://www.acr.org/-/media/ACR/Files/Clinical-Resources/Contrast_Media. pdf.

46. Nandwana SB, Moreno CC, Osipow MT, et al. Gadobenate dimeglumine administration and nephrogenic systemic fibrosis: is there a real risk in patients with impaired renal function? Radiology 2015;276(3):741–7.

47. Wang Y, Alkasab TK, Narin O, et al. Incidence of nephrogenic systemic fibrosis after adoption of restrictive gadolinium-based contrast agent guidelines. Radiology 2011;260(1):105–11.

48. Altun E, Martin DR, Wertman R, et al. Nephrogenic systemic fibrosis: change in incidence following a switch in gadolinium agents and adoption of a gadolinium policy—report from two U.S. universities. Radiology 2009;253(3):689–96.

49. Bashir MR, Bhatti L, Marin D, et al. Emerging applications for ferumoxytol as a contrast agent in MRI. J Magn Reson Imaging 2015;41(4):884–98.

50. Hope MD, Hope TA, Zhu C, et al. Vascular imaging with ferumoxytol as a contrast agent. AJR Am J Roentgenol 2015;205(3):W366–73.

51. Toth GB, Varallyay CG, Horvath A, et al. Current and potential imaging applications of ferumoxytol for magnetic resonance imaging. Kidney Int 2017; 92(1):47–66.

52. Sun MR, Ngo L, Genega EM, et al. Renal cell carcinoma: dynamic contrast-enhanced MR imaging for differentiation of tumor subtypes—correlation with pathologic findings. Radiology 2009;250(3):793–802.

53. Pandey A, Yoruk U, Keerthivasan M, et al. Multiresolution imaging using golden angle stack-of-stars and compressed sensing for dynamic MR urography. J Magn Reson Imaging 2017;46(1):303–11.

54. Song T, Laine AF, Chen Q, et al. Optimal k-space sampling for dynamic contrast-enhanced MRI with an application to MR renography. Magn Reson Med 2009;61(5):1242–8.

55. Annet L, Hermoye L, Peeters F, et al. Glomerular filtration rate: assessment with dynamic contrast-enhanced MRI and a cortical-compartment model in the rabbit kidney. J Magn Reson Imaging 2004; 20(5):843–9.

56. Tofts PS, Cutajar M, Mendichovszky IA, et al. Precise measurement of renal filtration and vascular parameters using a two-compartment model for dynamic contrast-enhanced MRI of the kidney gives realistic normal values. Eur Radiol 2012;22(6):1320–30.

57. Yoruk U, Saranathan M, Loening AM, et al. High temporal resolution dynamic MRI and arterial input function for assessment of GFR in pediatric subjects. Magn Reson Med 2016;75(3):1301–11.

Infectious and Inflammatory Diseases of the Urinary Tract
Role of MR Imaging

João Cruz, MD[a,b], Filipa Figueiredo, MD[a],
António P. Matos, MD[a], Sérgio Duarte, MD[b],
Adalgisa Guerra, MD[c], Miguel Ramalho, MD[a,b],*

KEYWORDS

• MR imaging • Urinary tract infection • Acute pyelonephritis • Pyonephrosis • Cystitis • Abscess

KEY POINTS

- Noncontrast MR imaging is the best imaging modality for the evaluation of complicated urinary tract infection in pregnant patients.
- MR imaging is particularly helpful for the evaluation of complicated lower urinary tract infections and inflammatory disorders, including prostatic and urethral infections and inflammation.
- A limitation of MR imaging compared with CT in the evaluation of urinary tract infections is low sensitivity for the detection of stones and air, impairing the ability to detect obstructing stones and emphysematous pyelonephritis and pyelitis.

INTRODUCTION

Urinary tract infection (UTI) is defined as the bacterial invasion of the urinary tract, which can occur anywhere between the urethra and the kidney and is among the most common of all bacterial infections. Bacteria infect the usually sterile urinary tract either by traveling from the blood stream to the kidneys (hematogenous spread) or, more commonly, by infecting the urethra and traveling upward toward the bladder and kidneys (ascending infection). Less frequently, infection can arise from direct extension, in cases of fistulas with the surrounding organs.[1–4] Imaging studies are indicated for the evaluation of complicated UTIs, in patients who are septic or not responsive to initial antimicrobial therapy, and in patients with recurrent UTI episodes or atypical clinical presentation or atypical laboratory results, to look for complications (eg, obstruction, abscess, or perirenal fluid collection) and to identify rare forms of pyelonephritis.[4–11]

In this article, the role of MR imaging and MR imaging semiology is reviewed. For systematization purposes, infectious and inflammatory diseases are divided into upper urinary tract, including kidneys and ureters, and lower urinary tract, including the bladder, urethra, and prostate.

MR IMAGING EVALUATION OF THE URINARY TRACT

Ultrasound is routinely used as a first-line imaging method. It plays an important role in the detection of hydronephrosis, calculi, perinephric collections, congenital anomalies, or urinary tract wall thickening. This method has limited sensitivity,

The authors declare that they have no conflict of interest.

[a] Department of Radiology, Hospital Garcia de Orta, Av. Torrado da Silva, 2805-267 Almada, Portugal;
[b] Department of Radiology, Hospital da Luz, Estrada Nacional 10, km 37, Setúbal 2900-722, Portugal;
[c] Department of Radiology, Hospital da Luz, Avenida Lusíada, 100, Lisbon 1500-650, Portugal
* Corresponding author. Department of Radiology, Hospital Garcia de Orta, Av. Torrado da Silva, 2805-267 Almada, Portugal.
E-mail address: jmpmramalho@gmail.com

however, in the evaluation of urinary tract inflammation and infection.[4,5]

CT and MR imaging provide excellent anatomic detail and image quality, which improve the diagnostic work-up of the pathologic conditions of the urinary tract and surrounding tissues.[7,8,12,13]

Several investigators consider CT the gold standard for the imaging evaluation of UTIs because it allows the assessment of the renal parenchyma, urinary tract, and vasculature in a single examination and with extremely short acquisition times. CT has high accuracy in demonstrating changes in renal parenchymal perfusion, calculi, gas-forming infections, hemorrhage, obstruction, inflammatory masses, abscess, or retroperitoneal collections.[8,11,13] The absence of ionizing radiation of MR imaging is also relevant considering the commonly young age of patients with UTIs.[5,7,8,11,14] Also, MR imaging may improve the distinction between healing, fibrotic, and edematous (presumably active) infectious foci and improve imaging in kidney infections.[5,9] Specific disadvantages of MR imaging encompass the lesser spatial resolution as well as the lower sensitivity at showing calcifications (contrary to CT, which has a great accuracy at depicting calcification) and gas.[5,8,14–17]

One important aspect to consider is related to the use of intravenous (IV) contrast medium, because the high accuracy of CT depends greatly on the use of IV iodinated contrast agents, which allow the assessment of renal perfusion and the depiction and characterization of inflammatory lesions and abscesses. The administration of IV contrast is limited, however, in patients with renal impairment due to concerns of worsening the underlying renal impairment or of postcontrast acute kidney injury.[18–20] Dynamic contrast enhancement (DCE)–MR imaging has been used as an alternative to contrast-enhanced CT, because it is much less nephrotoxic, especially when used in appropriate clinical doses.[21,22] Iodinated contrast agents, however, may be used in patients underlying hemodialysis, where gadolinium-based contrast agents (GBCAs) are generally contraindicated due to potential triggering of nephrogenic systemic fibrosis or worsening gadolinium deposition in the body.[23] Furthermore, unenhanced MR imaging, combining morphologic and functional sequences, such as diffusion-weighted imaging (DWI), show high diagnostic value compared with unenhanced CT, particularly in pregnant patients in whom the use of GBCAs is not recommended.[10,24,25]

SEQUENCES

Despite modern software development, the basic MR imaging examination is still based on a combination of T1-weighted images (WI) and T2-WI and functional techniques, including DCE and DWI.

High spatial resolution is achieved by a combination of external pelvic phased-array coils, thin-section thickness (≤3 mm), no interslice gaps, and large matrix size.[26] Bowel peristalsis can be minimized with antiperistaltic agents.[26]

To image the kidneys, axial 3-D T1-WI in-phase and out-of-phase gradient-recalled-echo (GRE) and fat-suppressed (FS) T1-WI GRE imaging is performed before and after the IV GBCA administration.[27] Postcontrast sequences remain an integral part of most protocols. DCE images are acquired in a late arterial phase (35–40 seconds after contrast injection) and in nephrogenic phase (100 seconds after contrast injection), when all of the renal parenchyma, including the medulla, enhances. Interstitial phase and excretory phase are also usually acquired. Non-FS and FS single-shot (SS) echo-train spin-echo (ETSE) T2-WI in at least 2 planes are obtained. Damaged tissue tends to develop edema, which makes water-sensitive sequences sensitive for pathology and generally able to distinguish pathologic tissue from normal tissue.[27]

For the lower urinary tract, in addition to FS T1-WI GRE, at least 2 planes of 2-D T2-WI turbo spin-echo are obtained.[27]

MR imaging urography (MRU) can be performed with 2 different imaging strategies.

Unenhanced MR Imaging Urography

Unenhanced MRU, based on heavily (static-fluid) T2-weighted FSE or SS–fast spin-echo (FSE) sequences, is especially useful in the urinary tract, because water-containing structures, such as the collecting system and the bladder, are bright white, providing static hydrographic images of the urinary tract. Despite being useful and reliable to reveal hydronephrosis and perirenal high SI in acute urinary obstruction, its inability to fully visualize nondilated ureters is usually cited as a major disadvantage.[5,25,27]

Contrast-Enhanced Excretory MR Imaging Urography

Contrast-enhanced excretory MRU (CE-MRU) is performed with 3-D–GRE T1-weighted sequences after IV GBCA administration. In routine practice, the excretory CE-MRU is the technique most commonly used because the administration of a paramagnetic contrast agent permits the evaluation of renal excretory function and better visualization of the nondilated urinary tract.[25,27] Low-dose (5–20 mg) IV furosemide administration has been recommended for excretory CE-MRU.

because the increased urine flow leads to a rapid and uniform distribution of gadolinium, improving the visualization of the nondilated upper urinary tract.[25]

When IV contrast cannot be administered, DWI offers a viable alternative.[24] DWI is usually performed in 2 blocks covering the abdomen and pelvis separately. At least 2 b values (<100 s/mm^2 and ≥600 s/mm^2) should be used to enable the calculation of the apparent diffusion coefficient (ADC) maps. DWI, with a low b value (<100 s/mm^2), can be used as a surrogate for FS T2-weighted MR imaging sequences to save examination time.[27]

UPPER URINARY TRACT
Acute Pyelonephritis

Acute pyelonephritis (APN) is a nonspecific inflammatory process secondary to ascending (more frequently) or hematogenous bacterial infection.[5,11] *Escherichia coli* causes more than 80% of APN.[1] Patients with APN can present with all the symptoms of cystitis, flank pain, and fever, and they may be acutely ill with nausea, vomiting, and unstable vital signs.

Imaging studies are usually reserved for patients who do not improve to seek possible obstruction, urologic abnormalities, and perinephric and intrarenal abscesses.

On MR imaging, T1 and T2 baseline acquisitions may reflect the distribution of edema within the renal parenchyma, resulting in typically increased renal volume and nonhomogeneous hypointensity in T1-WI and hyperintensity in T2-WI (**Fig. 1**); however, these findings have low sensitivity to detect inflammatory foci. The decrease or loss of the corticomedullary differentiation is a nonspecific finding, which may be seen in a small percentage of cases.[11]

DCE study harbors the greatest accuracy of MR imaging because it enables the identification of inflammatory foci that were not detected at the baseline and increases the diagnostic confidence. On postcontrast FS T1-WI, a reduction of parenchymal contrast enhancement is observed in the affected area, allegedly resultant of poor functioning parenchyma due to vasospasm, tubular obstruction, or interstitial edema. The distribution of inflammatory foci is typically patchy with wedge-shaped areas radiating from the papilla to the cortical surface, with the renal parenchyma demonstrating a typical striated appearance due to interspersed areas of parenchyma spared—*striated nephrogram sign*. The most sensitive phase for identifying these nonenhancing areas is the nephrographic phase.[5,6,9,11,28,29] Differentiation of striated nephrogram sign from renal infarction is essential; however, it seldom represents a diagnostic challenge due to different clinical contexts.

The presence of perinephric heterogeneity and T2 hyperintensity immediately adjacent to the abnormal areas in the renal parenchyma, equivalent to CT perinephric fat-stranding sign, is also

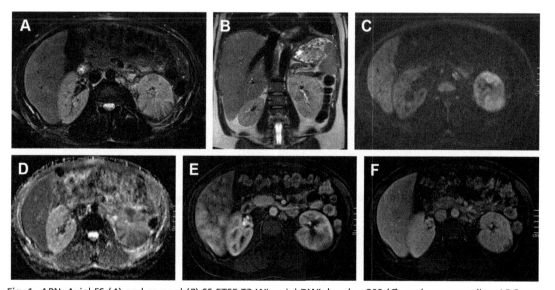

Fig. 1. APN. Axial FS (*A*) and coronal (*B*) SS-ETSE T2-WI; axial DWI, b value 800 (*C*), and corresponding ADC map (*D*); axial postcontrast FS 3-D–GRE T1-WI in the arterial (*E*) and interstitial phases (*F*). A 36-year-old woman with dysuria, left lumbar pain, and fever. The left kidney is enlarged, with diffuse nonhomogeneous SI on T2-WI (*A*, *B*), showing high SI on DWI and low SI on ADC map (*C*, *D*). A wedge-shaped reduction of parenchymal contrast enhancement is observed in the affected area (*E*, *F*), with a typical striated appearance due to interspersed areas of spared parenchyma—*striated nephrogram sign*.

seen in a moderate amount of cases and is due to inflammatory infiltration that has spread beyond the renal capsule. This is better appreciated on FS T2-WI. The spread of these inflammatory changes also results in thickening of the Gerota fascia as well as of the urothelium of the renal sinuses.[29,30]

The high blood flow and water transport functions of the kidney make it a particularly interesting organ to study with DWI.[6,9,12] Some studies have shown good agreement between DWI and CE–MR imaging for the diagnosis of APN, with good sensitivity for DWI to detect the focal areas of pyelonephritis and to demonstrate the disappearance of inflammatory foci, providing evidence of complete healing. It still lacks specificity and clinical validation, however.[7,9–12,31,32] Faletti and colleagues[7] reported superiority of DCE–MR imaging over DWI in identifying complications of APN, including focal abscesses.

Isolated pyelitis and pyeloureteritis may rarely occur and are depicted as circumferential thickening of the walls of the collecting system, with T2 hyperintensity due to the presence of mural edema and increased contrast-enhancement and stranding of the periureteral fat due to the presence of inflammation.

Renal Abscess

Untreated or inadequately treated APN may progress to tissue necrosis and liquefaction, resulting in the coalescence of suppurative foci into a larger focal collection, especially in diabetics (75% of the cases), immunocompromised patients, and patients with obstruction.[5]

Although initially, abscesses appear as small wedge-shaped or rounded nonenhancing areas with irregular and poorly defined margins, the mature abscesses instead are sharply marginated. Abscesses typically show low, inhomogeneous signal intensity (SI) on T1-WI and high SI on T2-WI depending on the amount of protein, fluid, and cellular debris. When debris are present, a fluid-fluid level may be seen.[5] Postcontrast images show a peripheral halo enhancement, which usually progresses through different phases (**Fig. 2**).[9] The delayed phase occasionally reveals itself critical to identify the abscess foci and differentiate them from nonabscessed foci and infarction scars.[11] The external part of the capsule of the abscess can appear irregular due to associated inflammatory infiltration.[5,6] Abscesses usually show high signal on DWI and low ADC values. One possible explanation for the decreased ADC

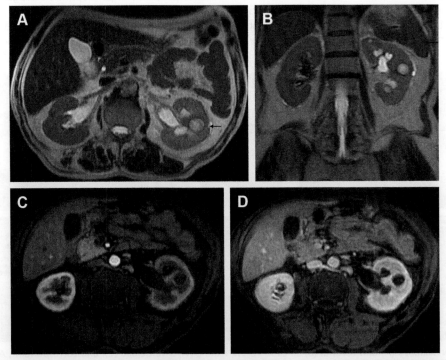

Fig. 2. Renal abscess. Axial (*A*) and coronal (*B*) SS-ETSE T2-WI; axial postcontrast FS 3-D–GRE T1-WI in the arterial (*C*) and interstitial phases (*D*). A 66-year-old man admitted with APN resistant to antibacterial treatment. On the left kidney (*arrow* [*A*]), a heterogeneously high T2 SI lesion is seen with a thick wall that shows progressive enhancement after contrast injection. Weaker corticomedullary renal enhancement and pyelic urothelial enhancement was present (*C*). A small amount of perinephric fluid is depicted on T2-WI (*A*).

values within the abscess cavity is the conglomeration of white blood cells with intact cell membranes, which leads to high viscosity and cellularity.

The presence of gas may be seen as areas of susceptibility artifact within an inflammatory mass, strongly implying abscess. It is an uncommon finding, however, and differentiation from calcific foci may be difficult or even impossible.[6]

Abscesses may spread through the renal parenchyma and rupture its capsule into the perirenal space and remain contained by Gerota fascia or may diffuse into other retroperitoneal space and the abdominal wall, well evaluated by multiplanar MR imaging.[5,6,33]

Emphysematous Pyelonephritis

Emphysematous pyelonephritis (EPN) is a potentially serious fulminant bacterial infection of the kidneys characterized by gas in the collecting system, renal parenchyma, and perinephric tissues. Most commonly, it occurs in diabetic patients with urinary tract obstruction and often carries adverse outcomes, with a mortality rate of 20%.[34] Glucose-fermenting *E coli* is responsible for 70% of EPN cases, followed by *Klebsiella pneumonia*, and *Proteus mirabilis*.[35] Nevertheless, nondiabetic patients also get EPN.[36]

CT is very sensitive and allows an accurate staging of the disease and is considered the gold standard for diagnosis.[37]

A diagnosis of EPN is challenging on MR imaging and is characterized by the presence of gas in the renal parenchyma, the urinary tract, or perirenal tissue. The free gas manifests as signal voids on both T1- and T2-WI, with blooming artifact recognized better on GRE sequences. Contrast injection may be useful to assess the extent of renal parenchyma destruction.[38] The presence of gas limited to the collecting system may be related to emphysematous pyelitis, which has a less severe prognosis. A potential pitfall may be the presence of gas in the collecting system due to recent catheterization or a urointestinal fistula.[6,34]

Hydronephrosis and Pyonephrosis

Hydronephrosis is important in the context of UTI because it makes the urinary tract vulnerable to infection and permanent dysfunction. Obstruction predisposes to and usually precedes the infection but the reverse can also occur.[5,6,39] The differentiation of pyonephrosis and hydronephrosis is important because pyonephrosis needs immediate intervention due to the high risk of sepsis and loss of kidney function.[12]

MR imaging is more sensitive than CT for the diagnosis of sources of urinary obstruction other than urolithiasis; nevertheless, MR imaging still has a high sensitivity (>90%) for the detection of obstructive ureteral calculi.[27] The relative absence of protons within urinary calculi makes them incapable of generating signal on MR imaging; thus, calculi is only detected by the surrounding signal-generating urine on T2-WI (**Fig. 3**). Having said that, it is understandable that the sensitivity for renal stones increases in relation to the size of the calculus and the use of thin sections.[40] Balanced gradient-echo sequences are also particularly effective for the depiction of larger stones as hypointense filling defects surrounded by hyperintense urine, with the advantage of being insensitive to flow-related artifacts (present on SS-FSE T2-WI).

Other signs of urinary tract obstruction include swelling of the ipsilateral kidney, periureteric and perinephric edema, and urothelial wall thickening. Hyperenhancement after contrast injection renders the presence of inflammatory hyperemia. After contrast administration, there is a delayed nephrogram because of decreased renal perfusion. If delayed images are obtained, a persistent nephrogram can be seen on the obstructed side.[29,41]

Pyonephrosis is defined as the presence of pus in a dilated renal collecting system. With pus under pressure, patients may deteriorate rapidly and become septic, prompting differential diagnosis between hydronephrosis and pyonephrosis, which has a vital clinical significance. Pyonephrosis may be caused by a broad spectrum of pathologic conditions involving either an ascending infection of the urinary tract or the hematogenous spread of a bacterial pathogen.[39]

MR imaging findings in pyonephrosis include thickening of the renal pelvic wall (>2 mm) and dilatation and obstruction of the collecting system, which appears hypointense on T1-WI and hyperintense on T2-WI unless the dependent portion of the collecting system contains high-protein content material or debris (and fluid-debris level) (**Fig. 4**),[5] A striated nephrogram in the renal parenchyma similar to that seen in pyelonephritis can occur in both pyonephrosis and obstructive uropathy, although, in pyonephrosis, changes appear more severe. Some studies refer the potential of DWI in demonstrating changes in perfusion and diffusion during acute renal obstruction with significant lower ADC values of the pyonephrotic renal pelvis compared with the hydronephrotic renal pelvis (**Fig. 5**).[12,32,42]

Pregnant women are a special subset of patients in whom MR Imaging harbors substantial

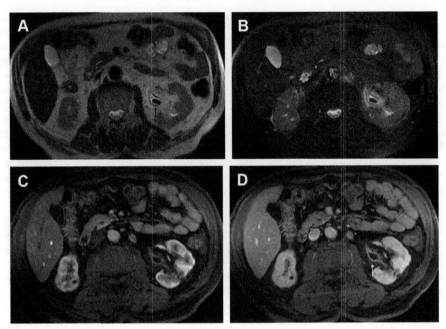

Fig. 3. Obstructive lithiasis. Axial non-FS (*A*) and FS (*B*) SS-ETSE T2-WI; axial postcontrast FS 3-D–GRE T1-WI in the arterial (*C*) and nephrographic phase (*D*). A 74-year-old man with prior cystectomy and left percutaneous nephrostomy due to obstructive lithiasis. A sizable calculus (*arrow* [*A*]) is seen as a filling defect with low SI in all sequences surrounded by urine with high T2 signal. There is associated thickening and hyper-enhancement of the urothelial wall (*arrow* [*D*]), as well as marked parapelvic edema due to associated inflammation, best seen on FS T2-WI. This edema is indicative of acute obstruction. There is an area of cortical scarring from previous nephrostomy.

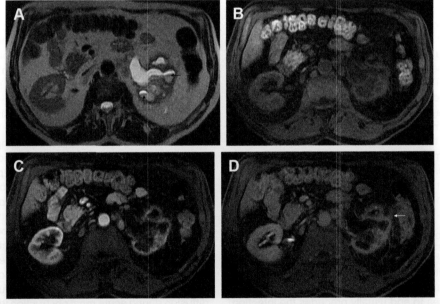

Fig. 4. Pyonephrosis. Axial (*A*) SS-ETSE T2-WI; axial precontrast (*B*) and postcontrast FS 3-D–GRE T1-WI in the arterial (*C*) and excretory phase (*D*). A 69-year-old man with a known invasive bladder tumor and recurrent UTIs. There is pyelocalyceal ectasia of the left kidney with fluid levels depicted on T2-WI (*arrows* [*A*]). There is associated thickening of the pelvic urothelium, which shows increased enhancement after contrast injection as well as heterogeneous perinephric enhancement due to extracapsular spread of inflammatory changes (*arrow* [*D*]). These findings are consistent with pyonephrosis. The kidney shows diffuse cortical thinning due to chronic obstruction.

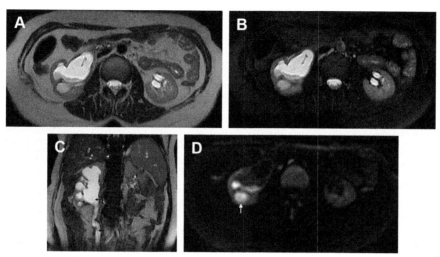

Fig. 5. Pyonephrosis. Axial non-FS (*A*) and FS (*B*) SS-ETSE T2-WI; coronal steady-state free precession (*C*) and axial DWI, b value 800 (*D*). A 57-year-old woman with history of chronic obstructive lithiasis and onset of right lumbar pain and fever, who refused IV contrast medium administration. There is right uretero-hydronephrosis with diffuse renal cortical thinning due to chronic obstruction. Despite the absence of IV contrast, fluid-fluid level in the right kidney pelvis is seen on the T2-WI, with high SI on DWI (*arrow* [*D*]), compatible with pyonephrosis. The high DWI SI is explained by the conglomeration of inflammatory cells, causing restricted diffusion of water molecules. A stent in the urinary tract is noticed (*arrows* [*C*]).

advantages.[14,43,44] The incidence of ureteric stones is up to 1 in 1500 pregnancies, and 80% to 90% of these cases occur during the second and third trimesters.[40] With a positive predictive value of 80%, MR imaging allows for the differentiation of the physiologic dilatation (seen in up to 90% of pregnant women in the third trimester of pregnancy) from the pathologic dilatation caused by an obstructive stone. DWI might be important in the diagnosis of eventual pyonephrosis, because there is a tendency to not administer GBCAs even in the third trimester.

Xanthogranulomatous Pyelonephritis

Xanthogranulomatous pyelonephritis (XGP) is a rare, chronic granulomatous inflammatory disorder of the kidney characterized by a destructive mass that invades the renal parenchyma.[45] XGP is most commonly associated with *P mirabilis* or *E ooli* infection, usually due to long-standing urinary tract obstruction, classically due to a staghorn calculus, seen in 80% of cases. The kidney is usually nonfunctional. Most cases of XGP involve a diffuse process; however, up to 20% are focal. Pathologically, there is parenchymal destruction and replacement with lipid-laden macrophages.

On MR imaging, it manifests most commonly as a diffuse form with nephromegaly, hydronephrosis, peripelvic fibrosis, and destruction of renal architecture often extending to the perirenal and pararenal space and adjacent structures. The renal cortical thickness is reduced. The cortex may contain multiple abscesses surrounded by the xantoid tissue. Reports on the signal characteristics of the XGP differ to some extent. Some investigators described a hyperintense appearance of the solid component of XGP on T1-WI compared with the renal parenchyma,[46–48] whereas other investigators reported a more isointense appearance of the solid component on T1-WI.[49–51] It is possible that the SI of the solid component of XGP on T1-WI depends on the amount of xanthoma cells involved in the granulomatous process. On T2-WI, the solid component of XGP tends to show isointensity with the normal kidney.[52] The content of the locular spaces or cavities is variable and may reflect the heterogeneous composition of the content. Extensive reactive sinus replacement lipomatosis has been reported in XGP and is well-recognized and characterized with MR imaging.[47] Perirenal inflammatory infiltration and enhancement of the perirenal fascia are usually present. Fistulization with the gastrointestinal tract or skin may be occasionally seen. Focal XGP may demonstrate findings similar to those seen in the diffuse form (with sparing of part of the kidney), but others may present as focal pseudotumor and mimic the features of bacterial abscess or renal cell carcinoma

(Fig. 6).[53] Obstruction by lithiasis is usually present in both cases.[5,6]

OTHER FORMS OF UPPER URINARY TRACT INFECTION
Infected Renal Cyst

Kidney cysts are extremely frequent; however, infection of a renal cyst is uncommon in otherwise healthy patients. Patients with autosomal dominant polycystic kidney disease are a special subset of patients, having a higher incidence of renal cyst infection (which accounts for 15% of all causes of hospitalizations of these patients), in whom MR imaging plays an important role on the evaluation of suspected infected cyst.[54,55]

Usually infected cysts present with heterogeneous intracystic SI on T1-WI, instead of the homogeneously very low SI of cystic lesions, with bright heterogeneous SI on T2-WI, wall thickening, and enhancement after contrast injection (Fig. 7). If intralesional septa are present, they usually enhance as well. These findings, however, should not be confused with high T1 SI due to intracystic protein or hematic content neither with contrast enhancement lining the cyst wall due to surrounding functional parenchyma.[54,55] High SI on DWI

(and consequent low SI on ADC) may be seen due to the presence of intracystic inflammatory cells/pus.[54]

LOWER URINARY TRACT
Acute Infectious Cystitis

Cystitis is an inflammation of the bladder and in most cases caused by a bacterial infection. Uncomplicated acute infectious cystitis is usually treated without imaging, as discussed previously. On MR imaging, it is perceived as uniform circumferential wall thickening, with high SI on T2-WI and low SI on T1-WI due to edema. Hyperenhancement of the bladder urothelium is similar to that seen in inflammatory conditions of the urothelium in the remaining urinary tract. Another common feature is the perivesical fat stranding, better depicted on FS sequences, due to the extension of the inflammatory process and perivesical edema.[17]

Inflammation of the bladder may also occur due to the direct extension of the inflammatory processes occurring elsewhere in the pelvic cavity, especially gastrointestinal tract (eg, appendicitis, colitis, and diverticulitis) or gynecologic disorders (eg, pelvic inflammatory disease). Ileovesical or

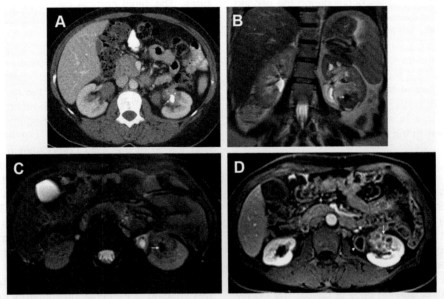

Fig. 6. XGP. Axial contrast-enhanced CT (*A*); coronal SS-ETSE T2-WI (*B*); axial FS SS-ETSE T2-WI (*C*) and axial post-contrast FS 3-D–GRE T1-WI in the nephrographic phase (*D*). A 47-year-old woman presenting with mild fever, dysuria and left-sided back and flank pain for the past 2 to 3 weeks. Contrast-enhanced CT scan demonstrates inferior pelvic calculi (*arrow* [*A*]), with focal parenchymal atrophy and an extensive peri-nephric inflammatory infiltrate. On MR imaging, moderate dilatation of the collecting system was seen but the depiction of the calculi was more problematic appearing low in SI (*arrows* [*B* and *C*]). Postcontrast images showed a masslike lesion (*arrow* [*D*]) with multiple discrete abscesses indistinguishable from a neoplasm. This patient underwent partial nephrectomy confirming the diagnosis of focal XGP. Note the mild pyelitis with increased contrast enhancement (*short arrow* [*D*]) and adjacent soft tissue edema.

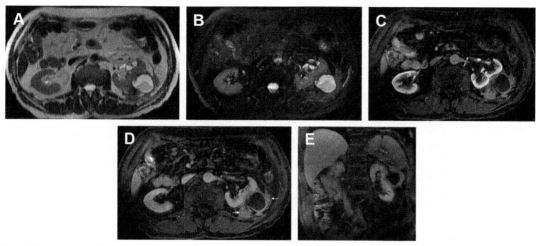

Fig. 7. Infected renal cyst. Axial non-FS (*A*) and FS (*B*) SS-ETSE T2-WI; axial postcontrast FS 3-D–GRE T1-WI in the arterial (*C*) and nephrographic phase (*D*); coronal postcontrast FS 3-D–GRE T1-WI on the interstitial phase (*E*). A 66-year-old man with a prolonged history of lumbar pain, fever and weight loss. There is a complex cystic lesion in left kidney showing intracavitary dependent debris. It demonstrates irregularly thickened walls, with progressive enhancement after contrast injection. There is perinephric edema and progressive enhancement of the thickened paranephric tissues (*arrows* [*D*]). Percutaneous biopsy was performed, revealing inflammatory tissue without evidence of neoplastic cells. After antibiotic therapy, CT (not shown) showed reduction in size of this cystic lesion.

colovesical fistulas represent a possible complication of ileocolic disorders, most frequently Crohn disease and diverticulitis, and commonly present with pseudonodular thickening of the bladder wall (**Fig. 8**). Vesicovaginal fistula may follow direct tumoral invasion or radiation therapy for gynecologic malignancies.

MR imaging depicts bladder wall thickening adjacent to the fistulous track, demonstrating high SI on T2-WI due to the presence of edema, with increased contrast enhancement of the inflamed mucosa. Fistulous tracks can be seen as a layered tram track configuration or as a linear enhancing structure. Debris and gas inside the bladder lumen may be depicted, the latter seen as signal voids or blooming artifacts, as discussed previously (**Fig. 9**).[56]

Rarely, infectious cystitis can lead to mural bladder abscess formation, which generally develops at the bladder dome, without appreciable communication with the bladder lumen.[17]

Radiation and Chemotherapy Cystitis

MR imaging findings of chemotherapy and radiation-induced cystitis are nonspecific and cannot be distinguished from other causes of cystitis. Diffuse or focal irregular bladder wall thickening and decreased bladder volume is characteristic. High T2 SI within the bladder wall and perivesical fat may be shown due to edema. In the chronic phase, a small fibrosed bladder with a thick wall, hydronephrosis, fatty replacement of the pelvic musculature, and widening of the presacral space may be seen (**Fig. 10**).[56,57]

Increased SI of the mucosa on T1-WI may also be seen and is likely due to mucosal hemorrhage. Hemorrhagic cystitis is not only associated with some chemotherapy agents (namely intravesical use of mitomycin C or cyclophosphamide, ifosphamide, busulfan, and cabazitaxel) but also to radiotherapy due to the denudation of the urothelium.[57] Severe radiation injuries cause bladder wall necrosis and fistula development, as discussed previously.

Emphysematous Cystitis

Emphysematous cystitis is a rare condition, almost invariably occurring in diabetic patients, in which gas produced by microorganisms dissects within the bladder wall. This air content may be depicted as signal voids in all MR imaging sequences, possibly with blooming artifact on GRE sequences with longer echo times.[5,17]

Cystitis Cystica et Glandularis and Papillary-Polypoid Cystitis

Cystitis cystica et glandularis and papillary-polypoid cystitis are chronic reactive inflammatory disorders that occur in the setting of chronic irritation of the bladder wall.

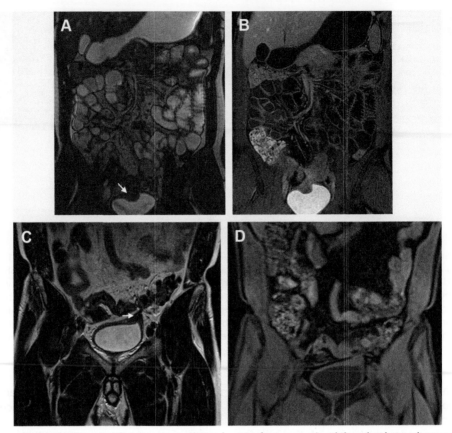

Fig. 8. Ileovesical and colovesical fistulas. Coronal steady-state free precession (*A*) and enhanced coronal FS 3-D–GRE T1-WI at the interstitial phase (*B*) in a patient with Crohn disease complicated with ileovesical fistula (*arrow* [*A*]). Coronal non-FS SS-ETSE T2-WI (*C*) and unenhanced coronal FS 3-D–GRE T1-WI (*D*) in a patient with a history of previous diverticulitis and resultant colovesical fistula (*arrow* [*C*]). Note the typical bladder pseudomass appearance in cases of bowel to bladder fistulas.

Cystitis cystica et glandularis are common and usually together at presentation and their development has been linked to long-standing mucosal irritation (urethral reimplantation, neurogenic bladder, and bladder exstrophy).[58]

Papillary-polypoid cystitis is an uncommon nonspecific chronic cystitis, usually after long-standing catheterization.[59]

Their imaging appearance is nonspecific and is usually characterized as an exophytic lesion of the bladder.[60,61]

On MR imaging, it is usually present with low-to iso-signal intensity on T1-WI and low SI on T2-WI, with a central branching high SI pattern corresponding to the vascular stalk.[62] One feature that may help distinguishing these entities from bladder carcinoma is the sparing of muscular layer of the bladder wall. Nevertheless, obliteration of the bladder wall and stranding of perivesical fat also may be seen, reflecting the extension of the inflammatory process. Due to the nonspecificity of their radiological appearances, the differential diagnosis with bladder carcinoma is difficult and biopsy is necessary for a definitive diagnosis (**Fig. 11**).[4,17,56,61]

Urachal Inflammatory and Infectious Conditions

The abnormal persistence of the embryologic communication between the bladder and the umbilicus is often recognized in adults and infection is its most commonly encountered complication. These urachal anomalies usually present with nonspecific symptoms as abdominal pain and tenderness, fever, purulent urinary discharge, and occasionally a palpable mass.[63,64]

Infection presents as heterogeneous SI on T1 and T2-WI in the lumen of the urachal remnant, possibly with liquid-liquid levels, and hyperenhancement of the remnant walls after contrast injection, similar to infection seen elsewhere in the urinary tract.

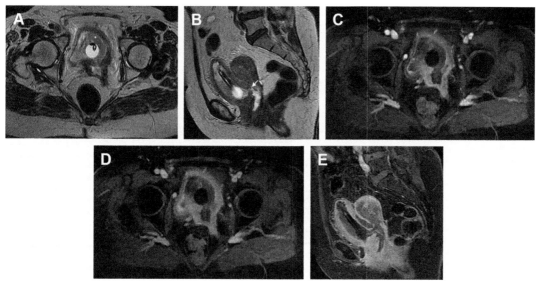

Fig. 9. Vesicovaginal fistula. Axial (*A*) and sagittal (*B*) FSE T2-WI; axial postcontrast FS 3-D–GRE T1-WI in the arterial (*C*) and interstitial phase (*D*); sagittal postcontrast FS 3-D–GRE T1-WI in the interstitial phase (*E*). A 61-year-old woman with history of cervical cancer submitted to radiotherapy, admitted in the authors' institution with pelvic pain, fetid vaginal discharge, vomiting and fever. A fistulous tract is depicted between the anterior wall of vagina and the bladder (*arrow* [*B*]). The bladder shows heterogeneous intraluminal content (*asterisk* [*A*]). There is marked enhancement of the thickened bladder wall, uterus, vagina and surrounding tissues, due to extensive inflammation.

Although it is unusual, severe infection can result in the formation of complex fistulas and abscesses, with the attendant risk of potential intraperitoneal rupture causing peritonitis and sepsis (**Fig. 12**).[63,64]

Other less frequently reported complications (beyond malignancy) include urachal granulomas, calcifications, and stone formation that result from chronic urinary stasis.[63]

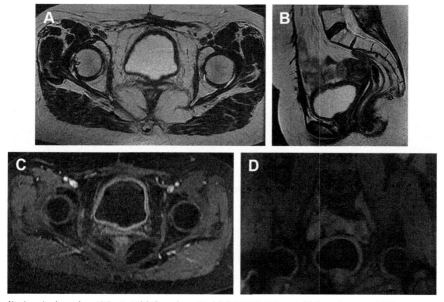

Fig. 10. Radiation-induced cystitis. Axial (*A*) and sagittal (*B*) FSE T2-WI; axial (*C*) and coronal (*D*) postcontrast FS 3-D–GRE T1-WI in the nephrographic phase. Follow-up MR imaging in a 58-year-old woman with cervical canal squamous cell carcinoma, submitted to chemotherapy and radiotherapy 1 year before. There is diffuse thickening with increased enhancement after contrast injection of the bladder wall, due to the radiation-induced inflammation.

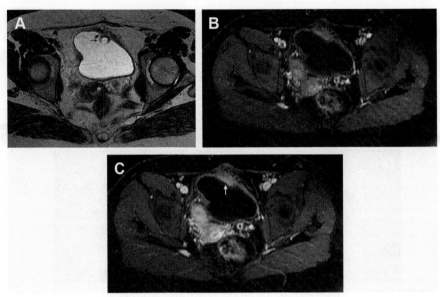

Fig. 11. Chronic cystitis. Axial (*A*) FSE T2-WI; axial postcontrast FS 3-D–GRE T1-WI in the arterial (*B*) and interstitial phase (*C*). A 29-year-old woman with long-term catheterization due to ureteric calculi and history of recurrent UTIs. There is irregular focal thickening of the bladder wall (*arrow* [*C*]), which shows hyper-enhancement after contrast injection. This thickened are was in close contact to the tip of the urethral catheter (*arrow* [*A*]). It is important however to exclude malignancy. A layer of intraluminal sediment is depicted on T2-WI.

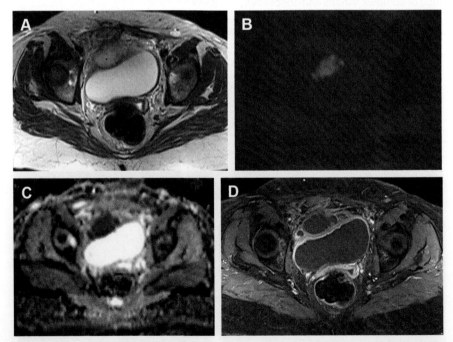

Fig. 12. Urachal abscess. Axial (*A*) FSE T2-WI; axial DWI, b value 800 (*B*), and ADC map (*C*); and axial postcontrast FS 3-D–GRE T1-WI in the nephrographic phase (*D*). A 57-year-old woman presents with urinary frequency, dysuria and recurrent UTI's. There is a midline fluid collection adjacent to the dome of the bladder wall (*asterisk* [*A*]), with thickened hyper-enhancing walls, in keeping with urachal abscess. The pus inside the abscess shows characteristic restricted diffusion with low SI on the ADC map. The bladder also shows diffuse wall thickening and hyperenhancement due to inflammatory reaction to the adjacent process.

Urethral Diverticula Infection

Classically, urethral diverticula arise from the posterolateral wall of the midurethra at the level of the pubic symphysis, with various degrees of extension around the circumference of the urethra, from a simple round or oval structure located lateral or posterior to the urethra to a U-shaped or circumferential diverticulum extending around the urethra.

A history of recurrent UTIs is seen in 30% to 50% of patients with urethral diverticula. Inflamed urethral diverticula may show thick wall or multiple septa, heterogeneous SI on T1-WI, and high signal on T2-WI, with enhancement after contrast injection. A fluid-fluid level may be seen in the presence of intradiverticular debris (**Fig. 13**).[65–67]

Diverticula with hemorrhagic or proteinaceous contents appear hyperintense on T1-WI and hypointense on T2-WI. Calculus formation may also be associated with urethral diverticula (in 1.5%–10% of cases) due to stagnation of the infected urine. Its MR imaging appearance is similar to that of calculi elsewhere in the urinary tract, showing as a filling defect with low SI on T1-W1 and T2-WI in the dependent portion of a diverticulum.[65,68,69]

Differentiation must be made between urethral diverticula and cysts or abscesses of Skene glands, another type of periurethral cystic masses that usually lie lower and closer to the external urethral meatus. On MR imaging, Skene cyst infection has a similar appearance of that of urethral diverticula infection.[69]

Prostatic Abscess

Prostatic abscesses occur in 2.7% of patients with acute bacterial prostatitis and require urology consultation for drainage.[70] Typical MR imaging findings of abscess is an iso-low T1 SI poorly defined nodule, with heterogeneous high T2 SI and peripheral enhancement on postgadolinium images, usually with low ADC value (**Fig. 14**). The central gas sign may be seen as central low SI in all sequences, with blooming artifact.

Granulomatous Prostatitis

Granulomatous prostatitis is an uncommon benign inflammatory condition, which often presents with a firm nodule on digital rectal examination and elevated prostate-specific antigen, thus clinically mimicking prostate cancer. It may be idiopathic or associated with previous intravesical bacille Calmette-Guérin (BCG) therapy for bladder cancer, tuberculous prostatitis, or previous intervention, such as transurethral resection of the prostate.

Granulomatous prostatitis may appear as a discrete mass with markedly low T2 SI, with moderate enhancement, which is usually lower than prostate cancer, and low ADC values due to its highly increased cellular density that causes restriction of water diffusion, which may be more pronounced than observed for other inflammatory or infectious processes (**Fig. 15**). There may be associated infiltration of the periprostatic fat by inflammation, thus mimicking extraprostatic tumor

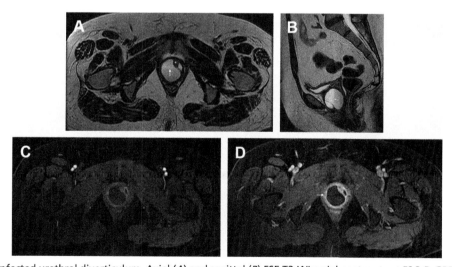

Fig. 13. Infected urethral diverticulum. Axial (A) and sagittal (B) FSE T2-WI; axial postcontrast FS 3-D-GRE T1-WI in the arterial (C) and venous phase (D). A 51-year-old woman with history of recurrent UTIs and complaints of stress urinary incontinence and dysuria. A cystic structure is seen surrounding the midurethra (asterisk [A]), showing thick walls and an internal septum. Fluid-fluid levels are depicted (arrows [A and B]) due to the presence of debris. Progressive enhancement of the walls and septum of the diverticulum is seen on postcontrast images (arrow [D]).

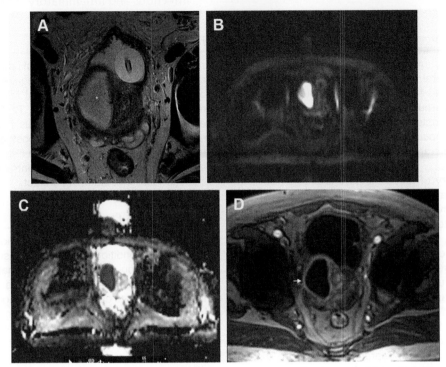

Fig. 14. Prostatic abscess. Axial (*A*) high-resolution FSE T2-WI; axial DWI, b value 1600 (*B*), and ADC map (*C*); axial postcontrast FS 3-D–GRE T1-WI in the interstitial phase (*D*). A 78-year-old man with history of benign prostatic hyperplasia, presents to the emergency department with complaints of dysuria, pelvic tenderness, urinary frequency and persistent high fever. A large lobulated fluid collection (*asterisk* [*A*]) is seen in the right central hemi-prostate, with slightly inhomogeneous T2 signal and increased marginal enhancement (*arrow* [*D*]), compatible with prostatic abscess. There is marked restriction to water diffusion with very high SI on b value 1600 (*B*) and low very low ADC signal (*arrow* [*C*]), due to the presence of inflammatory cells.

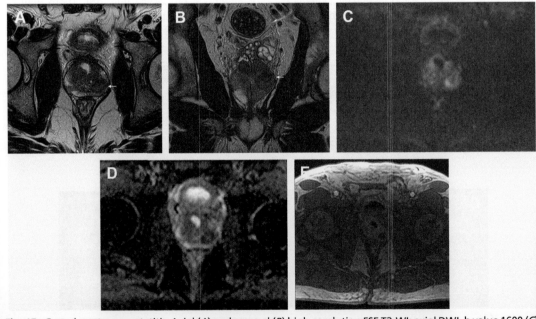

Fig. 15. Granulomatous prostatitis. Axial (*A*) and coronal (*B*) high-resolution FSE T2-WI; axial DWI, b value 1600 (*C*), and ADC map (*D*); axial postcontrast FS 3-D–GRE T1-WI in the arterial phase (*E*). A 72-year-old man with prior history of bladder cancer treated with intravesical BCG therapy, as well as prostatic benign hyperplasia, evaluated for high prostate-specific antigen (PSA) value. A well-defined low T2 signal nodule (*arrows* [*A* and *B*]) is depicted in the left hemi-prostate, showing peripheral enhancement and restricted diffusion (PI-RADS 5). Differentiation from prostatic cancer is not possible by imaging. Tranrectal ultrasound guided biopsy revealed granulomatous prostatitis.

extension. Histologic confirmation usually is needed not only to exclude cancer but also because patients with BCG-related granulomatous prostatitis should be treated with antituberculosis drugs.[71–73]

SUMMARY

In conclusion, MR imaging is a robust imaging technique for the evaluation of complicated UTIs. MR imaging may be the recommended imaging modality for the assessment of lower UTIs and performs with at least similar diagnostic accuracy to CT in upper UTIs, except for the identification of calculi and EPN. The absence of the ionizing radiation of MR imaging is an advantage in the evaluation of younger patients and in cases of required follow-up studies. Furthermore, MR imaging high-contrast resolution is a suitable alternative for the unenhanced evaluation when IV contrast cannot be administered.

REFERENCES

1. Foxman B. Epidemiology of urinary tract infections: incidence, morbidity, and economic costs. Am J Med 2002;113(Suppl 1A):5S–13S.
2. Gupta K, Hooton TM, Naber KG, et al. Executive summary: international clinical practice guidelines for the treatment of acute uncomplicated cystitis and pyelonephritis in women: a 2010 update by the Infectious Diseases Society of America and the European Society for Microbiology and Infectio. Clin Infect Dis 2011;52(5):561–4.
3. Wagenlehner FME, Hoyme U, Kaase M, et al. Uncomplicated urinary tract infections. Dtsch Arztebl Int 2011;108(24):415–23.
4. Lane DR, Takhar SS. Diagnosis and management of urinary tract infection and pyelonephritis. Emerg Med Clin North Am 2011;29(3):539–52.
5. Browne RFJ, Zwirewich C, Torreggiani WC. Imaging of urinary tract infection in the adult. Eur Radiol 2004;14(3):168–83.
6. Ifergan J, Pommier R, Brion M-C, et al. Imaging in upper urinary tract infections. Diagn Interv Imaging 2012;93(6):509 10.
7. Faletti R, Cassinis MC, Fonio P, et al. Diffusion-weighted imaging and apparent diffusion coefficient values versus contrast-enhanced MR imaging in the identification and characterisation of acute pyelonephritis. Eur Radiol 2013;23(12):3501–8.
8. Hiorns MP. Imaging of the urinary tract: the role of CT and MRI. Pediatr Nephrol 2011;26(1):59–68.
9. Piccoli GB, Consiglio V, Deagostini MC, et al. The clinical and imaging presentation of acute "non complicated" pyelonephritis: a new profile for an ancient disease. BMC Nephrol 2011;12:68.
10. Rathod SB, Kumbhar SS, Nanivadekar A, et al. Role of diffusion-weighted MRI in acute pyelonephritis: a prospective study. Acta Radiol 2014;56(2):244–9.
11. Martina MC, Campanino PP, Caraffo F, et al. Dynamic magnetic resonance imaging in acute pyelonephritis. Radiol Med 2010;115(2):287–300.
12. Thoeny HC, De Keyzer F. Diffusion-weighted MR imaging of native and transplanted kidneys. Radiology 2011;259(1):25–38.
13. Yoo JM, Koh JS, Han CH, et al. Diagnosing acute pyelonephritis with CT, 99mTc-DMSA SPECT, and Doppler ultrasound: a comparative study. Korean J Urol 2010;51(4):260–5.
14. Blanco LT, Socarras MR, Montero RF, et al. Renal colic during pregnancy: diagnostic and therapeutic aspects. Literature review. Cent European J Urol 2017;70(1):93–100.
15. Kalb B, Indik JH, Ott P, et al. MRI of patients with implanted cardiac devices. J Magn Reson Imaging 2017;1–9. https://doi.org/10.1002/jmri.25824.
16. Ramalho M, Hithaya I, Alobaidy M, et al. MRI Evaluation of cooperative and non-cooperative patients with non-traumatic acute abdominal pain – preliminary observations. Clin Imaging 2016;40(4):707–13.
17. Tonolini M, Ippolito S. Cross-sectional imaging of complicated urinary infections affecting the lower tract and male genital organs. Insights Imaging 2016;7(5):689–711.
18. James HE, Matthew SD, Jonathan RD, et al. ACR Manual on Contrast Media. 2017. Version 10.3 2017 ACR Committee on Drugs and Contrast Media. Available at: http://www.t2star.com/ewExternalFiles/ACR%20Contrast_Media%20ver10.3_2017.pdf.
19. Tao SM, Wichmann JL, Schoepf UJ, et al. Contrast-induced nephropathy in CT: incidence, risk factors and strategies for prevention. Eur Radiol 2016;26(9):3310–8.
20. Samadian F, Dalili N, Mahmoudieh L, et al. Contrast-induced nephropathy: essentials and concerns. Iran J Kidney Dis 2018;12(3):135–41.
21. Ramalho M, Ramalho J, Burke LM, et al. Gadolinium retention and toxicity—an update. Adv Chronic Kidney Dis 2017;24(3):138–46.
22. Morzycki A, Bhatia A, Murphy KJ. Adverse reactions to contrast material: a canadian update. Can Assoc Radiol J 2017;68(2):187–93.
23. Joffe P, Thomsen HS, Meusel M. Pharmacokinetics of gadodiamide injection in patients with severe renal insufficiency and patients undergoing hemodialysis or continuous ambulatory peritoneal dialysis. Acad Radiol 1998;5(7):491–502.
24. Vivier PH, Sallem A, Beurdeley M, et al. MRI and suspected acute pyelonephritis in children: comparison of diffusion-weighted imaging with gadolinium-enhanced T1-weighted imaging. Eur Radiol 2014;24(1):19–25.

25. Roy C, Ohana M, Host P, et al. MR urography (MRU) of non-dilated ureter with diuretic administration: static fluid 2D FSE T2-weighted versus 3D gadolinium T1-weighted GE excretory MR. Eur J Radiol Open 2014;1(1):6–13.

26. De Haas RJ, Steyvers MJ, Fütterer JJ. Multiparametric MRI of the bladder: ready for clinical routine? Am J Roentgenol 2014;202(6):1187–95.

27. Chung AD, Schieda N, Shanbhogue AK, et al. MRI evaluation of the urothelial tract: pitfalls and solutions. Am J Roentgenol 2016;207(6):W108–16.

28. Yuh BI, Cohan RH. Different phases of renal enhancement: role in detecting and charaterizing renal masses during helical CT. AJR Am J Roentgenol 1999;173:747–55.

29. Thornton E, Mendiratta-Lala M, Siewert B, et al. Patterns of fat stranding. Am J Roentgenol 2011;197(1):1–14.

30. Yu TY, Kim HR, Hwang KE, et al. Computed tomography findings associated with bacteremia in adult patients with a urinary tract infection. Eur J Clin Microbiol Infect Dis 2016;35(11):1883–7.

31. De Pascale A, Piccoli GB, Priola SM, et al. Diffusion-weighted magnetic resonance imaging: new perspectives in the diagnostic pathway of non-complicated acute pyelonephritis. Eur Radiol 2013; 23(11):3077–86.

32. Düzenli K, Öztürk M, Yıldırım İO, et al. The utility of diffusion-weighted imaging to assess acute renal parenchymal changes due to unilateral ureteral stone obstruction. Urolithiasis 2017;45(4):401–5.

33. Haddad MC, Hawary MM, Khoury NJ, et al. Radiology of perinephric fluid collections. Clin Radiol 2002;57(5):339–46.

34. Kua C, Abdul Aziz Y. Air in the kidney: between emphysematous pyelitis and pyelonephritis. Biomed Imaging Interv J 2008;4(4):e24.

35. Kuo C-Y, Lin C-Y, Chen T-C, et al. Clinical features and prognostic factors of emphysematous urinary tract infection. J Microbiol Immunol Infect 2009; 42(5):393–400.

36. Michaeli J, Mogle P, Perlberg S, et al. Emphysematous pyelonephritis. J Urol 1984;131(2):203–8.

37. Craig WD, Wagner BJ, Travis MD. Pyelonephritis: radiologic-pathologic review. Radiographics 2008; 28(1):255–76.

38. Brown JA, Maharaj P, Khan O, et al. A rare case of emphysematous pyelonephritis within a horseshoe kidney. West Indian Med J 2011;60(2):229–31.

39. St Lezin M, Hofmann R, Stoller ML. Pyonephrosis: diagnosis and treatment. Br J Urol 1992;70(4):360–3.

40. Masselli G, Weston M, Spencer J. The role of imaging in the diagnosis and management of renal stone disease in pregnancy. Clin Radiol 2015;70(12):1462–71.

41. Wasnik AP, Elsayes KM, Kaza RK, et al. Multimodality imaging in ureteric and periureteric

pathologic abnormalities. Am J Roentgenol 2011;197(6):1083–92.

42. Kalayci TO, Apaydin M, Sönmezgöz F, et al. Diffusion-weighted magnetic resonance imaging findings of kidneys with obstructive uropathy: differentiation between benign and malignant etiology. ScientificWorldJournal 2014;2014:980280.

43. Ray JG, Vermeulen MJ, Bharatha A, et al. Association between MRI exposure during pregnancy and fetal and childhood outcomes. JAMA 2016;316(9):952.

44. Kanal E, Barkovich AJ, Bell C, et al. ACR guidance document for safe MR practices: 2007. Am J Roentgenol 2007;188(6):1447–74.

45. Çaliskan S, Özsoy E, Kaba S, et al. Xanthogranulomatous pyelonephritis. Arch Iran Med 2016;19(10):712–4.

46. LiPuma JP. Magnetic resonance imaging of the kidney. Radiol Clin North Am 1984;22(4):925–41.

47. Laugareil P, Bléry M, Despoisse, et al. Xanthogranulomatous pyelonephritis with fatty proliferation of the renal space. Aspects in x-ray computed tomography and MRI. J Radiol 1989;70(4):295–7 [in French].

48. Joërg A, Cussenot O, Houlle D, et al. Xanthogranulomatous pyelonephritis. Value of magnetic resonance imaging. Ann Urol (Paris) 1989;23(3):232–5 [in French].

49. Ramboer K, Oyen R, Verellen S, et al. Focal xanthogranulomatous pyelonephritis mimicking a renal tumor: CT- and MR-findings and evolution under therapy. Nephrol Dial Transplant 1997;12(5):1028–30.

50. Mulopulos GP, Patel SK, Pessis D. MR imaging of xanthogranulomatous pyelonephritis. J Comput Assist Tomogr 1986;10(1):154–6.

51. Feldberg MA, Driessen LP, Witkamp TD, et al. Xanthogranulomatous pyelonephritis: comparison of extent using computed tomography and magnetic resonance imaging in one case. Urol Radiol 1988; 10(2):92–4.

52. Verswijvel G, Oyen R, Van Poppel H, et al. Xanthogranulomatous pyelonephritis: MRI findings in the diffuse and the focal type. Eur Radiol 2000;10(4):586–9.

53. Inouye BM, Chiang G, Newbury RO, et al. Adolescent xanthogranulomatous pyelonephritis mimicking renal cell carcinoma on urine cytology: an atypical presentation. Urology 2013;81(4):885–7.

54. Jouret F, Lhommel R, Devuyst O, et al. Diagnosis of cyst infection in patients with autosomal dominant polycystic kidney disease: attributes and limitations of the current modalities. Nephrol Dial Transplant 2012;27(10):3746–51.

55. Chicoskie C, Chaoui A, Kuligowska E, et al. MRI isolation of infected renal cyst in autosomal dominant polycystic kidney disease. Clin Imaging 2001; 25(2):114–7.

56. Wong-You-Cheong JJ, Woodward PJ, Manning MA, et al. Inflammatory and nonneoplastic bladder

masses: radiologic-pathologic correlation. Radiographics 2006;26(6):1847–68.

57. Jia JB, Lall C, Tirkes T, et al. Chemotherapy-related complications in the kidneys and collecting system: an imaging perspective. Insights Imaging 2015;6(4):479–87.

58. Smith AK, Hansel DE, Jones JS. Role of cystitis cystica et glandularis and intestinal metaplasia in development of bladder carcinoma. Urology 2008;71(5):915–8.

59. Abu-Yousef MM, Narayana AS, Brown RC. Catheter-induced cystitis: evaluation by cystosonography. Radiology 1984;151(2):471–3.

60. Roh JE, Cho BS, Jeon MH, et al. Polypoid cystitis in an adult without history of catheterization. Iran J Radiol 2011;8(3):173–5.

61. Ozaki K, Kitagawa K, Gabata T, et al. A case of polypoid and papillary cystitis mimicking an advanced bladder carcinoma with invasion of perivesical fat. Urol Ann 2014;6(1):72.

62. Kim SH, Yang DM, Kim NR. Polypoid and papillary cystitis mimicking a large transitional carcinoma in a patient without a history of catheterization: computed tomography and magnetic resonance findings. J Comput Assist Tomogr 2004;28(4):485–7.

63. Parada Villavicencio C, Adam SZ, Nikolaidis P, et al. Imaging of the urachus: anomalies, complications, and mimics. Radiographics 2016;36(7):2049–63.

64. Qureshi K, Maskell D, McMillan C, et al. An infected urachal cyst presenting as an acute abdomen - A case report. Int J Surg Case Rep 2013;4(7):633–5.

65. Chaudhari VV, Patel MK, Douek M, et al. MR imaging and US of female urethral and periurethral disease. Radiographics 2010;30(7):1857–74.

66. Dwarkasing RS, Dinkelaar W, Hop WCJ, et al. MRI evaluation of urethral diverticula and differential diagnosis in symptomatic women. Am J Roentgenol 2011;197(3):676–82.

67. Ryu J, Kim B. MR imaging of the male and female urethra. Radiographics 2001;21(5):1169–85.

68. Chou C-P, Levenson RB, Elsayes KM, et al. Imaging of female urethral diverticulum: an update. RadioGraphics 2008;28(7):1917–30.

69. Hahn WY, Israel GM, Lee VS. MRI of female urethral and periurethral disorders. Am J Roentgenol 2004;182(3):677–82.

70. Millán-Rodríguez F, Palou J, Bujons-Tur A, et al. Acute bacterial prostatitis: two different subcategories according to a previous manipulation of the lower urinary tract. World J Urol 2006;24(1):45–50.

71. Rosenkrantz AB, Taneja SS. Radiologist, be aware: ten pitfalls that confound the interpretation of multiparametric prostate MRI. Am J Roentgenol 2014;202(1):109–20.

72. Sah VK, Wang L, Min X, et al. Multiparametric MR imaging in diagnosis of chronic prostatitis and its differentiation from prostate cancer. Radiol Infect Dis 2015;1(2):70–7.

73. Bour L, Schull A, Delongchamps N-B, et al. Multiparametric MRI features of granulomatous prostatitis and tubercular prostate abscess. Diagn Interv Imaging 2013;94(1):84–90.

Magnetic Resonance Imaging of the Perirenal Space and Retroperitoneum

Jorge Elias Jr, MD, PhD*, Valdair Francisco Muglia, MD, PhD

KEYWORDS

- Retroperitoneum • Perirenal space • Magnetic resonance imaging • Diagnostic imaging

KEY POINTS

- Previous knowledge of certain underlying diseases helps to identify the most likely diagnosis and can even preclude biopsy.
- Many retroperitoneal lesions may mimic each other in magnetic resonance appearance, and histopathologic confirmation is needed.
- Age, mass location, and characterization of tissue components are crucial to narrow the differential diagnosis of a retroperitoneal lesion.
- The presence of macroscopic fat indicates a narrow list of fat-containing tumors, among them the liposarcoma, which is the most common retroperitoneal tumor.

INTRODUCTION

Evaluation of retroperitoneum is essential in all abdominal imaging studies, such as ultrasonography, computed tomography (CT), and magnetic resonance (MR) imaging, for any given clinical indication. Although retroperitoneal pathologic processes could be asymptomatic with indolent biological behavior, some diseases and lesions can manifest as acute pain syndrome, such as back or abdominal pain, prompting for imaging assessment. These pathologic processes include a wide range of neoplastic, proliferative, and inflammatory/infectious conditions that may present similar clinical features and overlapping imaging findings.[1,2] The precise location and tissue characterization are the main goals of imaging evaluation, which is needed to define biopsy planning, and to help the surgical approach, whenever possible. To the best of our knowledge, there is no new evidence driven by direct comparison between CT and MR imaging for the assessment of performance in the evaluation of retroperitoneum. Although CT is usually the preferred modality for the retroperitoneum in routine clinical practice, MR imaging has been reported to be the most accurate modality for adrenal and pancreas evaluation, and CT and MR imaging have been reported to have comparable accuracy for kidney disease.[3–5] MR imaging has superior soft tissue contrast resolution compared with CT because of its multiple techniques, which permit detection of the free water molecules (as in edema and large masses of cytoplasm), macroscopic and microscopic fat, and differences between compact/dense tissues and loose/sparse soft tissue. Moreover, postcontrast MR imaging sequences are more sensitive to depict differential tissue vascularization compared with CT. A disadvantage of MR imaging is the low sensitivity for the detection of calcifications compared with CT. Despite these advantages of MR imaging

Disclosure: Dr J. Elias Jr carried out the present work with the support of CNPq, National Council of Scientific and Technological Development - Brazil (311023/2015-0). Dr V.F. Muglia has nothing to disclose.
Internal Medicine Department, Imaging and Physics Science Center, Clinical Hospital of Ribeirao Preto Medical School, University of Sao Paulo, Second Floor, Av. Bandeirantes, 3900, Ribeirao Preto, Sao Paulo CEP 14049-900, Brazil
* Corresponding author.
E-mail address: jejunior@fmrp.usp.br

Magn Reson Imaging Clin N Am 27 (2019) 77–103
https://doi.org/10.1016/j.mric.2018.08.007

compared with CT, MR imaging evaluation also usually does not permit a definitive diagnosis in the lesions of retroperitoneum except in a few specific disease entities, but imaging is very important in most cases to narrow the differential diagnosis.

NORMAL ANATOMY AND IMAGING TECHNIQUE

Detailed knowledge of the compartmental anatomy of the retroperitoneum is essential to understand the origin and dissemination of retroperitoneal diseases and lesions as well as pathologic process from adjacent spaces that may involve the retroperitoneum. The retroperitoneum is defined anteriorly by the posterior parietal peritoneum and posteriorly by the transversalis fascia, extending from diaphragm to the pelvic inlet level. It has 5 compartments: 2 lateral, 2 symmetric posterior ones containing the psoas major muscle, and 1 central vascular compartment containing the great vessels and neural and lymphatic structures. The lateral compartments are asymmetrical and divided by anterior and posterior renal fascia, which creates 3 spaces: anterior and posterior pararenal and perirenal spaces.

The perirenal space is defined by the anterior and posterior sheets of renal fascia, known as anterior renal fascia (ARF) or Gerota fascia and posterior renal fascia (PRF) or Zuckerkand fascia, respectively (Fig. 1A). It is larger superiorly and delimited by the diaphragm, and thinner inferiorly, where both ARF and PRF adhere to the ureter, assuming an inverted, closed cone shape.[6] Although cadaveric studies have shown the closed feature of perirenal space, interfascial planes exist and may permit fluid collection extension toward other spaces, including the pelvis.[6,7]

Both perirenal spaces contain the kidneys, renal pelvis and proximal ureters, adrenal glands, and perirenal fat.[7] Moreover, there is a fine bridging septa network comprising 3 different septa types that supports the kidney,[6] which is seen on imaging evaluation only when it accumulates fluid (Fig. 1B) or cellular tissue caused by pathologic processes. The focus here is the perirenal space and the most common lesions arising from this compartment. Besides the kidney and hilum components (renal artery, vein, and pelvis), adipose tissue, lymph nodes, and adrenal are the main structures in this space.

IMAGING PROTOCOLS

MR imaging evaluation of retroperitoneum can be reliably assessed using a phased-array receiver coil with the patient placed in supine position in a 1.5-T or 3-T scanner. A combination of breath-hold and breathing-independent T1-weighted and T2-weighted sequences acquired in at least 2 different planes is present in virtually any MR protocol.[8] A complete and comprehensive MR imaging evaluation is achieved with gradient echo variations of precontrast and postcontrast T1-weighted sequences, mainly in-phase and out-of-phase spoiled gradient-echo, and fat-suppressed three-dimensional gradient echo. Also, non–fat-suppressed T2-weighted and different techniques of fat-suppressed T2-weighted sequences are needed.[8] Although postcontrast fat-suppressed T1-weighted sequences are important for delineation of many retroperitoneal disease processes and must be obtained, even with its preclusion, in selected cases because of renal impairment or other concerns, MR imaging findings still can evaluate size, location, and tissue characteristics of most lesions.[9] Diffusion-weighted imaging (DWI) has gained attention, mainly for the MR evaluation of oncologic patients, because some reported evidence has shown the added value of this technique to detect tumor deposits and tumor activity.[10,11] In current MR systems, addition of DWI sequences ultimately has very little impact on total time for

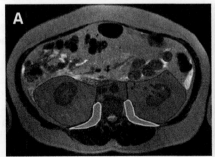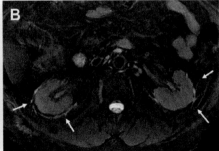

Fig. 1. Retroperitoneal anatomy. Axial T2-weighted MR image (A) of the midabdomen showing the perirenal space (red), the central vascular perirenal space (blue), and the psoas muscles (yellow). The perirenal space (arrows) is also shown on the axial T2-weighted fat-suppressed MR image (B).

Table 1
Parameters of basic generic abdominal/retroperitoneum magnetic resonance protocol

Sequence	Planes	Fat Suppression	IV Contrast	Repetition Time (ms)	Echo Time (ms)	Flip Angle (Degrees)	Section Thickness (mm)	Matrix Size
T1-weighted 2D SGE	Coronal	–	Pre	10	4.4	15	6–8	250 × 330
T2-weighted FSE/TSE	Coronal	–	–	1200–1500	80–90 90	6–8		330 × 330
T2-weighted FSE/TSE	Axial	–	–	1100–1300	160	90	6–8	330 × 330
T2-weighted STIR/SPAIR	Axial	+	–	1100	80	90	6–8	300 × 300
T1-weighted 2D SGE	Axial	–	Pre	110–140	2.2 and 4.4	80	6–8	300 × 380
Diffusion (b = 0, 150, 500, 1000)	Axial	–	Pre	4500–5000	70–80 90	4–6		200 × 200
T1-weighted 3D SGE	Axial/coronal/sagittal[a]	+	Pre and post[a]	4.3	1.7	3.5	10	250 × 250

b is b value, which determines the degree of diffusion weighting.
Abbreviations: 2D, two dimensional; 3D, three dimensional; FSE, fast spin echo; SGE, spoiled gradient echo; SPAIR, spectral attenuated inversion recovery; STIR, short-tau inversion recovery; TSE, turbo spin echo.
[a] Postcontrast images were acquired at hepatic arterial dominant, portal venous, and interstitial phases with the same injection protocol.

Table 2
Tissue component classification of retroperitoneal lesions

Tissue Component	
Fat containing	Lipomatosis
	Lipoma
	Low-grade liposarcoma[b]
	High-grade liposarcoma[a]
	Hibernoma
	Teratoma
Myxoid stroma	Schwannoma
	Neurofibroma
	Ganglioneuroma
	Pleomorphic sarcoma (myxoid malignant fibrous histiocytoma)[a]
	Leiomyosarcoma[a]
Small round cells	Lymphoma[b]
	Peripheral primitive neuroectodermic tumor[c]
Cystic or necrotic	Paraganglioma[a]
	Liposarcoma
	Lymphangioma
	Mucinous cystic lesion

[a] Hypervascular.
[b] Hypovascular.
[c] Necrosis is also a frequent feature.

the examination acquisition. **Table 1** shows the parameters of a basic generic abdominal/retroperitoneum MR protocol.

IMAGING FINDINGS/PATHOLOGY

The correct lesion localization, including its origin and extension, and the correct characterization of specific tissue components and vascularization, are the key features of the imaging evaluation of retroperitoneal masses.[8,12] However, large masses may pose some difficulty in determining its exact origin. Displacement of adjacent organs and structures and a series of described radiologic signs contribute to the correct evaluation in most cases.[12] The radiologic signs that indicate a specific organ origin are known as the beak sign, the phantom (invisible) organ sign, the embedded organ sign, and the prominent feeding artery sign.[2,12]

The most common retroperitoneal mass lesions are related to inflammatory/infectious or neoplastic lymph adenopathy, such as tuberculosis and lymphoma. Moreover, retroperitoneal primary neoplasms are rare.[13] Among them, sarcomas are the most common, although only 10% to 20% of sarcomas are located in retroperitoneum, corresponding with only 0.1% to 0.2% of all solid malignancies.[14] Nonetheless, retroperitoneal neoplasms are malignant in 70% to 80% of cases.[15]

Although the classic imaging description of retroperitoneal conditions is based on lesion location, a practical and comprehensive approach for diagnosis of retroperitoneal masses must be based on the evaluation of the tissue component of the lesion, with some added specific findings such as vascularization that permit to narrow the differential diagnosis (**Table 2**).[12] In this article, lesions are classified according to their main tissue component, which correlates to their histopathologic features: fat, myxoid stroma, necrosis, cystic nature/cystic components, and small round cells. A specific subset of infiltrative perivascular lesions with lymph nodes and retroperitoneal organ involvement is presented comparatively with lymphomas because they may mimic lymphoma presentation (**Table 3**). Vascularization features for each lesion are presented as well.

DIAGNOSTIC CRITERIA
Fat-Containing Lesions

A myriad of lesions arising from adipose tissue can be found in perirenal space, varying from benign to frankly malignant (**Table 4**). Benign lesions include

Table 3
Differential diagnosis of retroperitoneal/perivascular lesions

	Anterior Aortic Displacement	Ureter Involvement	IVC Involvement	Location in Retroperitoneum
Lymphoma	Typically present	Sporadically	Frequent	Anywhere
ECD	Absent	Sporadically	Usually spared	Anywhere
Idiopathic retroperitoneal fibrosis	Absent	Frequent	Frequent	Typically L4 to S1

Abbreviations: ECD, Erdheim-Chester disease; IVC, inferior vena cava.

Table 4
Differential diagnosis of fat-derived lesions in the retroperitoneum

	Incidence	Origin Type of Fat Tissue	Signal Intensity Pattern	Visible Fat	Typical Features
Lipomatosis	Rare	White	Homogeneous	Always	Diffuse. No mass formation
Lipoma	Rare	White	Homogeneous	Always	Round, well-defined small masses
Low-grade liposarcoma	Most common sarcoma	White	Homogeneous Mild heterogeneity	Very frequent Low proportion	Round, well-defined, large masses, thick septa
High-grade liposarcoma	Most common sarcoma	White	Heterogeneous	Usually scarce or not seen	Large and heterogeneous mass
Hibernomas	Very rare	Brown	Heterogeneous	Not seen	Heterogeneous Large-caliber vessels

the diffuse form of fat proliferation (lipomatosis) and the rarer focal lesions (lipomas).[16,17]

Lipomatosis is a rare condition defined as diffuse, increased proliferation of histologically benign adipose tissue in certain areas of the body. Although pelvis and intraperitoneal space/mesentery are common locations, lipomatosis is rare in the retroperitoneum.[17,18] Epidemiologically, they are more common in middle age, the fourth and fifth decades, with a clear male predominance in the literature. Clinical presentation varies from absence of symptoms (incidental finding) to urinary symptoms such as dysuria, urgency, and even hematuria. At imaging, typical fat findings such as bright signal on T1-weighted imaging are seen involving and distorting organs[18] without signs of invasion (**Fig. 2**).

Lipomas represent benign focal proliferation of mature fat tissue and are exceedingly rare in the retroperitoneum.[16,17] The assumption that a rounded, homogeneous fat mass represents a lipoma should be made with caution, because they cannot be confidently distinguished from well-differentiated liposarcomas based on imaging findings.

Although liposarcomas are the most common retroperitoneal sarcomas, the perirenal space is the preferred location for this neoplasm.[19,20] The peak of incidence occurs in sixth and seventh decades of life, with no gender predominance.[20,21] On histology, this neoplasia is usually divided into 5 subtypes, from well-differentiated to undifferentiated lesions, as follows: well-differentiated, myxoid, dedifferentiated, round

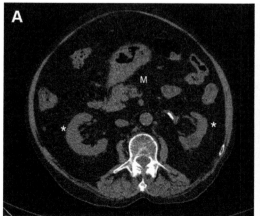
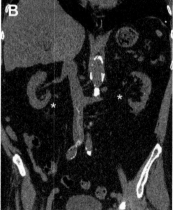

Fig. 2. Lipomatosis. Axial (*A*) CT scan and coronal reformation (*B*) show increased amount of abdominal fat within the peritoneal space (M) and in retroperitoneum, particularly in perirenal space (*asterisks*).

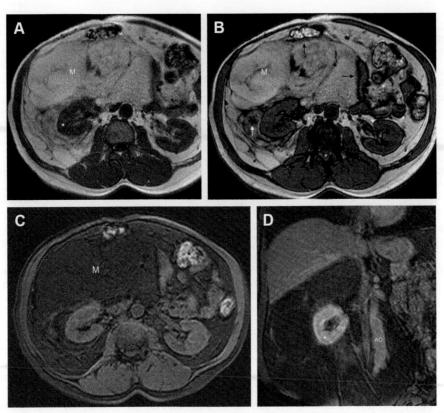

Fig. 3. Liposarcoma. Axial in-phase (*A*) and out-of-phase (*B*) SGE T1 images showing a huge perirenal mass (M), with high signal intensity, displacing the right kidney (*asterisks*) anteriorly. The colon and small bowel are also displaced by the mass (*black arrows* in *B*). The presence of chemical shift artifacts (*white arrow* in *B*) in the interface between soft tissue and areas of high signal indicates the adipose tissue origin of the mass. Axial T1 with fat suppression (*C*) showing diffuse loss of signal confirming that it is a fat-containing lesion. Coronal postgadolinium T1-weighted spoiled gradient echo (SGE) image (*D*) showing the enhancing soft tissue and septations in the lesion and its relationship to the aorta (AO) and to the kidney (*asterisk*).

cell, and pleomorphic lesions.[22] At diagnosis, they often present as a large, palpable mass, because no particular symptom is usually associated with this neoplasia. Cross-sectional imaging plays a major role for confirming the diagnosis, because fat can easily be confirmed by CT or MR imaging, and for staging (**Fig. 3**), when tumor extension is assessed, particularly if adjacent organs and/or vessels are involved.[19–21]

Mass characterization by imaging is important because large and heterogeneous lesions, usually presenting with areas of necrosis, are often associated with high-grade lesions on histology and poorer prognosis.[23] In the more aggressive lesions, adipose tissue may not be defined by imaging, and liposarcomas should be suspected by the location and heterogeneity of the lesion (**Fig. 4**).

Resectability should be assessed by checking any signs of invasion of adjacent organs and/or signs of major vessel encasement.[20,21]

An even rarer lesion derived from fat tissue that may occur in the retroperitoneum is hibernoma.[24]

These lesions are histologically benign and arise from brown adipose tissue but can show white fat, myxoid tissue, and spindled cells.[24,25] The most common locations are mediastinum, axilla, and neck, with the abdomen and retroperitoneum accounting for only 10% of cases. At MR imaging, hibernomas rarely show macroscopic fat. They tend to show intermediate signal between muscle and fat on T1 but typically show large intralesional vessels.[26]

Myxoid Stroma Lesions

Pathologically, myxoid stroma is characterized by mucoid matrix rich in mucopolysaccharide acid with variable vascularization. Most commonly, myxoid stroma has low signal on T1-weighted sequences and variable high signal on T2-weighted sequences. Usually, myxoid benign lesions present delayed to mild postgadolinium enhancement, and malignant lesions have accentuated enhancement on early phase.

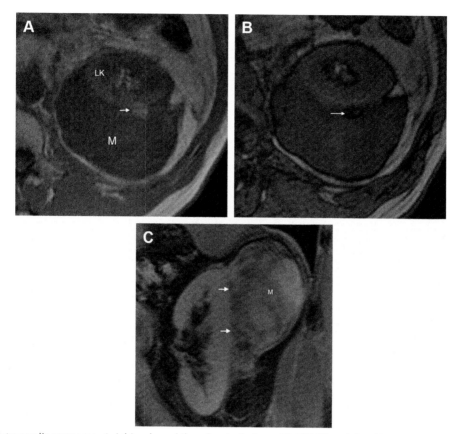

Fig. 4. Fat-poor liposarcoma. Axial in-phase (A) and out-of-phase (B) SGE T1-weighted images. A posterior perirenal mass (M) is seen displacing the left kidney (LK). The mass has the predominance of low signal intensity and only a small area of high signal on T1 is seen (arrow in A). In the opposed-phase image (B), this area shows chemical shift artifact indicating the presence of macroscopic fat (arrow in B). Small amount of macroscopic fat can be depicted easily on out-of-phase images when searching for India-ink (chemical shift) artifact. Sagittal postgadolinium T1-weighted imaging (C) clearly shows the heterogeneous enhancement. The interface between the mass and the kidney is smooth and regular and there is no notch sign suggesting the extrarenal origin (arrows in C).

Neurogenic tumors

Neurogenic tumors account for 10% to 20% of retroperitoneal neoplasm and are classified as ganglion cell origin (ganglioneuromas), paraganglionic system origin (paragangliomas), or nerve sheath origin (neurilemmomas/schwannomas, neurofibromas, and malignant nerve sheath tumors).[27,28] Ganglioneuromas, neurofibromas, and schwannomas are mainly myxoid stroma tumors because paragangliomas are classified as cystic/necrotic tumors.[2,12]

Overall, neurogenic tumors tend to show a fusiform shape, increased T2-weighted signal intensity, and highly intense contrast enhancement. There is no single imaging feature that can make the differentiation between benign and malignant neurogenic tumors, but the presence of distant metastasis and accelerated interval growth rate contribute to this differentiation when present. Classic findings of osseous remodeling are associated with benign slow-growing tumors, but, even so, some benign tumors may present malignant transformation. Detailed MR imaging findings, actuarial data, other diagnostic features and biological behavior of the main neurogenic tumors are presented in Table 5.

Pleomorphic sarcoma (malignant fibrous histiocytoma)

Pleomorphic sarcoma, formerly known as malignant fibrous histiocytoma (MFH), is considered the third most common retroperitoneal sarcoma, accounting for 6% to 15% of all cases.[20] This terminology and tumor classification were changed in 2002 by the World Health Organization, comprising fibrohistiocytic tumors grouped as undifferentiated pleomorphic sarcomas (storiform-pleomorphic, giant cell, angiomatoid, and inflammatory subtypes) and myxofibrosarcoma (or myxoid MFH).[33] Although rare, most of reported

Table 5
Neurogenic tumors: magnetic resonance imaging findings, actuarial data, other diagnostic features, and biological behavior

Neurogenic Tumors	MR Imaging Findings	Actuarial Data	Other Diagnosis Features	Biological Behavior
Ganglioneuroma (Fig. 5)	Homogeneous paravertebral mass (5–15 cm) with low signal on T1-weighted and marked high signal on T2-weighted images. Delayed heterogeneous enhancement may be seen. Extension along normal structures. Punctate calcifications may be seen. Necrosis is uncommon	20–40-y age group, with no sex predilection. Represent 0.7%–1.6% of all primary retroperitoneal tumors	Slow-growing tumor	Benign; rarely recur after surgical excision, rare description of malignant transformation
Ganglioneuroblastoma (Fig. 6)	Vary ranging from a predominantly solid mass to a predominantly cystic mass. Encapsulated. May contain granular calcification. MR features similar to neuroblastoma more than ganglioneuroma	2–4-y age group, with no sex predilection	The most common tumor site is the abdomen, followed by the mediastinum, neck, and lower extremities	Malignant
Neuroblastoma (Fig. 7)	Heterogeneous irregular and lobulated mass with low signal intensity on T1-weighted images and high signal intensity on T2-weighted images. Variable contrast enhancement. Hemorrhagic areas may manifest as areas of high signal intensity on T1-weighted images, and cystic change may appear bright on T2-weighted images. 85% of cases present with calcifications (coarse, amorphous, mottled). It may invade adjacent organs and encase vessels with luminal compression	Boys, first decade of life	Two-thirds located in the adrenal gland, and the remaining occur along the paravertebral sympathetic chain	Malignant; metastasis to bone, liver, lymph nodes, and skin (70% of cases at onset)

	Imaging findings	Demographics	Clinical associations	Comments
Paraganglioma (Fig. 8)	Paravertebral mass, hypointense or isointense to liver parenchyma on T1-weighted and markedly hyperintense on T2-weighted images; best appreciated with fat suppression. Intense early enhancement, which persists in the subsequent phases. Necrotic changes in up to 70%. 15% punctate calcification. Fluid-fluid level. Typically arise at the renal hila and near the inferior mesenteric artery origin (organ of Zuckerkandl)	40–60 y, with no sex predilection	Functional tumors are often associated with hypertension, tachycardia, headache, and diaphoresis because of high catecholamine levels. May be associated with von Hippel-Lindau syndrome, MEN type II, and NF-1	More aggressive than their adrenal counterpart. Malignant in up to 40% of cases on selected series
Schwannoma (Fig. 9)	Oval mass with low to intermediate T1 and high T2 signal intensity with slow but persistent postcontrast enhancement of solid components. Central enhancement in a targetlike fashion may be seen. Necrotic changes in only about 30% of cases. Frequently shows prominent cystic degeneration and calcification. Encapsulated. Compression of nerve to one side	Female predilection (2:1). 20–50 y. Accounts to 4%–5% of all retroperitoneal tumors	—	Benign; very low risk of malignant transformation

(continued on next page)

Table 5
(continued)

Neurogenic Tumors	MR Imaging Findings	Actuarial Data	Other Diagnosis Features	Biological Behavior
Neurofibroma	Well-circumscribed, round mass with low T1 and high T2 signal intensity; a central area of lower signal intensity may also be seen on T2-weighted images. Central enhancement in a targetlike fashion may be seen as homogeneous contrast enhancement. Occasionally, myxoid degeneration. Usually unencapsulated. Diffuse expansion of the entire nerve	Male predilection. 20–40 y (younger in NF-1). Accounts for 1% of retroperitoneal tumors	—	Degeneration to malignant peripheral nerve sheath tumor may be seen, more commonly in the setting of neurofibromatosis
Plexiform neurofibroma (Fig. 10)	Usually bilateral, mainly symmetric, elongated parapsoas masses with homogeneous low attenuation	—	Characteristic of NF-1	Up to 5% lifetime risk of malignant transformation
MNST	Aggressive sarcoma arising from a peripheral nerve (eg, sciatic nerve, brachial plexus, sacral plexus) or preexisting benign nerve sheath tumor (eg, neurofibroma). Include malignant schwannoma, neurogenic sarcoma, and neurofibrosarcoma. 50% of these tumors originate de novo, and the rest of them are derived from neurofibroma or ganglioneuroma or occur after exposure to radiation. Distant metastasis in 65% of cases. More common in the 20-year-old to 50-year-old group, with no sex predilection. In 25% to 50% of cases, these tumors are associated with NF-1			

Abbreviations: MEN, multiple endocrine neoplasia; MNST, malignant nerve sheath tumors; NF-1, type 1 neurofibromatosis.
Modified from Sangster GP, Migliaro M, Heldmann MG, et al. The gamut of primary retroperitoneal masses: multimodality evaluation with pathologic correlation. Abdom Radiol (NY) 2016;41:1411–30 with data compiled from Refs. [5,12,29–32]

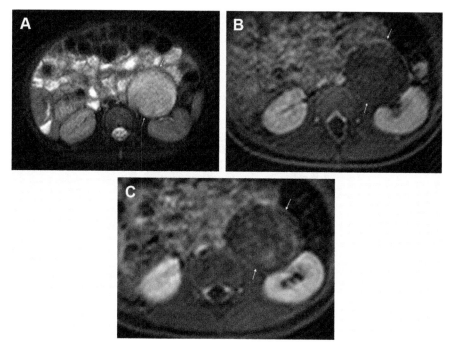

Fig. 5. Ganglioneuroma. Axial spectral attenuated inversion recovery (SPAIR) T2-weighted (*A*), intermediate (*B*), and late (*C*) postcontrast three-dimensional (3D) T1-weighted images show a round and well-defined paraverte-bral solid mass located in the left perirenal space (*arrows*), with high signal intensity on T2-weighted (*A*) and low signal on T1-weighted images, presenting slight initial enhancement with progressive delayed postcontrast enhancement at late phase (*B*, *C*).

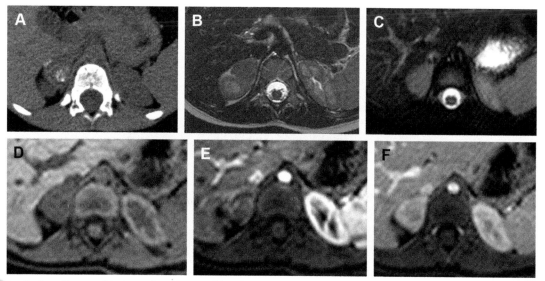

Fig. 6. Ganglioneuroblastoma in a 4-year-old girl. Precontrast CT scan (*A*) shows an oval soft tissue mass with granular calcifications located in the right suprarenal location. Axial turbo spin echo (TSE) T2-weighted MR (*B*), SPAIR fat-suppressed T2-weighted (*C*), precontrast (*D*), immediate postgadolinium (*E*), and interstitial-phase gadolinium-enhanced (*F*) fat-suppressed 3D SGE T1-weighted images show a slight high signal intensity of the mass on T2-weighted (*B*, *C*), low signal on T1-weighted (*D*), and progressive delayed enhancement (*E*, *F*) images.

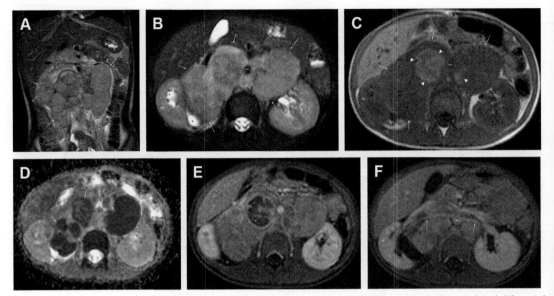

Fig. 7. Neuroblastoma in an 8-year-old girl. Coronal TSE T2-weighted (*A*), axial SPAIR T2-weighted (*B*), axial SGE T1-weighted (*C*), apparent diffusion coefficient (ADC) map (*D*), and interstitial-phase (*E, F*) postgadolinium 3D T1-weighted images show lobulated coalescent masses (*arrows*) with heterogeneous high signal intensity on T2-weighted and predominantly low signal intensity on T1-weighted images with spontaneous high signal intensity foci on T1-weighted imaging that may represent internal hemorrhage and/or necrosis (*C, arrowheads*). There is mass effect with compression of both kidneys, more accentuated in the right kidney (RK), which has hydronephrosis (*asterisks*). Accentuated restricted diffusion is seen on the ADC map (*D, arrows*). There is also encasement of the aorta (AO) with encasement and displacement of renal vessels (*F, arrows*).

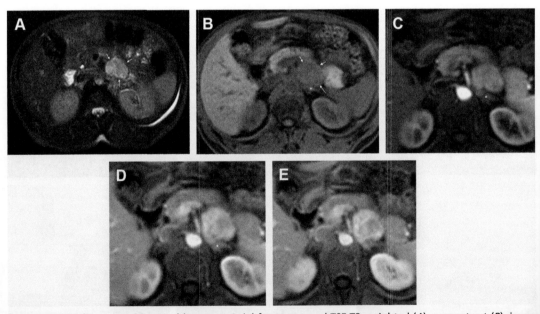

Fig. 8. Paraganglioma in a 66-year-old woman. Axial fat-suppressed TSE T2-weighted (*A*), precontrast (*B*), immediate (*C*), intermediate (*D*), and interstitial (*E*) postgadolinium fat-suppressed 3D SGE T1-weighted images show a left circumscribed lobulated retroperitoneal mass with heterogeneous high signal intensity on T2-weighted image (*A and B, arrows*), isointense to muscle on T1-weighted image, with intense immediate postcontrast enhancement (*C*) that persists in later postcontrast phases, although is possible to depict internal slight washout areas on interstitial phase (*E*). The mass is located anterior to the left adrenal, which can be depicted better on T1-weighted images (*B, C, and D, asterisks*).

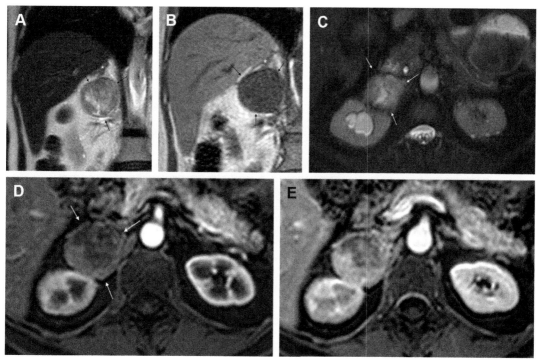

Fig. 9. Schwannoma in a 73-year-old woman. Coronal TSE T2-weighted (*A*), coronal SGE T1-weighted (*B*), axial SPAIR T2-weighted (*C*), immediate (*D*), and interstitial-phase (*E*) postgadolinium fat-suppressed 3D SGE T1 images show a round, circumscribed, solid mass (*arrows*), located in the right perirenal space, inferior to the ipsilateral adrenal (*A*, *B*, *asterisks*), with heterogeneous but predominantly high signal intensity on T2 weighting (*A*, *C*), homogeneous low signal intensity on T1 weighting, and with heterogeneous and progressive postgadolinium enhancement (*D*, *E*). A complete excision of the mass was performed with adrenalectomy, which showed that there was no involvement of the adrenal gland.

retroperitoneal cases are tumors composed of spindle-shaped and round histiocytes arranged in storiform pattern, or inflammatory subtypes.[20,34] They most frequently affect men at 50 to 60 years of age. They most commonly present as a large, well-defined soft tissue mass, with low to intermediate signal intensity on T1-weighted sequences and heterogeneous higher signal intensity on T2-weighted sequences compared with muscle (**Fig. 11**). Solid components, cystic degeneration, hemorrhage, myxoid stroma, and fibrous tissue may be present, which determine a heterogeneous enhancement and sometimes a so-called bowl-of-fruit sign.[20,34] Calcifications are described in up to 20% of cases.

Leiomyosarcoma

Leiomyosarcoma is a malignant neoplasm of mesenchymal origin that develops from the smooth muscle cells and it is the second most common retroperitoneal sarcoma in adults, accounting for 21.3% to 30% of cases.[20,21,33,35] It occurs most frequently related to major veins, mainly the inferior vena cava (IVC), and may develop as a mass completely external to the IVC lumen (62%), or with intraluminal and extraluminal components (33%), or as completely intraluminal (5%).[20,21,35] Overall, it occurs in the fifth to sixth decades and has a female predilection, with intravenous IVC tumors being overwhelmingly more frequent in middle-aged women (80%–90%).[20,21,35,36] Treatment options for leiomyosarcomas are surgical excision and chemotherapy, although only 25% of cases respond to chemotherapy.[33] Radiotherapy seems to have no role for treatment of leiomyosarcomas.[33] The craniocaudal and luminal localization of the mass related to the IVC dictate the signs and symptoms (such as Budd-Chiari syndrome, abdominal pain, renal insufficiency, lower extremity edema) directly affect the surgical resectability, middle-segment and lower-segment IVC tumors being more suitable for resection.

Most leiomyosarcomas are well-defined and heterogeneous masses because of internal hemorrhagic foci and necrosis, and rarely have a cystic appearance. Thus, MR imaging features are nonspecific and may vary according to these internal changes.[6] Nonetheless, the mass may

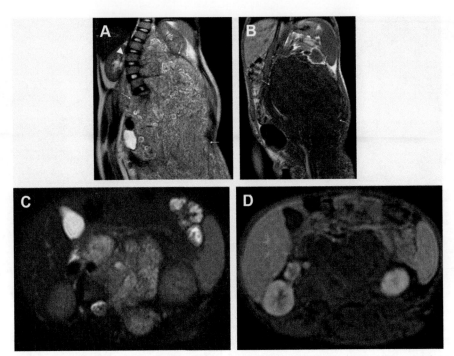

Fig. 10. Neurofibroma plexiforme. Coronal TSE T2-weighted (*A*) and SGE T1-weighted (*B*), axial fat-suppressed T2-weighted (*C*), and postgadolinium fat-suppressed 3D T1-weighted (*D*) images show an extensive left paravertebral mass with heterogeneous high signal intensity on T2-weighted images (*A, C*), low signal intensity on T1-weighted image (*B*), and very low postgadolinium enhancement (*D*) (*A, B, arrows*). The mass causes compression and displacement of adjacent structures. Lumbar scoliosis is appreciated (*A, arrowhead*).

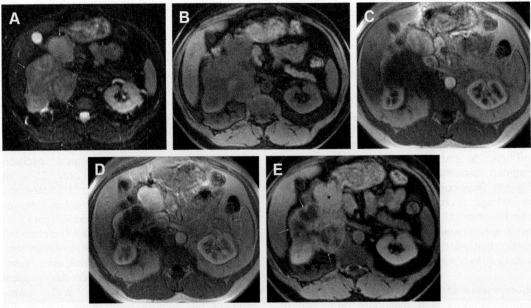

Fig. 11. Pleomorphic sarcoma with angiomatoid and inflammatory components. Axial fat-suppressed short-tau inversion recovery T2-weighted (*A*), fat-suppressed SGE 2D T1-weighted (*B*), immediate (*C*), and intermediate (*D*) postgadolinium SGE 2D T1-weighted, and interstitial postgadolinium fat-suppressed SGE 2D T1-weighted (*E*) images. Large lobulated right retroperitoneal mass, located superiorly to the right kidney (*A, arrows*) with heterogeneous high signal intensity on T2 weighting and isointense to low signal intensity on T1 weighting (*B*), and accentuated heterogeneous postgadolinium enhancement predominantly peripheric and centripetal (*E, arrows*), with solid areas presenting intense and persistent postgadolinium enhancement (*E, asterisks*). The mass invades the right kidney and shows partial encasement of inferior vena cava.

present low to intermediate signal intensity on T1-weighted sequence images, reported as isointense to muscle, and heterogeneous, with intermediate to high signal intensity on T2-weighted sequences (**Fig. 12**).[21,36,37] Usually these masses present heterogeneous restricted diffusion on high-b-value DWI images (see **Fig. 12**B, C). Postcontrast enhancement is also mostly heterogeneous, with predominance of hypervascular or hypovascular areas depending on internal changes, as well as the extent of muscular and fibrous components (see **Fig. 12**).[21,36,37] Collateral vessels are frequently depicted.[38] When small, it may be impossible to differentiate from bland thrombus, but an expansile nature, feeding arteries, and postcontrast enhancing foci are considered neoplastic characteristics differentiating the tumor from bland thrombus.[21,36,37]

Small Round Cell Lesions

Lymphomas

Lymphomas are the most common retroperitoneal masses. They may also spread to mesenteric lymph nodes and also may extend into perirenal space, following lymphatics vessels.[39]

Incidence of lymphoma varies according to histologic types, Hodgkin disease, and non-Hodgkin disease. Men show slight predominance and tend to be diagnosed at younger ages than women, with few exceptions.[39,40]

Imaging presentation is variable and, when the retroperitoneum is involved, the disease is usually advanced and is associated with poor prognosis.[39,41,42]

The diagnostic criteria for lymphadenopathy, which is the main imaging finding of lymphoma involvement, is based primarily on size and varies according to the different sites in the abdomen.[43] The short axis is the preferred parameter and the cutoff values are 10 mm for retroperitoneal perivascular nodes, 8 mm for mesenteric lymph nodes, and 8 to 9 mm for pelvic lymph nodes. However, size alone is an insensitive criterion and other parameters are usually taken into account when assessing potential lymphadenopathy.[43,44] Normal lymph nodes tend to preserve their elongated (ovoid) shape, whereas malignant ones are usually round. Normal or reactive lymph nodes also show preservation of internal architecture, with preserved fatty hilum and thin cortex that can easily be assessed by MR imaging.[45] Other sign of metastatic lymph nodes, with high specificity, is the irregular contour.[46] In addition, the presence of multiple lymph nodes with short axis in the upper limit of normality in a patient with previously diagnosed lymphoproliferative malignancy should be considered suspicious.[47]

The typical lymph nodes show an intermediate to slightly hyperintense signal on T1-weighted images and a discrete bright signal on T2-weighted images (**Fig. 13**).[43–45] The signal intensity of involved lymph nodes usually shows lower T1 signal and lower T2 signal. Necrosis and calcifications may occur in involved retroperitoneal lymph nodes, but it is not a common finding and usually occurs after treatment, radiation therapy, and/or chemotherapy.[43–46,48]

Compared with other locations, retroperitoneal lymphomatous lymph nodes tend to coalesce

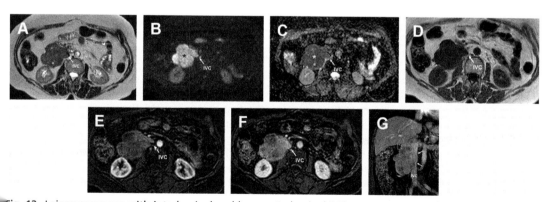

Fig. 12. Leiomyosarcoma with intraluminal and large extraluminal IVC components. Axial TSE T2-weighted (*A*), DWI (b = 1000) (*B*), ADC map (*C*), SGE T1-weighted (*D*), immediate (*E*), interstitial-phase axial (*F*), and coronal (*G*) postgadolinium fat-suppressed 3D T1-weighted images. Lobulated left retroperitoneal mass, located in the perirenal space, along and related to the IVC. The mass shows slight increased heterogeneous signal intensity with small, high-signal, scattered foci on T2 weighting (*A*) and accentuated restricted diffusion seen on DWI (*B*) and ADC map (*C*) (*asterisks*). As expected, the mass shows isointense to low signal intensity to muscle on T1 weighting (*D*) with heterogeneous postgadolinium enhancement. The small intraluminal IVC component is seen in all images (*arrows*).

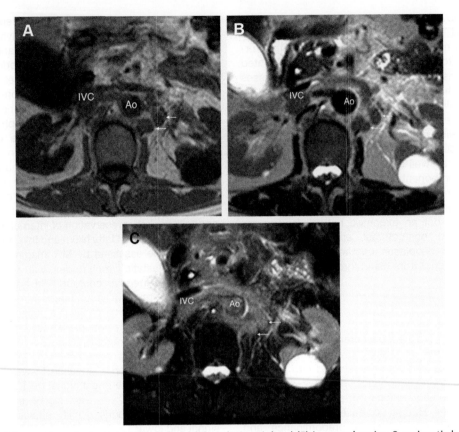

Fig. 13. Adenopathy criteria. Axial T1-weighted (*A*) and T2-weighted (*B*) images showing 2 periaortic lymph nodes (*arrows*). The more medial and posterior node is round, slightly enlarged, and there is no fat in the hilum. The more lateral and anterior node has a normal shape and size, but signal intensity is similar. Both have intermediate to low signal on T1, usually seen in lymphomatous nodes. Notice how difficult it is to define both nodes on T2 with fat suppression (*C*, *arrows*). T1 and T2 images without fat suppression techniques are preferable for lymph node detection.

and form confluent soft tissue masses (**Fig. 14**). Lymphomatous masses may also show very low signal on T2 images after treatment, which has been associated with the development of fibrosis.

Another pattern of growth is a mass involving the kidney and perirenal spaces, and retroperitoneal lymphomas can invade or encase the kidney and perinephric space. Primary lymphomas of the kidney are infiltrative masses and are seen as isolated mass lesions arising from the kidney.[40,49]

On histology, there is a predominance of non-Hodgkin lymphoma variants with most renal/perirenal lymphomas originating from B-cell precursors. Burkitt lymphoma should be considered when renal/perirenal involvement is seen in children.[50]

MR imaging appearance varies according to pathologic patterns, as described earlier.[43–45] A common finding to all forms is the low signal on T1 and T2 sequences, with the latter prompting

suspicion for lymphoproliferative disease. More undifferentiated and aggressive variants may show a more intermediate signal on T2 images (**Fig. 15**).

Although functional and hybrid imaging are beyond the scope of this article, it is important to state that 18F-fludeoxyglucose PET/CT is now the first option for initial staging of Hodgkin disease and non-Hodgkin lymphoma because of its high accuracy and also because it provides important prognostic information secondary to the detection of metabolic activity.[51] PET/CT has a central role in restaging, for monitoring therapy, and for recurrence detection.[51,52]

Recently, whole-body MR imaging using DWI has been assessed as a nonionizing imaging modality alternative to PET/CT for staging lymphoma. The technique relies on coronal T2-weighted images with fat suppression and DWI to show adenopathy and other areas of lymphomatous involvement (**Fig. 16**). Although the initial

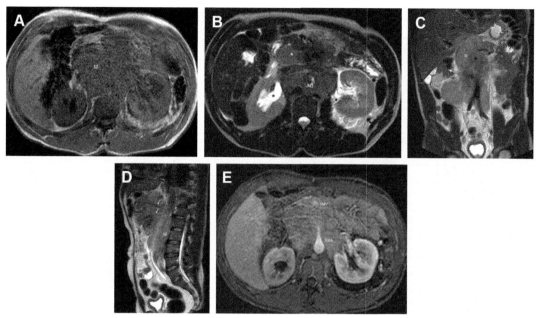

Fig. 14. Retroperitoneal and mesenteric coalescent lymphomatous mass. Axial T1-weighted image (*A*) showing a retroperitoneal and mesenteric mass (M) with intermediate signal. Axial (*B*), coronal (*C*), and sagittal (*D*) T2 images showing an extensive retroperitoneal mass, with an intermediate to high signal, displacing the aorta anteriorly and involving major aortic branches, celiac axis (*curved arrow* in D), and superior mesenteric artery (*straight arrow* in D). An isolated enlarged lymph node is seen (*asterisk* in B and *arrow* in C). Axial T1 postcontrast image (*E*) displays the superior mesenteric vein (SMV) displaced by the mass. A diffuse large B-cell lymphoma was confirmed at histology. SMA, superior mesenteric artery.

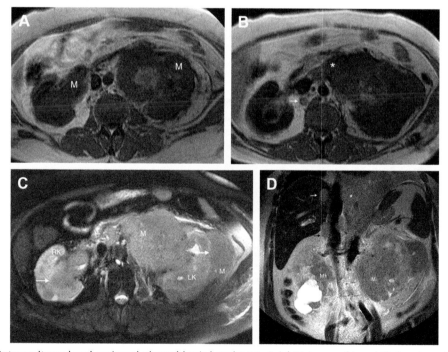

Fig. 15. Retroperitoneal and perirenal plasmablastic lymphoma. Axial T1 images (*A* and *B*) showing a heterogeneous mass (M), predominantly of low signal, with areas of high signal, in the left perirenal space, surrounding left kidney, with extension to midline (*asterisk* in B). Another mass (M) is seen in the right hilum, in (*A*). A round, enlarged, isolated lymph node is seen, adjacent to IVC in (*B*) (*arrow*). On axial (*C*) and coronal (*D*) T2 images, the lesion has intermediate signal. In (*C*), it is possible to depict the infiltrative pattern of the lesion with indistinct margins with both kidneys (*arrows*, C). In (*D*), a contiguous mass (*asterisk*) is seen extending cranially. Liver involvement (*white arrow*) and involved isolated lymph nodes (*black arrow*) are seen.

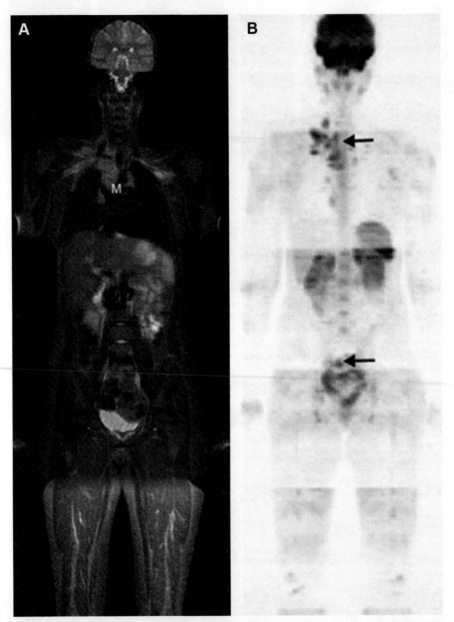

Fig. 16. Whole-body MR imaging lymphoma. Coronal T2-weighted image with fat suppression (*A*) showing a mass of coalescent lymph nodes (M) in this patient with non-Hodgkin, B-cell lymphoma. DWI (*B*) in coronal plane (shown in *black-white inversion*) of the same patient, in a slightly different plane, showing lymph nodes in the mediastinum and retroperitoneum (*arrows in B*). (*Courtesy of* Rubens Choniajk, MD, AC Camargo Cancer Center, Sao Paulo, Brazil.)

results are promising, the technique requires state-of-art scanners and coils, but results are encouraging.[53–55]

Peripheral primitive neuroectodermal tumors

Peripheral primitive neuroectodermal tumors (pPNETs) are tumors composed of primitive undifferentiated small round cells originating from the neuroectoderm and derived from tissues outside the central and autonomic nervous system.[56] These tumors are related to the Ewing sarcoma because most of them present the same chromosomal translocation (t(11;22) (q24;q12)).[57] pPNETs are rare but can occur in unusual locations, including the peritoneum cavity and retroperitoneum in approximately 14% of cases.[56,58]

Treatment alternatives for pPNET comprise surgical excision of the mass, with or without radiotherapy and neoadjuvant or adjuvant chemotherapy. Imaging evaluation plays an important role to support the therapeutic plan.

Most retroperitoneal primitive neuroectodermal tumors (PNETs) present as a solitary solid mass, and rarely may presents as a mixed solid cystic mass, but necrosis occurs in more than 70% of cases.[56,59] It can be located anywhere in the retroperitoneum, ranging from 3 cm to more than 10 cm, although tumors as larger as 30 cm have been reported.[59] Half of the cases reported by Yi and colleagues,[56] in 2014, presented well-defined margins.

Usually, pPNETs are heterogeneous on CT and MR imaging, and show heterogeneous enhancement. Less frequently they show arterial encasement and venous invasion, as well as organ invasion and calcification. Larger tumors present heterogeneous signal intensity on T1-weighted and T2-weighted sequences, mainly because of necrotic foci and less frequently because of cystic components. Solid portions of the tumor show enhancement, with no enhancement of necrotic foci, which can be seen as a ringlike enhancement pattern in some cases.[56,59]

Infiltrative Perivascular Lesions

Xanthogranulomatosis or Erdheim-Chester disease

Erdheim-Chester disease (ECD) is a rare systemic-type non-Langerhans cell histiocytosis,[60] in which the deposition of lipids in non-Langerhans cell histiocytes is seen (xanthogranulomatosis).[61] The bones, lungs, and retroperitoneum are the most commonly involved sites.[61,62] The bony involvement is characterized by medullary infarcts, periostitis and osteosclerosis. The most common presentation in the retroperitoneum is the presence of soft tissue masses around the kidneys, occurring in 67% of patients, which could be associated with hydronephrosis in 38% of patients.[62,63] Periaortic involvement is seen in about 40% (usually sparing the IVC), and adrenal gland infiltration is seen in 50% of patients. The diagnosis is made by clinical and radiological findings, which prompt histologic sampling for confirmation.[63,64]

At MR images, the typical ECD infiltration shows discrete hypointense signal on T1 and T2, with homogeneous enhancement after gadolinium-based contrast media (**Fig. 17**).[30,64]

Idiopathic retroperitoneal fibrosis

Idiopathic retroperitoneal fibrosis (IRF) is defined by the presence of chronic inflammatory and fibrotic processes in the retroperitoneum. In about 30% of cases, it is associated with secondary causes, such as infection, malignancy, and/or drug exposure.[65] When no cause can be found, the condition is called idiopathic, and it is also known as Ormond disease, referring to its first description in 1948.[66] The fibrotic changes ultimately lead to compression of vessels and ureters. IRF has been reported more often in men (2:1), after the fifth decade of life.[65]

However, the idiopathic form has recently been associated with immunoglobulin (Ig) G4–related

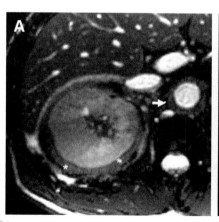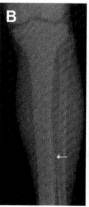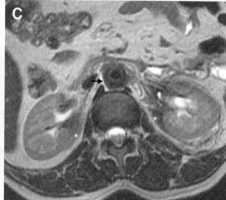

Fig. 17. ECD. Axial steady state free precision image (*A*) showing a right perirenal soft tissue with intermediate signal (*asterisks*). A similar finding is seen involving aorta (*arrow*). Calf radiograph (*B*) shows sclerotic changes in the proximal tibia. A continuous periosteal reaction is seen laterally, in midthird of tibia (*arrow*). Axial T2 image (*C*) from another patient. A soft tissue mass is seen involving both kidneys (*asterisks*). There is thick periaortic tissue (*arrow*) associated with thickening of aortic wall. Of note, there is no anterior displacement of aorta, a sign useful for excluding lymphomas. Also, there is no IVC involvement, a distinguishing feature from idiopathic retroperitoneal fibrosis (IRF). (*Courtesy of* Antonio Westphalen, MD, University of California at San Francisco, San Francisco, CA).

disease.[67] On histology, the features of IgG4-related disease are lymphoplasmacytic infiltrate, storiform fibrosis, and tissue eosinophilia, and these have also been described for most of patients with IRF.[68]

The secondary forms have been related to some specific drugs, such as ergot alkaloid derivatives (eg, ergotamine, methysergide) and L-dopa–derived agents (eg, methyldopa). The latter association has led to an increasing number of patients with Parkinson disease and IRF development.[69] IRF secondary to malignancy is thought to be derived from metastatic foci eliciting an inflammatory response, and a desmoplastic reaction, also leading to fibrotic changes.[70] The most common malignancy associated with IRF is lymphoma, but other primary sites can be involved, such as breast, colorectum, and kidney.

The classic imaging presentation of IRF is a mass surrounding the aorta and IVC at L4 to L5 level, or just above aortic bifurcation, with homogeneous low signal on T1-weighted images.[71] At T2-weighted images, signal is variable, reflecting the phase and degree of inflammation, but it is often homogeneous (**Fig. 18**). Early phase (immature) shows high T2 signal, whereas a low T2 signal is seen on the later mature phase. The degree of enhancement decreases from mature to immature phases but usually it is homogeneous.[70,71] Malignant IRF tend to show heterogeneous signal on T1 and T2, with variable enhancement. IgG4-related IRF is indistinguishable from other forms of retroperitoneal fibrosis in terms of isolated retroperitoneal imaging findings.[72]

Several conditions may show similar appearance to IRF and are important in the differential. ECD can be differentiated based on lack of IVC involvement, which is often seen on IRF.[30,73] Malignancy-related IRF, especially those associated with lymphoma, can be distinguished because the latter usually shows larger masses,

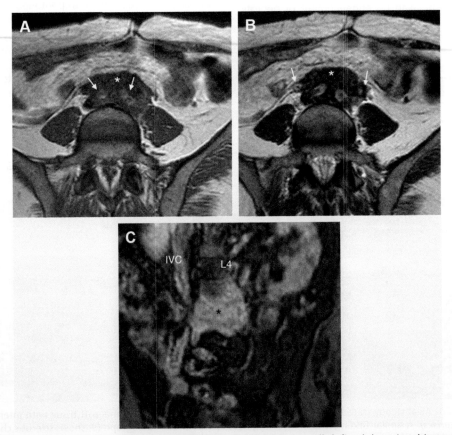

Fig. 18. Retroperitoneal fibrosis. Axial T1-weighted image (*A*) shows a well-defined, low-signal-intensity lesion (*asterisk*) surrounding common iliac arteries (*arrows*). Axial T2 image (*B*) showing the same lesion (*asterisk*) with marked hypointense signal. Two high-signal, circular structures are seen at periphery of the mass corresponding with dilated ureters (*arrows*). The right ureter shows a low-signal central dot that represents a pigtail catheter. Coronal T1 postcontrast image (*C*) shows the intense and homogeneous signal of the lesion. The location of IRF is typical, extending from L4 vertebral body to S1 (*asterisk*).

perirenal extension, anterior aortic displacement and signal heterogeneity.[73]

Rosai-Dorfman disease

A specific form of sinus histiocytosis associated to extensive lymphadenopathy was first reported in 1969 and is named Rosai-Dorfman disease (RDD) following its first description.[74] RDD is non-neoplastic histiocytic disorder typically with massive lymphadenopathy caused by infiltration of sinuses of the lymph node by large histiocytes, with a clear predominance in the cervical area.[75] Children and adolescents are the group with the highest incidence. There is a slight male predominance. Typical presentation includes fever, cervical lymphadenopathy, leukocytosis, increased erythrocyte sedimentation rate, and hypergammaglobulinemia.[75–77]

Extranodal disease is also frequent (40%), especially in skin and bones, but abdominal manifestations are not common (4% of patients with RDD), occurring later in the course of disease.[76,77]

Kidneys are the most common organ affected by RDD and are involved in half of patients with abdominal manifestations. The common finding is a renal sinus mass extending to perirenal space (**Fig. 19**), with a subcapsular spread. These lesions usually show as hypointense on T1-weighted images and low to intermediate signal on T2-weighted images with associated postgadolinium scarce enhancement.[78] Rarely, a disseminated mass infiltrates renal parenchyma, leading to acute renal failure.[79]

Cystic or Necrotic Lesions

Paragangliomas may have cystic foci and this is discussed earlier with regard to neurogenic tumors.

Lymphangioma

Retroperitoneal lymphangiomas represent malformations, presumed linked to failure of communication between retroperitoneal lymphatic vessels and lymphatic trunks of the abdomen.[80] There is

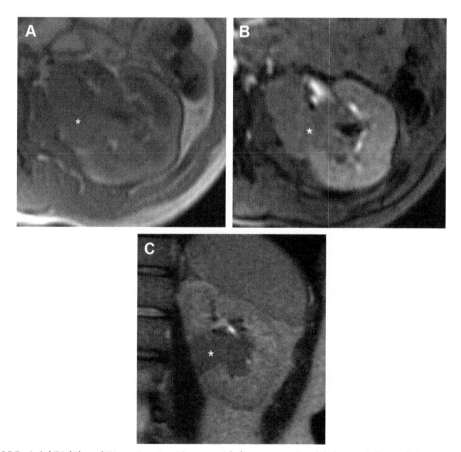

Fig. 19. RDD. Axial T1 (*A*) and T1 postcontrast image with fat suppression (*B*) show a left renal sinus mass extending to perirenal space with discrete low signal on T1 and poor enhancement (*asterisks*). Coronal T2-weighted image (*C*) showing the low-signal, homogeneous sinus mass protruding outside the renal pelvis to perirenal space (*asterisk*). (*Courtesy of* Antonio Westphalen, MD, University of California at San Francisco, San Francisco, CA.)

no age predominance, occurring at any age, but a male predominance is described. At histology, 3 types are described (capillary, cystic, and cavernous), but the capillary type has not been reported in retroperitoneum.[81]

Retroperitoneal lymphangiomas are rare and account for only 1% of all lymphangiomas. Perirenal spaces are the most common location, either surrounding kidney or adjacent to adrenals. At MR imaging, they often present as single loculated simple cysts, with homogeneous signal on T1-weighted and T2-weighted images.[81,82] However, septa may be present and usually are thin. Lymphangiomas may have a chylous content and, in these cases, they may show a typical high signal on T1 images.[81–83]

Other (Uncommon) Perirenal Conditions

Extramedullary hematopoiesis is rare condition in the retroperitoneum, because liver and spleen are the preferred locations in the abdomen.[84] However, when occurring in retroperitoneum, perirenal spaces are the most common location.[84,85] A perirenal well-defined mass with products of hemoglobin degradation is usually seen with associated high signal on T1-weighted and low signal on T2-weighted images.[85]

Table 6
Summary of characteristics of the Castleman disease subtypes

	Unicentric	HHV-8 Association	Idiopathic
Age	Fourth decade	Sixth decade	—
Symptoms	Mostly asymptomatic, incidental, or compressive symptoms	Constitutional flulike symptoms, POEMS syndrome	Constitutional flulike symptoms, fluid accumulation (edema, anasarca, ascites, pleural effusion), renal dysfunction, and/or proteinuria
Organomegaly	Rare	—	Large liver and/or spleen
Distribution of lymphadenopathy	Central (mediastinal, abdominal) most common	Peripheral + central	Peripheral + central
Diagnosis	Histologic examination of an excised lymph node	Histologic examination of an excised lymph node	Must meet both major criteria (characteristic lymph node histopathology and multicentric lymphadenopathy) and at least 2 of the 11 minor criteria[85,a]
Therapy	Surgical removal of the enlarged lymph node is usually curative	Treatment with rituximab is highly effective	Treatment with siltuximab effective in 34% of cases, various other therapeutic drugs have been used
Progression to lymphoma	Rare	Increased risk of Kaposi sarcoma, non-Hodgkin lymphoma, and Hodgkin lymphoma	Increased risk of non-Hodgkin lymphoma, Hodgkin lymphoma, and POEMS syndrome
Clinical course	Benign	Good prognosis when treated with rituximab, with >90% 5-y overall survival	Usually aggressive

Abbreviations: CRP, C-reactive protein; ESR, erythrocyte sedimentation rate; POEMS, polyneuropathy, organomegaly, endocrinopathy, monoclonal gammopathy, and skin changes.

[a] The minor diagnostic criteria comprise constitutional symptoms; hepatosplenomegaly; anasarca, edema, or effusions; eruptive cherry hemangiomatosis or violaceous papules, lymphocytic interstitial pneumonitis; increased CRP and/or ESR level, anemia; thrombocytopenia or thrombocytosis, hypoalbuminemia; renal dysfunction; polyclonal hypergammaglobulinemia.

Modified from Konen O, Rathaus V, Dlugy E, et al. Childhood abdominal cystic lymphangioma. Pediatr Radiol 2002;32:88–94.

Perirenal myelolipomas are rare lesions that may occur outside of adrenals in perirenal spaces.[86] They usually are single lesions but may be bilateral and diffuse. At MR imaging, they often appear as circumscribed masses with heterogeneous signal, caused by the presence of macroscopic fat and erythropoietic tissue showing corresponding MR signal on T1-weighted and T2-weighted images, or low T1 signal with intermediate T2 signal.[86] The differentiation from liposarcoma is a diagnostic dilemma and usually requires histopathologic confirmation.

Miscellanea

Castleman disease
The main finding of Castleman disease (CD) is an enlarged lymph node or nodes caused by hyperplasia, as first described in the 1950s.[87] The pathogenesis is unknown, but there is evidence of a disruptive immune regulation with B-lymphocyte excess and plasma-cell proliferation in lymphatic tissue.[88] Three pathologic variants of CD have been described: (1) hyaline-vascular variant, which is the most frequent and is composed of atrophic germinal centers, follicular dendritic cells prominence, small hyaline-vascular follicles, and capillary proliferation; (2) the plasma-cell variant, in which hyperplastic germinal centers with large lymphoid follicles are separated by sheets of plasma cells; and (3) mixed, with lymph nodes presenting features of both the hyaline-vascular and plasma-cell variants.[88,89] More recently, CD has been classified into unicentric or multicentric types. The multicentric CD has been associated with human herpesvirus 8 (HHV-8), although it could also be idiopathic.[90] A summary of the subtypes' characteristics is presented in **Table 6**. Although CD can occur anywhere along the lymphatic chain, the mediastinum is most

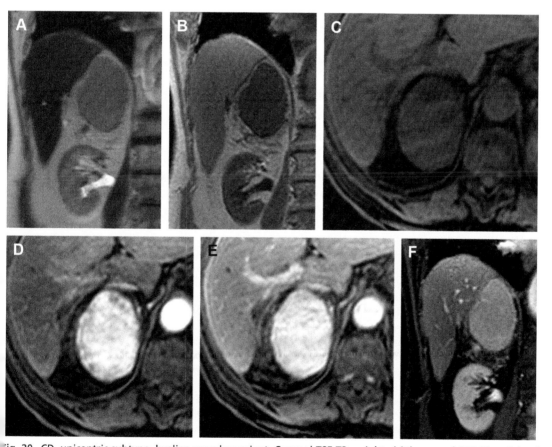

Fig. 20. CD, unicentric subtype, hyaline-vascular variant. Coronal TSE T2-weighted (*A*), coronal SGE T1-weighted (*B*), axial precontrast (*C*), immediate (*D*), intermediate (*E*), and coronal delayed (*F*) postgadolinium fat-suppressed 3D T1-weighted images. Oval, circumscribed, solid mass, located at right retroperitoneal space, superiorly to the right kidney with slight increase signal intensity to muscle on T2 weighting and low signal intensity on T1 weighting. There is an accentuated immediate postgadolinium enhancement, which persists through subsequent postcontrast phases. There was no involvement of the adjacent adrenal gland.

frequently affected (70%), whereas a retroperitoneal location is rarer, accounting for less than 10% of cases. There are more reported retroperitoneal cases in unicentric CD because of its higher incidence; however, multicentric CD has more abdominal/retroperitoneal involvement.[91]

The description of imaging characteristics of CD has been limited to case reports, review articles, and smaller retrospective reviews.[91] MR imaging features of CD show that the enlarged lymph nodes or masses are homogeneously hypointense to isointense to muscle on T1-weighted images; mostly hyperintense to muscle on T2-weighted images; in a few cases, isointense; and show homogeneous enhancement.[91] The presence of a more intense postcontrast enhancement seems to be associated most frequently with the hyalinevascular variant (Fig. 20).[91,92] Intralesional flow voids may be seen on T1-weighted and T2-weighted images, reflecting the vascularity of the lesion.[92] Rarely, it mimics a paraspinal neurogenic tumor.[93] Once CD is confirmed, whole-body imaging is indicated to identify unicentric or multicentric involvement.[92,94]

SUMMARY

Retroperitoneal diseases are frequently a great clinical challenge because of nonspecific presentation. Diseases may be asymptomatic with indolent biological behavior, and often show a large mass at initial imaging evaluation. MR imaging is a powerful diagnostic technique for assessment of detailed disease location and for characterization of tissue components and vascularization of lesions, which is critical for diagnostic assessment and treatment decisions, including surgical planning.

REFERENCES

1. Glockner JF, Lee CU. Magnetic resonance imaging of perirenal pathology. Can Assoc Radiol J 2016; 67:149–57.
2. Scali EP, Chandler TM, Heffernan EJ, et al. Primary retroperitoneal masses: what is the differential diagnosis? Abdom Imaging 2015;40:1887–903.
3. Noone TC, Semelka RC, Chaney DM, et al. Abdominal imaging studies: comparison of diagnostic accuracies resulting from ultrasound, computed tomography, and magnetic resonance imaging in the same individual. Magn Reson Imaging 2004; 22:19–24.
4. Servaes S, Khanna G, Naranjo A, et al. Comparison of diagnostic performance of CT and MRI for abdominal staging of pediatric renal tumors: a report from the Children's Oncology Group. Pediatr Radiol 2015;45:166–72.
5. Goenka AH, Shah SN, Remer EM. Imaging of the retroperitoneum. Radiol Clin North Am 2012;50: 333–55, vii.
6. Coffin A, Boulay-Coletta I, Sebbag-Sfez D, et al. Radioanatomy of the retroperitoneal space. Diagn Interv Imaging 2015;96:171–86.
7. Molmenti EP, Balfe DM, Kanterman RY, et al. Anatomy of the retroperitoneum: observations of the distribution of pathologic fluid collections. Radiology 1996;200:95–103.
8. AlObaidy M, Altun E, Semelka RC. Retroperitoneum and body wall. In: Semelka RC, Brown M, Altun E, editors. Abdominal-pelvic MRI. 4th edition. Hoboken (NJ): Wiley-Blackwell; 2015. p. 1005–95.
9. Mohd Zaki F, Moineddin R, Grant R, et al. Accuracy of pre-contrast imaging in abdominal magnetic resonance imaging of pediatric oncology patients. Pediatr Radiol 2016;46:1684–93.
10. Low RN, Gurney J. Diffusion-weighted MRI (DWI) in the oncology patient: value of breathhold DWI compared to unenhanced and gadolinium-enhanced MRI. J Magn Reson Imaging 2007;25: 848–58.
11. Mosavi F, Laurell A, Ahlstrom H. Whole body MRI, including diffusion-weighted imaging in follow-up of patients with testicular cancer. Acta Oncol 2015; 54:1763–9.
12. Nishino M, Hayakawa K, Minami M, et al. Primary retroperitoneal neoplasms: CT and MR imaging findings with anatomic and pathologic diagnostic clues. Radiographics 2003;23:45–57.
13. American Cancer Society. Cancer facts & figures 2017. Atlanta (GA): American Cancer Society; 2017.
14. Francis IR, Cohan RH, Varma DG, et al. Retroperitoneal sarcomas. Cancer Imaging 2005;5:89–94.
15. Elsayes KM, Staveteig PT, Narra VR, et al. Retroperitoneal masses: magnetic resonance imaging findings with pathologic correlation. Curr Probl Diagn Radiol 2007;36:97–106.
16. Craig WD, Fanburg-Smith JC, Henry LR, et al. Fat-containing lesions of the retroperitoneum: radiologic-pathologic correlation. Radiographics 2009;29:261–90.
17. Shaaban AM, Rezvani M, Tubay M, et al. Fat-containing retroperitoneal lesions: imaging characteristics, localization, and differential diagnosis. Radiographics 2016;36:710–34.
18. Heyns CF. Pelvic lipomatosis: a review of its diagnosis and management. J Urol 1991;146:267–73.
19. Chang IY, Herts BR. Retroperitoneal liposarcoma. J Urol 2013;189:1093–4.
20. Shiraev T, Pasricha SS, Choong P, et al. Retroperitoneal sarcomas: a review of disease spectrum, radiological features, characterisation and management. J Med Imaging Radiat Oncol 2013;57:687–700.
21. Messiou C, Moskovic E, Vanel D, et al. Primary retroperitoneal soft tissue sarcoma: Imaging

appearances, pitfalls and diagnostic algorithm. Eur J Surg Oncol 2017;43:1191–8.

22. Skubitz KM, Cheng EY, Clohisy DR, et al. Differential gene expression in liposarcoma, lipoma, and adipose tissue. Cancer Invest 2005;23:105–18.

23. Baldini EH. The conundrum of retroperitoneal liposarcoma–to be more aggressive or less aggressive? Int J Radiat Oncol Biol Phys 2017;98:269–70.

24. Fritchie KJ. Diagnostically challenging "fatty" retroperitoneal tumors. Surg Pathol Clin 2015;8:375–97.

25. Furlong MA, Fanburg-Smith JC, Miettinen M. The morphologic spectrum of hibernoma: a clinicopathologic study of 170 cases. Am J Surg Pathol 2001;25:809–14.

26. Colville J, Feigin K, Antonescu CR, et al. Hibernoma: report emphasizing large intratumoral vessels and high T1 signal. Skeletal Radiol 2006;35:547–50.

27. Shen Y, Zhong Y, Wang H, et al. MR imaging features of benign retroperitoneal paragangliomas and schwannomas. BMC Neurol 2018;18:1.

28. Sangster GP, Migliaro M, Heldmann MG, et al. The gamut of primary retroperitoneal masses: multimodality evaluation with pathologic correlation. Abdom Radiol (NY) 2016;41:1411–30.

29. Brennan C, Kajal D, Khalili K, et al. Solid malignant retroperitoneal masses–a pictorial review. Insights Imaging 2014;5:53–65.

30. Rajiah P, Sinha R, Cuevas C, et al. Imaging of uncommon retroperitoneal masses. Radiographics 2011;31:949–76.

31. Lonergan GJ, Schwab CM, Suarez ES, et al. Neuroblastoma, ganglioneuroblastoma, and ganglioneuroma: radiologic-pathologic correlation. Radiographics 2002;22:911–34.

32. Tu A, Ma R, Maguire J, et al. MPNST after radiosurgery: a report and review of the literature. Can J Neurol Sci 2014;41:74–81.

33. Pham V, Henderson-Jackson E, Doepker MP, et al. Practical issues for retroperitoneal sarcoma. Cancer Control 2016;23:249–64.

34. Hsiao PJ, Chen GH, Chang YH, et al. An unresectable retroperitoneal malignant fibrous histiocytoma: a case report. Oncol Lett 2016;11:2403–7.

35. Hartman DS, Hayes WS, Choyke PL, et al. From the archives of the AFIP. Leiomyosarcoma of the retroperitoneum and inferior vena cava: radiologic-pathologic correlation. Radiographics 1992;12:1203–20.

36. Cyran KM, Kenney PJ. Leiomyosarcoma of abdominal veins: value of MRI with gadolinium DTPA. Abdom Imaging 1994;19:335–8.

37. Bretan PN Jr, Williams RD, Hricak H. Preoperative assessment of retroperitoneal pathology by magnetic resonance imaging. Primary leiomyosarcoma of inferior vena cava. Urology 1986;28:251–5.

38. Huang J, Liu Q, Lu JP, et al. Primary intraluminal leiomyosarcoma of the inferior vena cava: value of MRI

with contrast-enhanced MR venography in diagnosis and treatment. Abdom Imaging 2011;36:337–41.

39. Roman E, Smith AG. Epidemiology of lymphomas. Histopathology 2011;58:4–14.

40. Swerdlow SH, Campo E, Pileri SA, et al. The 2016 revision of the World Health Organization classification of lymphoid neoplasms. Blood 2016;127:2375–90.

41. Hedgire SS, Kudrimoti S, Oliveira IS, et al. Extranodal lymphomas of abdomen and pelvis: imaging findings and differential diagnosis. Abdom Radiol (NY) 2017;42:1096–112.

42. Kulkarni NM, Pinho DF, Narayanan S, et al. Imaging for oncologic response assessment in lymphoma. AJR Am J Roentgenol 2017;208:18–31.

43. Dorfman RE, Alpern MB, Gross BH, et al. Upper abdominal lymph nodes: criteria for normal size determined with CT. Radiology 1991;180:319–22.

44. Ramirez M, Ingrand P, Richer JP, et al. What is the pelvic lymph node normal size? Determination from normal MRI examinations. Surg Radiol Anat 2016;38:425–31.

45. Grubnic S, Vinnicombe SJ, Norman AR, et al. MR evaluation of normal retroperitoneal and pelvic lymph nodes. Clin Radiol 2002;57:193–200 [discussion: 201–4].

46. Brown G, Richards CJ, Bourne MW, et al. Morphologic predictors of lymph node status in rectal cancer with use of high-spatial-resolution MR imaging with histopathologic comparison. Radiology 2003;227:371–7.

47. Ganeshalingam S, Koh DM. Nodal staging. Cancer Imaging 2009;9:104–11.

48. Fajardo L, Ramin GA, Penachim TJ, et al. Abdominal manifestations of extranodal lymphoma: pictorial essay. Radiol Bras 2016;49:397–402.

49. Foley RW, Aworanti OM, Gorman L, et al. Unusual childhood presentations of abdominal non-Hodgkin's lymphoma. Pediatr Int 2016;58:304–7.

50. Schmitz R, Young RM, Ceribelli M, et al. Burkitt lymphoma pathogenesis and therapeutic targets from structural and functional genomics. Nature 2012;490:116–20.

51. Wu LM, Chen FY, Jiang XX, et al. 18F-FDG PET, combined FDG-PET/CT and MRI for evaluation of bone marrow infiltration in staging of lymphoma: a systematic review and meta-analysis. Eur J Radiol 2012;81:303–11.

52. Cronin CG, Swords R, Truong MT, et al. Clinical utility of PET/CT in lymphoma. AJR Am J Roentgenol 2010;194:W91–103.

53. Gu J, Chan T, Zhang J, et al. Whole-body diffusion-weighted imaging: the added value to whole-body MRI at initial diagnosis of lymphoma. AJR Am J Roentgenol 2011;197:W384–91.

54. Koh DM, Blackledge M, Padhani AR, et al. Whole-body diffusion-weighted MRI: tips, tricks, and pitfalls. AJR Am J Roentgenol 2012;199: 252–62.

55. Littooij AS, Kwee TC, de Keizer B, et al. Whole-body MRI-DWI for assessment of residual disease after completion of therapy in lymphoma: a prospective multicenter study. J Magn Reson Imaging 2015;42: 1646–55.

56. Yi X, Liu W, Zhang Y, et al. Radiological features of primitive neuroectodermal tumors in intra-abdominal and retroperitoneal regions: a series of 18 cases. PLoS One 2017;12:e0173536.

57. de Alava E, Gerald WL. Molecular biology of the Ewing's sarcoma/primitive neuroectodermal tumor family. J Clin Oncol 2000;18:204–13.

58. Khong PL, Chan GC, Shek TW, et al. Imaging of peripheral PNET: common and uncommon locations. Clin Radiol 2002;57:272–7.

59. Kim MS, Kim B, Park CS, et al. Radiologic findings of peripheral primitive neuroectodermal tumor arising in the retroperitoneum. AJR Am J Roentgenol 2006;186:1125–32.

60. Gottlieb R, Chen A. MR findings of Erdheim-Chester disease. J Comput Assist Tomogr 2002;26:257–61.

61. Ozkaya N, Rosenblum MK, Durham BH, et al. The histopathology of Erdheim-Chester disease: a comprehensive review of a molecularly characterized cohort. Mod Pathol 2018;31:581–97.

62. Campochiaro C, Tomelleri A, Cavalli G, et al. Erdheim-Chester disease. Eur J Intern Med 2015;26: 223–9.

63. Veyssier-Belot C, Cacoub P, Caparros-Lefebvre D, et al. Erdheim-Chester disease. Clinical and radiologic characteristics of 59 cases. Medicine (Baltimore) 1996;75:157–69.

64. Nikpanah M, Kim L, Mirmomen SM, et al. Abdominal involvement in Erdheim-Chester disease (ECD): MRI and CT imaging findings and their association with BRAF(V600E) mutation. Eur Radiol 2018;28(9): 3751–9.

65. Heckmann M, Uder M, Kuefner MA, et al. Ormond's disease or secondary retroperitoneal fibrosis? An overview of retroperitoneal fibrosis. Rofo 2009;181: 317–23.

66. Ormond JK. Bilateral ureteral obstruction due to envelopment and compression by an inflammatory retroperitoneal process. J Urol 1948;59:1072–9.

67. Yildiz H. Retroperitoneal fibrosis and immunoglobulin G4. Am J Med 2018;131:e177.

68. Koo BS, Koh YW, Hong S, et al. Clinicopathologic characteristics of IgG4-related retroperitoneal fibrosis among patients initially diagnosed as having idiopathic retroperitoneal fibrosis. Mod Rheumatol 2015;25:194–8.

69. Sanchez-Chapado M, Angulo Cuesta J, Guil Cid M, et al. Retroperitoneal fibrosis secondary to treatment with L-dopa analogues for Parkinson disease. Arch Esp Urol 1995;48:979–83 [in Spanish].

70. Caiafa RO, Vinuesa AS, Izquierdo RS, et al. Retroperitoneal fibrosis: role of imaging in diagnosis and follow-up. Radiographics 2013;33:535–52.

71. Cohan RH, Shampain KL, Francis IR, et al. Imaging appearance of fibrosing diseases of the retroperitoneum: can a definitive diagnosis be made? Abdom Radiol (NY) 2018;43:1204–14.

72. Forestier A, Buob D, Mirault T, et al. No specific imaging pattern can help differentiate IgG4-related disease from idiopathic retroperitoneal fibrosis: 18 histologically proven cases. Clin Exp Rheumatol 2018;36:371–5.

73. Rosenkrantz AB, Spieler B, Seuss CR, et al. Utility of MRI features for differentiation of retroperitoneal fibrosis and lymphoma. AJR Am J Roentgenol 2012;199:118–26.

74. Rosai J, Dorfman RF. Sinus histiocytosis with massive lymphadenopathy. A newly recognized benign clinicopathological entity. Arch Pathol 1969; 87:63–70.

75. Abla O, Jacobsen E, Picarsic J, et al. Consensus recommendations for the diagnosis and clinical management of Rosai-Dorfman-Destombes disease. Blood 2018;131(26):2877–90.

76. Gumeler E, Onur MR, Karaosmanoglu AD, et al. Computed tomography and magnetic resonance imaging of peripelvic and periureteric pathologies. Abdom Radiol (NY) 2018;43(9):2400–11.

77. Xu Q, Fu L, Liu C. Multimodality imaging-based evaluation of Rosai-Dorfman disease in the head and neck: a retrospective observational study. Medicine (Baltimore) 2017;96:e9372.

78. Mar WA, Yu JH, Knuttinen MG, et al. Rosai-Dorfman disease: manifestations outside of the head and neck. AJR Am J Roentgenol 2017;208:721–32.

79. Lai FM, To KF, Szeto CC, et al. Acute renal failure in a patient with Rosai-Dorfman disease. Am J Kidney Dis 1999;34:e12.

80. Makni A, Chebbi F, Fetirich F, et al. Surgical management of intra-abdominal cystic lymphangioma. Report of 20 cases. World J Surg 2012;36:1037–43.

81. Shanbhogue AK, Fasih N, Macdonald DB, et al. Uncommon primary pelvic retroperitoneal masses in adults: a pattern-based imaging approach. Radiographics 2012;32:795–817.

82. Ferrero L, Guana R, Carbonaro G, et al. Cystic intra-abdominal masses in children. Pediatr Rep 2017;9: 7284.

83. Konen O, Rathaus V, Dlugy E, et al. Childhood abdominal cystic lymphangioma. Pediatr Radiol 2002;32:88–94.

84. Georgiades CS, Neyman EG, Francis IR, et al. Typical and atypical presentations of extramedullary hemopoiesis. AJR Am J Roentgenol 2002;179: 1239–43.

85. Roberts AS, Shetty AS, Mellnick VM, et al. Extramedullary haematopoiesis: radiological imaging features. Clin Radiol 2016;71:807–14.

86. Temizoz O, Genchellac H, Demir MK, et al. Bilateral extra-adrenal perirenal myelolipomas: CT features. Br J Radiol 2010;83:e198–9.

87. Castleman B, Iverson L, Menendez VP. Localized mediastinal lymphnode hyperplasia resembling thymoma. Cancer 1956;9:822–30.

88. Saeed-Abdul-Rahman I, Al-Amri AM. Castleman disease. Korean J Hematol 2012;47:163–77.

89. Talat N, Belgaumkar AP, Schulte KM. Surgery in Castleman's disease: a systematic review of 404 published cases. Ann Surg 2012;255:677–84.

90. Fajgenbaum DC, Uldrick TS, Bagg A, et al. International, evidence-based consensus diagnostic criteria for HHV-8-negative/idiopathic multicentric Castleman disease. Blood 2017;129:1646–57.

91. Hill AJ, Tirumani SH, Rosenthal MH, et al. Multimodality imaging and clinical features in Castleman disease: single institute experience in 30 patients. Br J Radiol 2015;88:20140670.

92. Madan R, Chen JH, Trotman-Dickenson B, et al. The spectrum of Castleman's disease: mimics, radiologic pathologic correlation and role of imaging in patient management. Eur J Radiol 2012;81: 123–31.

93. Nagano S, Yokouchi M, Yamamoto T, et al. Castleman's disease in the retroperitoneal space mimicking a paraspinal schwannoma: a case report. World J Surg Oncol 2013;11:108.

94. Barker R, Kazmi F, Stebbing J, et al. FDG-PET/CT imaging in the management of HIV-associated multicentric Castleman's disease. Eur J Nucl Med Mol Imaging 2009;36:648–52.

MR Imaging of the Urinary Bladder
Added Value of PET-MR Imaging

Ersan Altun, MD[1]

KEYWORDS

- MR imaging • PET • Bladder cancer • Staging

KEY POINTS

- MR imaging has been reported to be particularly successful in the differentiation of Ta-T1 tumors from T2 and higher staged tumors with 90% sensitivity and 88% specificity in a recent metaanalysis.
- MR imaging is still limited in the accuracy for the identification of involved lymph nodes, and the sensitivity and specificity of MR imaging in the identification of involved lymph nodes are 56% and 94 in a recent metaanalysis.
- PET-MR imaging could be helpful for staging of bladder cancer; however, there are very limited data in the literature to determine the added value of PET-MR imaging in bladder cancer staging, although it has the potential to improve the accuracy for T and N staging.

INTRODUCTION

Multidetector computed tomography (CT) techniques including CT urography have been the most commonly used cross-sectional imaging modality for the evaluation of urinary bladder for the last 2 decades.[1,2] However, CT scanning is limited in the assessment of bladder owing to low soft tissue contrast resolution and this particularly prevents the detection of small lesions, including but not limited to sessile or flat lesions.[1–3] The lack of adequate distension and inability to differentiate inflammatory and post-biopsy treatment changes from the tumor and normal bladder wall in addition to low soft tissue contrast resolution lead to a low accuracy of CT scanning in T staging of bladder cancer ranging from 35% to 55% with associated 10% to 39% understaging and 6% to 34% overstaging.[1,6]

MR imaging has been recently getting increasing attention for the evaluation of bladder cancer not only due to the limitations of CT scans, but also due to its higher soft tissue contrast resolution, and the use of functional MR imaging techniques, including diffusion-weighted imaging (DWI) and dynamic contrast enhanced (DCE) techniques, which have the potential to increase the accuracy of MR imaging compared with previously used conventional sequences.[4–6] However, adequate bladder distension is necessary to be able to achieve greater accuracy on MR imaging, similar to CT scanning.[4]

Bladder cancer is the sixth most common among all cancers, the fourth most common cancer among men, and the second most common in the genitourinary tract after prostate cancer.[7–9] Although cystoscopy and transurethral resection of bladder tumor have been reported to be the most accurate ways of detection and characterization of muscle invasiveness of the bladder tumors, these techniques still can understage and overstage the bladder cancer and approximately

The author has nothing to disclose.
Department of Radiology, The University of North Carolina at Chapel Hill, 101 Manning Drive, , Chapel Hill, NC 27514, USA
[1] Also holds a degree of Associate Professorship of Radiology in Turkey.
E-mail address: ersan_altun@med.unc.edu

one-third of invasive cancers have been reported to be understaged.[10,11] Although the specific role of MR imaging staging has not been defined yet, MR imaging has been reported to provide encouraging results to stage bladder cancer.[4,8,11,12] Additionally, PET-MR hybrid imaging has the potential to contribute to staging of bladder cancer, although there have been no sufficient data in the literature, to date.

Thus, in this review article, the role of MR imaging in the assessment of urinary bladder, particularly bladder cancer with possible potential role of PET-MR imaging in staging, is discussed.

BLADDER CANCER
Epidemiology

Bladder cancer is the most common malignancy of urinary tract. About 81,190 new cases of bladder cancer (4.7% of all new cancers) and 17,240 deaths from bladder cancer (2.8% of all cancer deaths) are expected in 2018.[7] The 5-year survival rate for bladder cancer is 76.8% between 2008 and 2014.[7]

Urothelial carcinoma, formerly known as transitional carcinoma, is the most common subtype, accounting for 90% of the bladder cancers; the remaining subtypes include squamous cell carcinomas and adenocarcinomas, forming 6% to 8% and 2% of all bladder cancers, respectively, in the Western world.[1,10] In the developing world, nonurothelial etiologies have a higher incidence compared with the Western world, at least partly owing to schistosomiasis.[1]

Histopathology and TNM Staging

Urothelial carcinoma has been classified into subgroups based on the extent of invasion into the deep layers of bladder wall and surrounding tissues, including non–muscle-invasive urothelial carcinoma and muscle-invasive urothelial carcinoma, because this differentiation has significant therapeutic and prognostic implications.[9]

Bladder cancer is staged according to 2017 American Joint Committee on Cancer TNM staging system https://www.cancer.net/cancer-types/bladder-cancer/stages-and-grades.[13]

Non–muscle-invasive urothelial carcinoma is more common and constitutes 70% of urothelial cancers, whereas muscle-invasive urothelial cancer constitutes 30%.[5] In addition to depth of invasion, urothelial carcinoma was classified into low grade or high grade based on the degree of nuclear anaplasia and architectural abnormalities.[10]

Non–muscle-invasive tumors arise from the urothelium and do not invade the muscularis propria. This subtype includes Ta lesions, which are papillary (exophytic), and low-grade lesions arising from the mucosa; Tis lesions, which are known as carcinoma in situ representing high-grade lesions located in the mucosa; and T1 lesions, which are usually high-grade superficial tumors invading the lamina propria or submucosa of the bladder wall.[10]

Muscle-invasive tumors are almost always high-grade tumors, and include T2 tumors characterized by invasion into the muscularis propria, T3 tumors characterized by invasion into the perivesical fat, and T4 tumors characterized by invasion into the prostate, vagina, uterus, bowel, abdominal/pelvic walls, and other distant organs.[10]

Squamous cell carcinomas and adenocarcinomas are aggressive tumors and usually present with advanced disease.[14]

Initial Approach to the Diagnosis and the Role of Imaging

Gross or microscopic hematuria is the initial typical presentation of bladder cancer, although lower urinary tract symptoms including frequency, urgency, or dysuria could also be the presenting symptoms, albeit less commonly.[10,14] Evaluation of the bladder and upper urinary tract is essential in the clinical assessment and workup of these symptoms to exclude a urinary tract malignancy.[10,14]

Cystoscopy is the gold standard for the evaluation of the bladder in these groups of patients to identify and exclude bladder cancer, and is usually combined with urine cytology.[10,14] Cystoscopy is particularly helpful for the detection of small lesions including flat lesions, which would not be identified with imaging techniques.[10,14] However, its main advantage is not only the ability to do histopathologic sampling, but also the ability to do transurethral resection of the tumors to determine the depth of invasion, and for therapeutic purposes.[10,14] Non–muscle-invasive urothelial carcinoma is usually an indolent tumor and can be treated with transurethral resection, intravesical immunotherapy, or intravesical chemotherapy.[10,14] However, muscle-invasive urothelial carcinoma requires more extensive treatment including cystectomy or multimodality treatment including chemotherapy and radiation therapy followed or preceded by cystectomy.[10,14]

Cross-sectional imaging with CT urography or MR imaging urography with intravenous contrast is performed to identify concurrent upper tract disease in all patients with bladder cancer.[10] If the bladder cancer is muscle-invasive urothelial cancer or other rare types of bladder cancer are present, cross-sectional imaging is also performed with additional purposes including the assessment of the extension of the pelvic disease, that is, locoregional staging and distant metastases.[10,14] However, local T staging is very limited with CT scanning and the purpose of CT scanning is usually to evaluate regional lymph nodes for involvement and distant organ metastases.[2,3,5] Although promising results have been obtained with MR imaging for local staging of bladder cancer, its specific role in the diagnostic and staging algorithm has not been determined yet.[1,2,4,6,8,11,12]

MR imaging has been recently reported to differentiate non–muscle-invasive urothelial carcinoma from the muscle-invasive urothelial carcinoma with 94% accuracy, and this process could be helpful for treatment planning because understaging remains a problem with biopsy and transurethral resection.[4,11] Therefore, the differentiation of muscle-invasive tumors from non–muscle-invasive tumors may lead to the use of timely and appropriate treatment of muscle-invasive tumors.[10]

MR IMAGING STAGING OF BLADDER CANCER
MR Imaging Technique

No specific patient preparation is needed. The patient should not void 2 hours before the examination and/or drink 500 mL of water 1 hour before the examination.

Staging MR imaging could be performed at 1.5 T or 3.0 T with phased-array body coils. Although there are still no sufficient data for the comparison of 1.5 T versus 3.0 T for local staging of bladder cancer, it has been reported that 3.0 T may provide higher accuracy in imaging of bladder cancer compared with 1.5 T, which likely results from higher signal-to-noise ratio compared with 1.5 T, particularly for high-resolution T2-weighted imaging and DWI.[15–17]

MR imaging protocol includes transverse, coronal, and sagittal single shot echo train spin echo T2-weighted sequences; transverse fat-suppressed single shot echo train spin echo T2-weighted sequence; transverse in-phase and out-of-phase dual echo spoiled gradient echo sequence; transverse, coronal, and sagittal high-resolution T2-weighted turbo spin echo (TSE); transverse breathing-independent DWI at b values of 0 and 1000 s/mm^2, and transverse DCE 3-dimensional gradient echo sequence at arterial phase (at 20–25 seconds after the injection), venous phase (at 60 seconds after the injection), and interstitial phase (at 120 seconds after the injection) followed by coronal and sagittal

Table 1
Pelvic MR imaging protocol for the evaluation of urinary bladder

Sequence	Plane	TR	TE	Flip Angle	Thickness/Gap	FOV	Matrix
Localizer	3-plane						
SS-ETSE	Coronal	1500[a]	85	170	6 mm/20%	350–400	192 × 256
SS-ETSE	Axial	1500[a]	85	170	6 mm/20%	350–400	192 × 256
SS-ETSE	Sagittal	1500[a]	85	170	6 mm/20%	350	192 × 256
SS-ETSE fat suppressed	Axial	1500[a]	85	170	8–10 mm/20%	350–400	192 × 256
T1 SGE in/out of phase	Axial	170	2.2/4.4	70	7 mm/20%	350–400	192 × 320
T2 3D TSE	Axial	1200	120	150	1.5 mm	250	256 × 256
T2 TSE	Axial/ coronal/ sagittal	5000	80	90	3 mm	230	256 × 256
Diffusion-weighted imaging	Axial	4500	88	90	3 mm	270	128 × 128
T1 3D GE FS pre	Axial	3.8	1.7	10	3 mm	350–400	160 × 256
Postgadolinium sequences							
T1 3D GE fat suppressed	Axial/ coronal/ sagittal	3.8	1.7	10	3 mm	350–400	160 × 256

Abbreviations: 3D GE, 3-dimensional gradient echo; FOV, field of view; FS, fat-suppressed; SGE, spoiled gradient echo; SS-TSE, single shot echo train spin echo; TE, echo time; TR, repetition time; TSE, turbo spin echo.
[a] TR between slice acquisitions.

acquisitions. The details of the MR imaging protocol are given in **Table 1**.

Except for high-resolution T2-weighted imaging and DWI, the remaining sequences cover the lower abdomen and pelvis with a large field of view from the level of the aortic bifurcation to the level of the symphysis pubis. High-resolution T2-weighted TSE sequences and DWI sequences should be acquired with high image matrix, 3-mm slice thickness without any intersection gap, and a small field of view covering the bladder.

Postgadolinium sequences are acquired with 0.1 mmol/kg of extracellular gadolinium-based contrast agents at 2 mL/s with automatic injection followed by a 20-mL saline flush. Postgadolinium DCE imaging could also be obtained as perfusion imaging with a lower spatial resolution and higher temporal resolution.[4,18–20] However, the role of perfusion imaging has not been well-established yet in the evaluation and staging of bladder cancer.[4,18–20]

MR Imaging Staging

T2-weighted TSE sequences, DWI sequences, and DCE imaging are used for T staging of bladder cancer. The remaining sequences are used for the evaluation of lymph node involvement, possible distant metastases, and additional incidental findings.

T staging

The normal bladder wall consists of 5 layers, including the (i) mucosa (urothelium), (ii) lamina propria, (iii) submucosa, (iv) muscularis propria (detrusor muscle), and (v) adventitia.[1,4,9,14,21,22] The muscularis propria forms the bulk of the bladder wall and is hypointense on T2-weighted TSE (**Fig. 1**), mildly hyperintense on high-value DWI showing intermediate signal intensity on apparent diffusion coefficient (ADC) mapping, and hypointense on T1-weighted images. The mucosa and submucosa are not visible on T2-weighted TSE and DWI images.[4,11,12,21,22] The mucosa and submucosa demonstrate early enhancement on the arterial phase DCE images, but the muscularis propria demonstrates late enhancement on the venous and interstitial phase DCE images.[4,11,12,18–20]

The tumor demonstrates intermediate signal on T2-weighted TSE images compared with

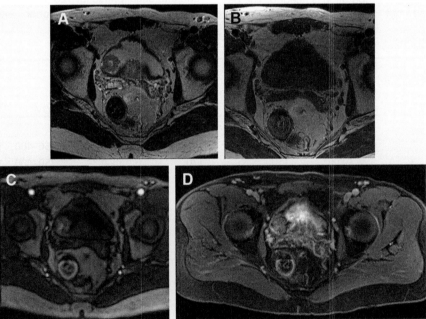

Fig. 1. T2-weighted high-resolution axial turbo spin echo (TSE) (*A*), T1-weighted high-resolution axial TSE (*B*), T1-weighted axial dynamic contrast enhanced postgadolinium 3-dimensional gradient echo (3D-GE) (*C*) with low spatial resolution and high temporal resolution and T1-weighted axial fat-suppressed postgadolinium excretory phase 3D-GE (*D*) images demonstrate a polypoid mass with a stalk at the right posterolateral wall of the urinary bladder extending into the bladder lumen. No evidence is found of disruption of the normal bladder wall underlying the tumor on high-resolution T2 TSE imaging. The normal bladder wall demonstrates uninterrupted low signal intensity and the tumor shows intermediate T2 signal. The tumor demonstrates early increased enhancement on the arterial phase compared with the background muscularis propria. The stalk demonstrates high T2 signal centrally in the tumor and increased enhancement compared with the remaining peripheral part of the tumor. This tumor does not demonstrate muscularis propria invasion and is staged as a T1 tumor.

background hypointense muscularis propria (see **Fig. 1**), and could be differentiated from the normal bladder wall.[4,11,12,21] The tumor shows a high signal intensity on DWI with a corresponding low signal intensity on ADC compared with the muscularis propria.[4,11,21–23] The tumor displays prominent enhancement compared with a nonenhancing or minimally enhancing muscularis propria on the arterial phase of DCE imaging[4,18–21,24] (see **Fig. 1**).

The tumor can be identified and staged with the help of these differential signal features compared with the underlying bladder wall.[4,11,15,17,21] The extension of tumor into the muscularis propria and extravesical fat tissue can be recognized and the differentiation between T1 versus T2, and T2 versus T3 tumors can be performed.[4,11,15,17,21] However, MR imaging has been reported to be particularly successful in the differentiation of Ta and T1 tumors from T2 and higher staged tumors with 90% sensitivity and 88% specificity in a recent metaanalysis.[15] Additionally, it has also been reported that DWI and 3.0 T imaging improved sensitivity and specificity to 92% and 96%, respectively.[15]

Ta and T1 tumors are usually associated with a fibrotic and/or inflammatory stalk arising from the submucosa with no evidence of malignancy.[4,11,15,16,21,22,24] The stalk demonstrates variable T2 signal from a low signal to a high signal (see **Fig. 1**), although it is usually intermediate to low in signal intensity and the stalk may be isointense to the tumor on T2 TSE images.[4,11,15,16,21,22,24,25] The stalk usually shows low signal on high b values images with associated high signal on ADC map without diffusion restriction.[4,11,15,16,21,22,24,25] The stalk usually shows early enhancement on DCE similar to the tumor[21,24] (see **Fig. 1**). Therefore, DWI is critical for the identification of stalk.[21,22,25] If the stalk is detected on DWI, the tumor is usually a non–muscle-invasive tumor and the tumor signal does not extend or disrupt the muscularis propria.[4,11,21,22] Additional findings that are helpful for the differentiation of non–muscle-invasive tumor from muscle-invasive tumor include tenting of the bladder wall and uninterrupted submucosal enhancement just beneath the tumor.[4,11,21,22] The submucosa sometimes can be seen as a thickened layer under the tumor and the absence of diffusion restriction would be suggestive of inflammation and/or fibrosis. However, it should be noted that superficial T1 tumors may also invade the submucosa without the presence of stalk, and the stalk may occasionally show diffusion restriction without evidence of malignancy.[4,11,21,22] Additionally, if there is discordance between the findings of T2 TSE, DWI, or DCE, DWI should be the dominant sequence in staging owing to the potential to differentiate the tumor tissue from inflammation and/or fibrosis.[21,22]

A T2 tumor (**Fig. 2**) is confined to the bladder wall and the intermediate tumor signal should not completely disrupt the dark signal of muscularis propria on T2-weighted TSE images.[4,11,21] Associated high DWI signal and corresponding low ADC signal should be confined to the wall and should not extend to extravesicle fat.[4,11,21] Increased enhancement of the tumor on the arterial phase should be confined to the wall and not extend into extravesicle fat.[4,11,18–21] However, if there is discordance between the findings of T2 TSE, DWI, or DCE, DWI should be the dominant sequence in staging owing to the potential to differentiate the tumor tissue from inflammation and/or fibrosis.[4,21,22] If there is extravesicle inflammation and fibrosis owing to treatment or postprocedural changes, which may demonstrate similar signal to the tumor on T2-weighted images or similar enhancement to the tumor on DCE, DWI should be the dominant sequence in staging owing to the potential to differentiate the tumor tissue from inflammation and/or fibrosis.[4,21,22]

A T3 tumor extends to the extravesicle fat, and the intermediate tumor signal disrupts the muscularis propria signal and is seen beyond the confines of bladder wall on T2-weighted TSE images[4,11,12,21] (**Fig. 3**). Associated high DWI signal and corresponding low ADC signal, and increased enhancement of the tumor on the arterial phase extend into the extravesicle fat beyond the confines of the bladder wall.[4,11,12,21–23] However, if the abnormal tumor signal involves the whole bladder wall without definite extension into the extravesicle fat, minimal to mild extension into the extravesicle fat could still be present histopathologically although not definitely seen on MR imaging.[4,9,21]

A T4 tumor invades the adjacent organs including the prostate, uterus, vagina, and pelvic sidewalls and abdominal wall.[13] T2 TSE (**Fig. 4**) is the dominant sequence for the evaluation of invasion of adjacent organs with the help of DWI and DCE.[4,11,21]

A limitation of MR imaging is the identification of small tumors including the small flat or sessile lesions, which are usually Tis or tumors less than 1 cm.[3]

Postbiopsy and posttreatment changes can cause variable signal changes including high, intermediate, and low signal changes on T2-weighted TSE images representing edema, inflammation, and fibrosis.[4,11,21,22] DWI can be helpful for the differentiation of postbiopsy and posttreatment changes from the tumor because

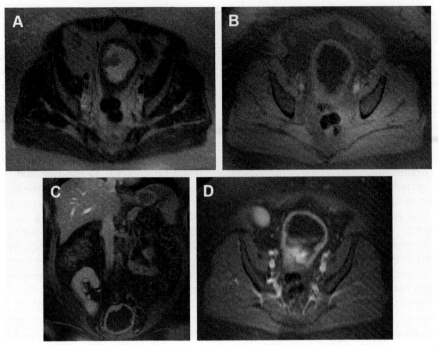

Fig. 2. T2-weighted axial single shot echo train spin echo (*A*), T1-weighted axial fat-suppressed 3-dimensional gradient echo (3D-GE) (*B*), T1-weighted coronal fat-suppressed coronal interstitial phase (*C*) and axial excretory phase (*D*) postgadolinium 3D-GE images demonstrate multiple polypoid enhancing masses extending into the bladder lumen. At least 1 of these masses demonstrate bladder wall invasion, particularly on the left side. The high signal intensity of the polypoid mass extends into the low signal normal bladder wall (*A*). This tumor demonstrates muscularis propria invasion and is staged as T2 tumor.

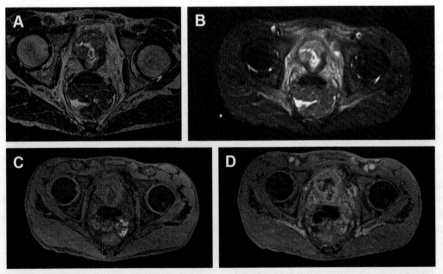

Fig. 3. T2-weighted axial high-resolution turbo spin echo (*A*), T2-weighted fat-suppressed single shot echo train spin echo (*B*), T1-weighted axial fat-suppressed 3-dimensinal gradient echo (3D-GE) (*C*), T1-weighted axial fat-suppressed postgadolinium 3D-GE (*D*) images demonstrate a large enhancing bladder mass that disrupts and extends beyond the confines of the normal bladder wall into the extravesicle fat. Normal low signal intensity of the muscularis propria is lost anteriorly and anterolaterally on both sides owing to tumor invasion. This tumor is staged as a T3 tumor.

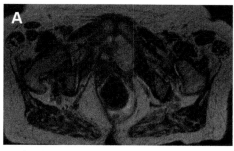
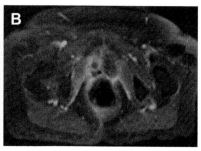

Fig. 4. T2-weighted axial high-resolution turbo spin echo (TSE) (*A*) and T1-weighted axial postgadolinium 3-dimensional gradient echo (*B*) images demonstrate a recurrent T4 tumor after cystectomy with associated invasion of the vaginal cuff.

these changes usually do not demonstrate diffusion restriction and, therefore, show either high to intermediate signal on DWI and ADC map, or low to intermediate signal on DWI and ADC map.[4,11,21,22]

N staging

The pelvic lymph nodes including internal iliac, external iliac, obturator, and presacral lymph nodes can be initially involved in N1 to N2 stage disease (https://www.cancer.net/cancer-types/bladder-cancer/stages-and-grades).[13] The common iliac chain lymph nodes are involved in the N3 stage.[13] More extensive retroperitoneal lymph node metastases above this level of are regarded as M1 disease.[13]

MR imaging remains limited in its accuracy for the identification of involved lymph nodes, and the sensitivity and specificity of MR imaging including DWI in the identification of involved lymph nodes are 76% to 79% and 79% to 89%.[4] However, it has also been recently reported in a metaanalysis covering the studies published since 2000 that the sensitivity and specificity of MR imaging are 56% and 94%, respectively.[16]

The inability to identify metastatic involvement in lymph nodes equal to or smaller than 8 to 10 mm owing to occult metastatic involvement or micrometastatic involvement, which do not change the normal morphology of the lymph nodes or cause the development of any obvious diffusion restriction is a significant limitation for the detection of malignant lymph nodes leading to false-negative results.[2–4,11,16,26,27] The inability to differentiate reactive and inflammatory changes from malignant involvement owing to overlapping MR imaging features, including but not limited to size increase, increased enhancement, or obvious diffusion restriction, is the other significant limitation leading to false-positive results.[2–4,11,16,26,27] Overall, these factors decrease the accuracy of MR imaging because of the overlap between the MR imaging appearance of lymph nodes with

occult or micrometastases and normal lymph nodes, and lymph nodes with inflammatory changes mimicking metastatic lymph nodes.[3,4,11,16,26,27]

Some morphologic features of lymph nodes and their combination could be a clue for involved lymph nodes, including diffusely increased heterogeneous T2 signal, focally increased homogeneous or heterogeneous T2 signal, focal or diffuse diffusion restriction, increased enhancement of lymph nodes including focal or diffuse heterogeneous enhancement of lymph nodes, asymmetrical increased cortical thickness, and the shape of the lymph nodes compared with the remaining lymph nodes for diffuse changes or remaining part of the background lymph node architecture for focal changes, although these details are not specific.

Ultrasmall particle superparamagnetic iron oxide (USPIO) also has been studied and has been reported to have the potential to identify metastatic involved lymph nodes measuring less than 8 to 10 mm, which otherwise could not be identified based on conventional size criteria.[16,26,27] These agents theoretically have the potential to identify normal lymph nodes or lymph nodes with benign inflammatory changes with the help of uptake of these agents by macrophages.[16,26,27] Therefore, normal lymph nodes are expected to demonstrate decreased signal and seem to be hypointense on T2- or T2*-weighted sequences owing to the uptake of USPIO by macrophages.[16,26,27] In contrast, the lymph nodes with metastatic involvement are expected to show increased signal and seem to be hyperintense on T2- or T2*-weighted sequences.[16,26,27]

Although promising results have been reported with the use of USPIO, the sensitivity and specificity of USPIO for nodal staging in the bladder cancer has been reported to be variable, at 55% to 96% and 71% to 95%, respectively.[4,16,26,27] The variability of the results demand more research studies to be performed to achieve better and more reproducible results. The variability could again be due to false-negative results secondary to micrometastases in lymph nodes or false-positive results secondary to reactive hyperplasia, nodal lipomatosis, and insufficient uptake of USPIO.

MR IMAGING-PET HYBRID IMAGING

PET-MR imaging could be helpful for staging of bladder cancer; however, there are very few data in the literature to determine the added value of PET-MR imaging in bladder cancer staging, although it has the potential to improve the accuracy for T and N staging.[28–32] Additionally, whole body M staging with limited evaluation of lung nodules could also be performed with PET-MR imaging, which is an important advantage.[28–32]

Challenges and Limitations

Adequate and standard distension of the bladder is an important issue that needs to be addressed for successful accurate fusion imaging of PET-MR imaging without misregistration.[28–32] PET-CT scanning has significant limitations for the evaluation of bladder cancer staging. One of these limitations is the inability of CT scans to differentiate the layers of bladder wall and the tumor from the normal bladder wall.[2] Another limitation of CT scanning is the inability to differentiate posttreatment effects from the tumor, and extravesical extension of the tumor from posttreatment effects.[2,3] Another limitation is the inability to reliably to determine the fludeoxyglucose (FDG) uptake of the tumor owing to the presence of excreted significant radioactivity in the bladder lumen.[28–32] The other limitation is the significant misregistration between CT and PET images owing to long acquisition time of PET with sequential very short acquisition time CT imaging, secondary to continuous excretion and increasing distension of the bladder between PET and CT acquisitions and the inability to do simultaneous acquisition.[28–32]

PET-MR imaging has the potential to overcome most of these limitations. As discussed elsewhere in this article, MR imaging has the potential and ability to differentiate the muscularis propria and tumor itself, the extension of the tumor into the muscularis propria and extravesicular fat, and the posttreatment effects from the tumor.[4,11,15,17,21,22,28–32]

Simultaneous acquisition is an important advantage PET-MR imaging systems, which has been demonstrated to eliminate the misregistration between MR imaging and PET images, and this is particularly shown to work with high-resolution T2-weighted images acquired simultaneously with PET imaging.[28–32]

Despite these advantages of PET-MR imaging compared with PET-CT scanning, the inability to identify the tumor or to differentiate it from the normal wall and posttreatment effects, owing to high radioactivity in the bladder lumen, is still a significant limitation of PET-MR imaging similar to PET-CT scanning.[28–32] To eliminate this limitation or minimize the effect of radioactivity in the lumen, particularly 2 different methods have been used, although the data are very limited in the literature regarding their use.[30–32] One of these methods is to catheterize the bladder and continuously drain the radioactivity from the bladder lumen. A variant of this method can also be used to drain the urine containing high amounts of radioactivity and subsequently to distend the bladder with 250 mL saline, diluting the radioactivity before simultaneous acquisition. However, the use of catheterization is invasive, increases radiation exposure to the personnel, and has also been demonstrated to result in significant residual activity in the bladder lumen.[31,32] Another technique is to use forced diuresis to excrete the radioactivity of the bladder noninvasively.[31–33] This technique uses hydration together with the diuresis in between the administration of FDG and simultaneous PET-MR imaging acquisition and has been demonstrated to have the potential to minimize the ^{18}F-FDG contrast in the lower urinary tract.[31–33] However, more research is needed to evaluate the use of the efficacy of these techniques, particularly the latter one.

T and N Staging

A few published pilot studies about the use of PET-MR imaging for bladder cancer T and N staging has reported that PET-MR imaging has the potential to improve the accuracy by providing metabolic information for the evaluation of equivocal findings seen on MR imaging alone.[29,32]

The sensitivity, specificity, and accuracy have been reported to be 72% to 94%, 0% to 100%, and 77% for tumor detection in the bladder on MR imaging alone, and has been reported to be 89%, 75%, and 86% on PET-MR imaging, respectively.[32] The sensitivity, specificity and accuracy have been reported to be 38% to 100%, 54% to 100%, and 71% to 76% for involved lymph node detection on MR imaging alone, and reported to be 88%, 100%, and 95% on PET-MR imaging, respectively.[32] PET-MR imaging has been reported to increase the accuracy for the detection of bladder tumors and involved lymph nodes in this pilot study.[3]

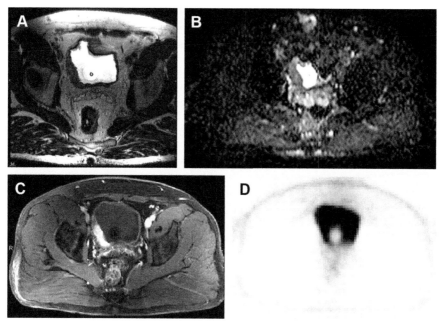

Fig. 5. T2-weighted axial high-resolution turbo spin echo (*A*), apparent diffusion coefficient map of an axial diffusion-weighted imaging sequence (*B*), axial arterial phase postgadolinium 3-dimensional gradient echo (*C*), and nonattenuation corrected simultaneously acquired axial PET image (*D*) show a right-sided bladder wall mass causing focal prominent bladder wall thickening associated with diffusion restriction and increased early enhancement. The normal signal intensity of the muscularis propria is lost and the tumor is a T3 tumor. However, no significant uptake is noted on the PET image, which is likely secondary to increased tracer accumulation in the bladder lumen.

PET-MR imaging has been reported to change the evaluations in 36% of the patients for the bladder tumor detection, 52% of the patients for pelvic lymph node evaluation, and 9% of the patients for other findings in the pelvis.[32] The rate of correct changes owing to PET-MR imaging evaluations over MR imaging alone according to the reference standard in this study has been reported to be 75% for bladder tumor detection, 91% for involved pelvic lymph node detection, and 100% for other findings in the pelvis.[32]

Despite the presence of significant technical limitations owing to the accumulated radioactivity in the bladder (**Fig. 5**), PET-MR imaging has the potential to increase the accuracy of T staging with its hypothetical role in the differentiation of posttreatment changes, which do not demonstrate FDG uptake, compared with the FDG avid tumoral tissue; in the determination of the presence of extravesical extension, particularly in patients with posttreatment changes; and in the determination of treatment response. PET-MR imaging has the potential to increase the accuracy of lymph node staging by determining FDG uptake in small, morphologically normal lymph nodes or the lack of FDG uptake in large, reactive pelvic lymph nodes. However, more research studies is needed to establish the role of PET-MR imaging in the detection and local T and N staging bladder tumors and the evaluation of treatment response.

SUMMARY

MR imaging has been increasingly getting attention for the evaluation of bladder cancer. Recent studies have been promising for the staging performance of MR imaging in the bladder cancer although its specific role has not been established yet. Additionally, the use of hybrid imaging with PET-MR imaging could has the potential to increase its accuracy although more research studies are needed.

REFERENCES

1. Hossein MM, Rajesh A. MR imaging of the urinary bladder. Magn Reson Imaging Clin N Am 2014;22: 129–34.
2. McKibben MJ, Woods ME. Preoperative imaging for staging bladder cancer. Curr Urol Rep 2015;16:22.
3. Moses KA, Zhang J, Hricak H, et al. Bladder cancer imaging: an update. Curr Opin Urol 2011;21:393–7.
4. Panebianco V, Barchetti F, de Haas RJ, et al. Improving staging in bladder cancer: the increasing

role of multiparametric magnetic resonance imaging. Eur Urol Focus 2016;2:113–21.

5. Lawrentschuk N, Lee TS, Scott AM. Current role of PET, CT, MR for invasive bladder cancer. Curr Urol Rep 2013;14:84–9.

6. Vargas HA, Akin O, Schoder H, et al. Prospective evaluation of MRI, ^{11}C-acetate PET/CT and contrast-enhanced CT for staging of bladder cancer. Eur J Radiol 2012;8:4131–7.

7. Surveillance, Epidemiology, and End Results Program. National Cancer Institute. Available at: https://seer.cancer.gov/statfacts/html/urinb.html. Accessed April 16th, 2018.

8. de Haas RJ, Stevyers MJ, Futerrer JF. Multiparametric MRI of the bladder: ready for clinical routine? Am J Roentgenol 2014;202:1187–95.

9. Raza SA, Jhaveri KS. MR imaging of urinary bladder carcinoma and beyond. Radiol Clin North Am 2012; 50:1085–110.

10. Lerner SP, Raghavan D. Overview of the initial approach and management of urothelial bladder cancer. 2017. Available at: https://www.uptodate.com/contents/overview-of-the-initial-approach-and-management-of-urothelial-bladder-cancer. Accessed April 16, 2018.

11. Panebianco V, De Berardinis E, Barchetti G, et al. An evaluation of morphological and functional multiparametric MRI sequences in classifying non-muscle and muscle invasive bladder cancer. Eur Radiol 2017;27:3759–66.

12. Rosenkrantz AB, Mussi TC, Melamed J, et al. Bladder cancer: utility of MRI in detection of occult muscle-invasive disease. Acta Radiol 2012;53: 695–9.

13. Bladder cancer. TNM staging. 2017. Available at: https://www.cancer.net/cancer-types/bladder-cancer/stages-and-grades. Accessed March 1, 2018.

14. Verma S, Rajesh A, Prasad SR, et al. Urinary bladder cancer: role of MR imaging. Radiographics 2012;32: 371–87.

15. Huang L, Kong Q, Liu Z, et al. The diagnostic value of MR imaging in differentiating T staging of bladder cancer: a meta-analysis. Radiology 2018;286: 502–11.

16. Woo S, Suh CH, Kim SY, et al. The diagnostic performance of MRI for detection of lymph node metastasis in bladder and prostate cancer: an updated systematic review and diagnostic meta-analysis. Am J Roentgenol 2018;2010:W95–109.

17. Woo S, Suh CH, Kim SY, et al. Diagnostic performance of MRI for prediction of muscle-invasiveness of bladder cancer: a systematic review and meta-analysis. Eur J Radiol 2017;95: 46–55.

18. Gupta N, Sureka B, Kumar MM, et al. Comparison of dynamic contrast-enhanced and diffusion weighted magnetic resonance image in staging and grading of carcinoma bladder with histopathological correlation. Urol Ann 2015;7:199–204.

19. Chabika C, Cornelis F, Descat E, et al. Dynamic contrast enhanced MRI-derived parameters are potential biomarkers of therapeutic response in bladder cancer. Eur J Radiol 2015;84:1023–8.

20. Nguyen HT, Jia G, Shah ZK, et al. Prediction of chemotherapeutic response in bladder cancer using K-means clustering of dynamic contrast-enhanced (DCE)-MRI pharmacokinetic parameters. J Magn Reson Imaging 2015;41:1374–82.

21. Panebianco V, Narumi Y, Altun E, et al. Multiparametric magnetic resonance imaging for bladder cancer: development of VI-RADS (vesicle imaging-reporting and data system). Eur Urol 2018. https://doi.org/10.1016/j.eururo.2018.04.029.

22. Takeuchi M, Sasaki S, Naiki T, et al. MR imaging of urinary bladder cancer for T-staging: a review and a pictorial essay of diffusion-weighted imaging. J Magn Reson Imaging 2013;38:1299–309.

23. Zhou G, Chen X, Zhang J, et al. Contrast-enhanced dynamic and diffusion-weighted MR imaging at 3.0T to assess aggressiveness of bladder cancer. Eur J Radiol 2014;83:2013–8.

24. Wang HJ, Pui MH, Guan J, et al. Comparison of early submucosal enhancement and tumor stalk in staging bladder urothelial carcinoma. AJR Am J Roentgenol 2016;9:1–7.

25. Kobayashi S, Koga F, Kajiono K, et al. Apparent diffusion coefficient value reflects invasive and proliferative potential of bladder cancer. J Magn Reson Imaging 2014;39:172–8.

26. Birkhauser FD, Studer UE, Froehlich JM, et al. Combined ultrasmall superparamagnetic particles of iron oxide-enhanced and diffusion-weighted magnetic resonance imaging facilitates detection of metastases in normal-sized pelvic lymph nodes of patients with bladder and prostate cancer. Eur Radiol 2013; 64:953–60.

27. Triantafyllou M, Studer UE, Birkhauser FD, et al. Ultrasmall superparamagnetic particles of iron oxide allow for the detection of metastases in normal sized pelvic lymph nodes of patients with bladder and/or prostate cancer. Eur J Cancer 2013;49:616–24.

28. Brendle CB, Schmidt H, Fleischer S, et al. Simultaneously acquired MR/PET images compared with sequential MR/PET and PET/CT: alignment quality. Radiology 2013;268:190–9.

29. Rosenkrantz AB, Friedman K, Chandarana H, et al. Current status of hybrid PET/MRI in oncologic imaging. Am J Roentgenol 2016;206:162–72.

30. Roy P, Lee JKT, Sheikh A, et al. Quantitative comparison of misregistration in abdominal and pelvic organs between PET/MRI and PET/CT: effect of mode of acquisition and type of sequence of different organs. Am J Roentgenol 2015;205: 1295–305.

31. Rosenkrantz AB, Balar AV, Huang WC, et al. Comparison of coregistration accuracy of pelvic structures between sequential and simultaneous imaging during hybrid PET/MRI in patients with bladder cancer. Clin Nucl Med 2015;40:637–41.

32. Rosenkrantz AB, Friedman KP, Ponzo F, et al. Prospective pilot study to evaluate the incremental value of PET information in patients with bladder cancer undergoing ^{18}F-FDG Simultaneous PET/MRI. Clin Nucl Med 2017;42:e8–15.

33. Kamel EM, Jichlinski P, Prior JO, et al. Forced diuresis improves the diagnostic accuracy of 18F-FDG PET in abdominopelvic malignancies. J Nucl Med 2006;47:1803–7.

Future Perspectives in Multiparametric Prostate MR Imaging

Aritrick Chatterjee, PhD, Aytekin Oto, MD, MBA*

KEYWORDS

• Prostate cancer • Multiparametric MR imaging • Quantitative • Future perspective

KEY POINTS

- Multiparametric MR imaging is increasingly being used for prostate cancer diagnosis. However, the performance of MR imaging needs to improve before it can be used for population-level screening.
- Despite attempts to standardize the reporting and interpretation of prostate MR imaging, adherence to the recommended standards remains a problem.
- The current state of prostate multiparametric MR imaging is based on subjective radiologist assessment. However, there is increasing evidence that quantitative measurements can improve the diagnosis of prostate cancer.
- The most widely accepted MR parameters used for prostate cancer detection clinically provide little information regarding the underlying histology and, therefore, the use of structural models may be useful in the future.
- Since, CAD is more sensitive to subtle changes, their role might be even more critical for focal therapy planning, especially to determine the optimal treatment option by differentiating between clinically significant and non-significant cancers and in determining the cancer tumor volume to reduce the number of recurrences due to incomplete ablation of cancer tissue.

INTRODUCTION

Prostate cancer is the most common noncutaneous cancer and among the leading cause of death among men in the United States.[1] Screening for elevated prostate-specific antigen has facilitated diagnosis of early stage clinical and pathologic stages of prostate cancer.[2] However, prostate-specific antigen testing has low sensitivity in prostate cancer detection. Transrectal ultrasound-guided biopsies prompted by elevated serum prostate-specific antigen levels are also limited in the accurate understanding of the aggressiveness of the disease. Although histology remains the reference standard for prostate cancer diagnosis, a transrectal ultrasound-guided biopsy samples a very small part of the prostate (approximately 1%) and often miss cancers, especially those located in the anterior of the prostate. Additionally, the Gleason score of the cancer diagnosed by transrectal ultrasound-guided biopsy is upgraded for an estimated 30% of patients undergoing repeat biopsy or radical prostatectomy.[3,4] Therefore, understanding the aggressiveness of cancer (distinguishing low-risk tumors from potentially life-threatening tumors) cannot be reliably determined, which causes many patients with low-risk tumors elect to undergo unnecessary surgery or radiation therapy. These limitations emphasize the need for a noninvasive and accurate evaluation method for the entire prostate for the detection,

Disclosures: Dr A. Chatterjee has no disclosures. Dr A. Oto has the following disclosures: Research Grant, Koninklijke Philips NV; Research Grant, Guerbet SA; Research Grant, Profound Medical Inc; Medical Advisory Board, Profound Medical Inc; Speaker, Bracco Group.
Department of Radiology, University of Chicago, 5841 South Maryland Avenue, Chicago, IL 60637, USA
* Corresponding author.
E-mail address: aoto@radiology.bsd.uchicago.edu

1064-9689/19/© 2018 Elsevier Inc. All rights reserved.

staging, and risk stratification of prostate cancer, which will lead to a better choice of treatment and decrease the overtreatment of indolent disease.[5]

Multiparametric MR imaging is increasingly used for prostate cancer diagnosis and guiding biopsies. It has a high negative predictive value[6] and good sensitivity and specificity in prostate cancer diagnosis.[7] It also has the potential to provide reliable information about the cancer grade, location, and volume for the selection of optimum therapy. Multiparametric MR imaging acquisition protocols and interpretation guidelines were recently recommended by American College of Radiology and European Society of Urogenital Radiology in the consensus guidelines entitled Prostate Imaging - Reporting and Data System (PI-RADS v2).[8] Recent studies such as the PROMIS[9] and PRECISION[10] trials support the concept of targeted biopsies, using multiparametric MR imaging for target selection. This approach is found to be more cost effective[11] and can lead to increased acceptance of multiparametric MR imaging for prostate cancer screening. Despite these promising results, 10% to 20% of clinically significant cancer can be missed on multiparametric MR imaging. Benign features such as prostatitis, prostatic hyperplasia, and atropy can mimic cancer, whereas cancer detection in the transition zone (site of approximately 30% of cancers) remains limited.[12] In addition, there is high interobserver variability in the interpretation of multiparametric MR imaging among radiologists,[13] and the lack of image acquisition standards along with a lack of quality control measures for these imaging sequences limits the reproducibility of the performance of prostate MR imaging studies. Therefore, the performance of MR imaging still needs to improve before it can be used for the screening of large populations. In this article, we briefly summarize the current state of prostate multiparametric MR imaging and its drawbacks, focusing on the future perspectives in multiparametric prostate MR imaging.

CURRENT STATE OF MULTIPARAMETRIC MR IMAGING OF THE PROSTATE

Prostate multiparametric MR imaging consists of T2-weighted imaging, diffusion-weighted imaging (DWI), precontrast T1-weighted imaging, and dynamic contrasted-enhanced (DCE) MR imaging. Multiparametric MR imaging is highly sensitive in the detection of prostate cancer compared with any individual sequence. A study[14] reported that individually T2-weighted MR imaging (58%), DWI (53%), and DCE-MR imaging (38%) sequences demonstrate lower sensitivity compared with multiparametric MR imaging (85%). The reported positive and negative predictive value for prostate cancer detection using multiparametric MR imaging is also much higher than that using either of these imaging sequences individually.

T2-Weighted Imaging

T2-weighted imaging allows excellent soft tissue contrast along with good spatial resolution and a high signal-to-noise ratio. It provides good visualization of the zonal anatomy, seminal vesicles, and neurovascular bundle. High-resolution T2-weighted imaging with 2-dimensional turbo/fast spin echo or 3-dimensional spin echo sequences with in plane resolution of less than or equal to 0.4 to 0.7 mm and a slice thickness of 3 mm or less is recommended. Images are acquired in the axial, sagittal, and coronal planes, whereas DWI, T1-weighted, and DCE-MR imaging are obtained in the same planes as axial T2-weighted imaging. Prostate cancer is hypointense on T2-weighted images compared with benign tissue[7,14–17] and quantitative T2 values are significantly lower in prostate cancer compared with benign prostate tissue.[18–22]

Diffusion-Weighted Imaging

DWI provides a signal sensitive to water movement and provides information about the tissue structure and density. A spin echo, echo planar imaging pulse sequence with a plane resolution of greater than 2.5 mm and slice thickness of 4 mm or less is generally used clinically. Images with at least 2 b-values are required to acquire an apparent diffusion coefficient (ADC) map using a monoexponential signal decay model. A lower b-value of 50 to 100 s/mm^2 and higher 800 to 1500 s/mm^2 is generally used. On high b-value (approximately 1500 s/mm^2 images) increased signal is seen in prostate cancer owing to reduced diffusivity. ADC is a measure of the magnitude of the diffusivity of water molecules and is used extensively clinically for the detection of cancer. ADC in cancer tissue is lower than in normal tissue and there is an inverse relation between ADC value and cancer Gleason grade.[23] A meta-analysis of 10 studies reported that the combined use of diffusion MR imaging, specifically ADC with traditional T2-weighted images demonstrated higher sensitivity (76%) and specificity (82%) compared with T2-weighted images alone.[24] In addition, tumor volumes estimated from DWI have been shown to demonstrate better correlation with histologic volume either than T2-weighted or DCE-MR imaging.[25]

T1-Weighted Imaging

Precontrast T1-weighted images are taken over a large field of view using spin or gradient echo pulse sequence either with or without fat suppression to observe postbiopsy changes. T1 hyperintensity in the prostate is usually due to hemorrhage in the prostate after biopsy.

Dynamic Contrasted-Enhanced MR Imaging

DCE-MR imaging involves the acquisition of serial T1-weighted images (fast/spoiled gradient echo sequence with fat suppression) of the prostate before and after the bolus injection of a chelated gadolinium molecule. Cancers show early focal signal enhancement owing to increased vascularity or angiogenesis.[26,27] Increased capillary permeability leads to higher uptake of contrast agent that shortens T1 relaxation time and therefore shows up as hyperintense region with respect to surrounding tissue. A temporal resolution of less than 10 seconds is recommended because the use of higher temporal resolution leads to increased diagnostic performance.[28]

A representative example of prostate cancer seen on multiparametric MR imaging currently used clinically is shown in **Fig. 1.**

FUTURE OF MULTIPARAMETRIC PROSTATE MR IMAGING
Standardization of Multiparametric MR Imaging

Prostate multiparametric MR imaging is continuously evolving. Initial consensus guidelines for prostate multiparametric MR imaging, the PI-RADS v1, was introduced by the European Society of Urogenital Radiology in 2012.[29] More recently, updated consensus guidelines by the American College of Radiology and European Society of Urogenital Radiology know as PI-RADS v2 were introduced in 2015.[8] MR spectroscopy, which was an integral part of PI-RADS v1, is not used

as a sequence in prostate multiparametric MR imaging any more. T2-weighted imaging and DWI are now the dominant sequence for PI-RADS scoring in the transition and peripheral zones, respectively, whereas the role of DCE-MR imaging is secondary. Despite attempts to standardize the reporting and interpretation of prostate MR imaging by PI-RADS, a recent investigation found that adherence to the recommended standards remains a problem.[30]

Moreover, there is a lack of consensus on the details of the imaging sequence parameters. Standardized imaging is particularly important for quantitative image analysis and multicenter trails. For example, it has been shown that the use of different b-values and its range and diffusion time affects ADC calculation and subsequent diagnostic performance among radiologists.[31–33] Most clinical scanners do not specify important diffusion parameters such as gradient strength and gradient time and how specific diffusion weighting is done, so different scanners using the same b-value might have different ADC values for the same tissue. Similarly, diagnostic results vary for T2-weighted imaging when different echo time are used.[34] The standardization is even more critical for DCE-MR imaging, where the variation for image acquisition is even greater. It has been shown that high temporal resolution tends to improve the performance of DCE-MR imaging in a prostate cancer diagnosis[28,35] and therefore PI-RADS v2 recommends a temporal resolution of less than 10 seconds. In addition, the use of different contrast agents with varying relaxivity affects the signal and image analysis.

There is a lack of quality control measures for these imaging sequences. In the future, clear standards and certifications need to be established. Imaging quality testing with phantom and patient

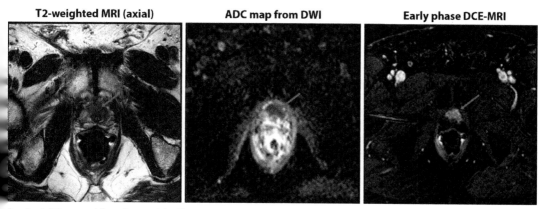

T2-weighted MRI (axial)   **ADC map from DWI**   **Early phase DCE-MRI**

Fig. 1. A 72-year-old patient with Gleason 4 + 3 prostate cancer. The cancer (*red arrows*) is hypointense on T2-weighted images and apparent diffusion coefficient (ADC) map, and demonstrates early focal enhancement on dynamic contrasted-enhanced MR imaging (DCE MRI). DWI, diffusion-weighted imaging.

imaging needs to be implemented such that prostate multiparametric MR imaging adheres to image quality assessment standards.

The variability in the imaging protocols and the lack of quality control measures limit the reproducibility of the performance of prostate MR imaging studies. It has been shown that the introduction of PI-RADS v2 provided only moderately reproducible MR imaging results for the detection of clinically significant cancer.[36] In light of these variations that affect multiparametric MR imaging interpretation, it might be judicious in the future for recommending the standardization of imaging protocols for more reproducible prostate multiparametric MR imaging results. The training and certification of radiologists interpreting prostate multiparametric MR imaging needs to be standardized to produce reproducible results.

Hardware Improvements

There have been substantial recent advances in MR hardware. More clinical centers are replacing their 1.5 T with 3 T MR systems, and some 7 T systems (primarily for research at this point) have recently been available clinically.[37] The main advantages of increased MR magnetic field strength are increased signal-to-noise ratio, which improves spatial resolution; decreased acquisition time; and increased temporal resolution for DCE-MR imaging. Studies have found that increased signal-to-noise ratio may lead to improvement in prostate cancer localization.[38] However, the tissue T1 relaxation times increase with high fields and may be mitigated by the loss in contrast enhancement in T1-weighted images owing to improved background suppression.[39]

Furthermore, the use of an endorectal coil in addition to a surface coil can be used to improve image quality. Barium sulfate suspension or perfluorocarbon fluid can be used to inflate the endorectal coil to squeeze air out to reduce susceptibility and motion artifacts. Endorectal coil increases the sensitivity and positive predictive value for prostate cancer detection over not using an endorectal coil.[39] The use of dedicated coils for prostate imaging and phase array coil with more receiver channels can lead to major improvements in signal-to-noise ratio as well as higher acceleration for parallel imaging.[40] Improved gradients coils can improve multiparametric MR imaging with DWI with higher *b*-values achievable. Newly designed coils using digital parallel transit/receive radiofrequency technology, compressed sensing, and so on have the potential to improve the performance of multiparametric MR imaging in the future.

Quantitative Multiparametric MR Imaging

The current state of prostate multiparametric MR imaging is based on subjective assessment by the radiologist. However, there is increasing evidence that quantitative measurements can improve the diagnosis of prostate cancer. ADC remains the backbone of prostate cancer diagnosis, with ADC values for prostate cancer being significantly lower than those for normal tissue. In addition, numerous studies have shown a negative correlation between ADC values and Gleason score; therefore, ADC values can be used as a predictor of tumor aggressiveness.[23] Although monoexponential models like ADC and T2 are used often, it has been shown that diffusion and T2-weighted signal are not monoexponential. Numerous models such as biexponential,[41,42] intravoxel incoherent motion,[43] kurtosis,[44] stretched exponential signal models,[45] and so on have been proposed. Although quantitative T2 numbers are not used clinically, they have been shown to be significantly lower in prostate cancer compared with normal tissue. A recent study has demonstrated that T2 maps have similar sensitivity but greater positive predictive value for detecting prostate lesions compared with standard T2-weighted images.[46] Quantitative and semiquantitative DCE-MR imaging metrics measured using Tofts'[47] or empirical mathematical model[48] have been shown to be effective in prostate cancer diagnosis. A representative example of prostate cancer seen on quantitative multiparametric MR imaging derived maps is shown in **Fig. 2**.

However, in addition to the absence of standard technique, the integration of quantitative multiparametric MR imaging is also challenging owing to the additional postprocessing and increased time involved. Despite these challenges, quantitative multiparametric MR imaging can lead to a major improvement over the subjective nature of qualitative assessment of prostate MR imaging. Therefore, with powerful computing capabilities, it will be possible to integrate quantitative analysis to prostate multiparametric MR imaging.

New Acquisition Methods

Another direction of numerous studies has been faster acquisition and reconstruction methods. The use of abbreviated protocol has also been investigated. MR spectroscopy was a recommended protocol earlier; however, with the introduction of the PI-RADS v2 guidelines, MR spectroscopy is not used any more. Few studies have shown that biparametric MR imaging, using only T2-weighted and DWI, offers similar diagnostic accuracy for prostate cancer detection in addition to a decrease in

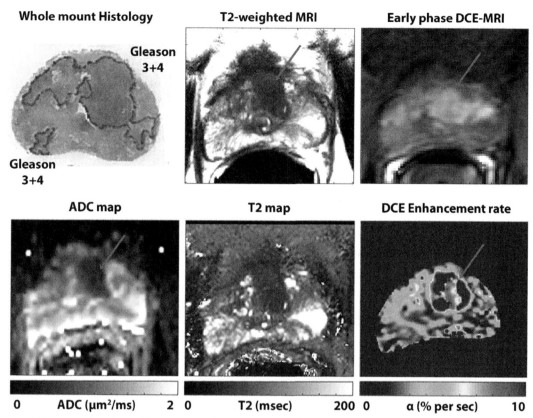

Fig. 2. A 67-year-old patient with a preoperative prostate-specific antigen level of 9.45 ng/mL. The Gleason 3 + 4 prostate cancer lesion (*red arrow*) is hypointense on T2-weighted images and apparent diffusion coefficient (ADC) mapping and demonstrates early focal enhancement on dynamic contrasted-enhanced MR imaging. Quantitate multiparametric MR imaging parameters from the lesion shows an apparent diffusion coefficient of 0.58 ± 0.09 μm²/ms, T2 = 60.6 ± 8.2 ms, and a dynamic contrasted-enhanced MR imaging (DCE-MRI) signal enhancement rate of 10.4% per second.

imaging time compared with that of conventional multiparametric MR imaging including DCE-MR imaging.[49–51] Other accelerated acquisition and reconstruction methods that have been investigated, including k-t-T2,[22] high temporal resolution or ultrafast DCE,[35] sensitivity encoding, and spiral or radial imaging. Another technique that has garnered a lot of attention is MR fingerprinting.[52] Although it allows rapid, simultaneous generation of quantitative maps of multiple physical properties such as T1 and T2, it has inherent drawbacks for prostate cancer diagnosis because it only provides similar images to standard multiparametric MR imaging.[53]

The most widely accepted MR parameters (eg, ADC, T2 and T1 values) used for prostate cancer detection clinically provide little information regarding the underlying complex microstructure or histology (Gleason grading), which remains the reference standard.[33,54] Tissue composition in prostate cancer is different from normal prostate.[55–58] Recently proposed prostate tissue structural models include the VERDICT model[59] and Luminal volume imaging,[60] which use increased cellularity

and reduced luminal fluid as the primary markers for cancer detection. Hybrid multidimensional MR imaging[61] was recently proposed, which exploits the distinct MR properties of tissue components,[62,63] to estimate fractional volumes of the prostate gland components. Prostate cancers show increased epithelium and reduced lumen and stroma volume compared with benign tissue, and these changes correlate with Gleason grade better than conventional ADC and T2. A representative example of tissue composition map estimated noninvasively through hybrid multidimensional MR imaging and its usefulness in prostate cancer detection is shown in **Fig. 3**.

There have been recent debates regarding the use of gadolinium-based contrast agents owing to the concerns with the deposition of gadolinium in tissue, especially in the brain, liver, bone, and skin.[64,65] Although there are no clinical consequences of gadolinium deposition, there are calls for improved and different approaches despite the diagnostic benefits of contrast agents.[66] Preliminary results suggest that DCE-MR imaging

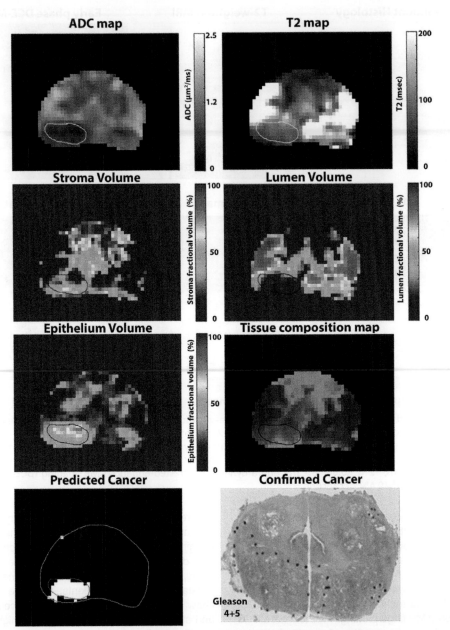

Fig. 3. Hybrid multidimensional MR imaging for the diagnosis of prostate cancer through noninvasive estimation of prostate tissue composition. A 60-year-old patient with a preoperative prostate-specific antigen level of 7.19 ng/mL. The Gleason 4 + 5 prostate cancer lesion (ROI) in the right peripheral zone shows elevated volume of epithelium (55%), reduced stroma (34%) and lumen (11%) volume, and reduced apparent diffusion coefficient (0.71 um²/ms) and T2 (105.6 ms) with respect to surrounding benign tissue.

with low gadolinium dose contrast agent[67] or high relaxivity agent[68] can distinguish prostate cancer from benign prostate tissue as effectively as the standard dose. A representative example showing a diagnosis of prostate cancer using low quantities (15% of standard clinical dose) of a high relaxivity contrast agent is shown in **Fig. 4**. Additionally, newly synthesized contrast agents such as iron[69] and vanadium based contrast agents[70] are being

investigated and will possibly be used in future multiparametric MR imaging protocols.

Interpretation

The findings from the recent studies such as the PROMIS[9] and PRECISION[10] clinical trials supports the use of multiparametric MR imaging before patients undergo biopsies to determine the location

Whole mount Histology

Gleason 3+4

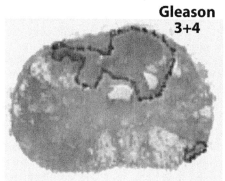

T2-weighted MRI

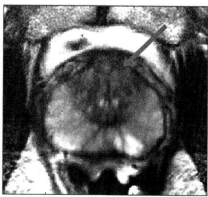

Standard clinical dose Early phase DCE-MRI

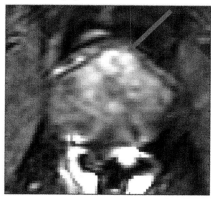

Low dose (15% of clinical dose) Early phase DCE-MRI

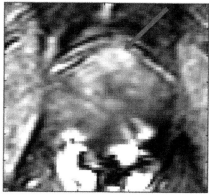

Fig. 4. Dynamic contrasted-enhanced MR imaging (DCE-MRI) using low dose (15% of standard clinical dose) gadolinium contrast agent (gadobenate dimeglumine, Multihance, Bracco) for a 44-year-old patient with a preoperative prostate-specific antigen level of 25.0 ng/mL. The Gleason 3 + 4 anterior prostate cancer lesion (*red arrow*) shows early enhancement on DCE MR imaging for both a low and standard clinical dose.

of the biopsy targets.[11] In addition, multiparametric MR imaging is more cost effective, which will lead to increased acceptance of multiparametric MR imaging for prostate cancer screening. However, numerous studies have shown high interobserver variability in the interpretation of multiparametric MR imaging among radiologists.[13] In addition, the experience of radiologists affects their performance.[13] However, the introduction of PI RADS v2 has led to the standardization of multiparametric MR imaging interpretation and improved reader agreement.[16] Another problem is that the prostate is a complex organ with different prostatic zones that appear differently on multiparametric MR imaging sequences and this property makes prostate cancer detection different in these zones.[12] Therefore, further standardization in the interpretation of multiparametric MR imaging (preferably with quantitative analysis) and training of radiologists will be an important consideration in the future.

There is no clear consensus about the definition of clinically significant cancer. Currently, the consensus is that any lesion with Gleason score 3 + 4 or greater and a volume of 0.5 mL or greater is considered clinically significant cancer. Although the Gleason grading system remains the standard, there are inherent problems with this system. For example, the Gleason grading system does not differentiate between 2 Gleason 3 + 4 cancer lesions, one with 40% volume covered with Gleason pattern 4 compared with another lesion with only 10% Gleason pattern. The lesion 40% with Gleason pattern 4 is likely to be more aggressive owing to the proliferative nature of higher Gleason pattern cancer. There is also substantial interobserver variation between pathologists for assigning Gleason score.

Computer-aided diagnosis (CAD) and artificial intelligence tools have recently been investigated for prostate cancer diagnosis using multiparametric MR imaging data to mitigate the problems with variability in prostate cancer diagnosis among radiologists. Numerous studies have shown promising results; however, a low specificity using CAD and lack of validation using multicenter studies remains as a major concern.[71–73] More recently, deep learning, neural networking, and risk map analysis tools have shown encouraging results (area under the receiver operating characteristic curve well over 0.8).[74–77] In addition, features such as lesion shape, size, heterogeneity, and histogram analysis may add additional useful diagnostic information. Because CAD is more sensitive to subtle changes, its role might be even more critical for focal therapy planning, especially to determine the optimal treatment option by differentiating between clinically significant and nonsignificant cancers and in determining the cancer tumor volume to decrease the number of recurrences owing to incomplete ablation of cancer tissue. **Fig. 5** shows a representative example of CAD risk map tool.

The biophysical basis of MR signal changes in prostate is still not clearly understood. The hypointense signal of prostate cancer on ADC maps and T2-weighted images is attributed to increased cellularity and a loss of extracellular space/fluid. However, new studies show that different tissue components have distinct MR properties[62] and these changes in tissue composition with the cancer including a different Gleason grade can explain the changes in MR signal.[58] In DCE-MR imaging, early focal signal enhancement of the cancer is attributed to angiogenesis.[26,27] However, new results support differential uptake of contrast by tissue components.[78] Hence, there is no clear consensus among the radiology community. A better understanding the underlying biophysical basis of signal changes and exploiting the distinctive MR properties of tissue components (specifically epithelium, because most cancers including prostate cancer are epithelial in nature) may be the key to the development of new clinical prostate cancer imaging techniques to detect prostate cancer and probe the tumor microenvironment.[79]

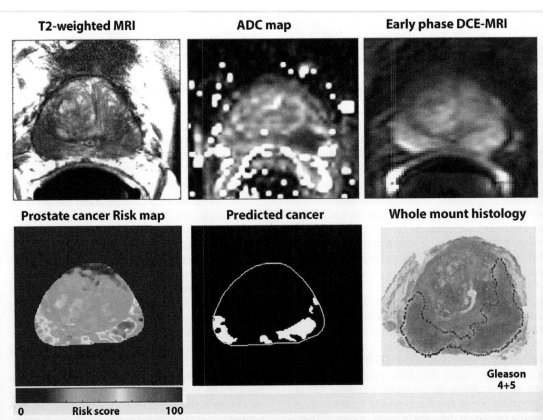

Fig. 5. A representative example of the use of computer-aided diagnosis for prostate cancer diagnosis in a 69-year-old patient with a preoperative prostate-specific antigen level of 26.13 ng/mL. The Gleason 4 + 5 prostate cancer lesion in both the left and right peripheral zones shows higher risk scores based on quantitative multiparametric MR imaging and is correctly predicted for prostate cancer presence. ADC, apparent diffusion coefficient; DCE-MRI, dynamic contrasted-enhanced MR imaging.

Integration of Clinical, Imaging, Pathology, and Genomics Data

In the future, it will be advantageous to integrate clinical data and other imaging techniques for improved prostate cancer diagnosis and for choosing the optimal treatment option for patients. New hybrid imaging techniques have potential for improving prostate cancer diagnosis. Positron emission tomography (PET), especially using prostate-specific membrane antigen tracers have shown great sensitivity for detecting aggressive cancers and for tumor staging. PET along with MR imaging combines the good soft tissue contrast, prostate anatomy, and high spatial resolution from MR imaging, along with the functional and molecular information provided by PET,[80] and provides improved accuracy for prostate cancer diagnosis than MR imaging alone.[81] New prostate-specific membrane antigen tracers will further improve the diagnostic accuracy in the future (**Fig. 6**).

Clinical data, in addition to MR imaging, have been shown to improve prostate cancer diagnosis and guide us in choosing the optimal treatment option.[82,83] Radiologists' interpretation of multiparametric MR imaging can be improved by correlating underlying tissue histology with their appearance on multiparametric MR imaging. Pathology results in addition to biopsy Gleason score, such as tissue composition estimated noninvasively using hybrid multidimensional MR imaging,[61] luminal volume imaging,[60] or VERDICT[59] can add to diagnosis using multiparametric MR imaging. An example of tissue composition estimated noninvasively using hybrid multidimensional MR imaging being validated by quantitative histology is shown in **Fig. 7**. While new molecular markers such Ki-67, hypoxia-inducible factor-1α, and vascular endothelial growth factor can used along with multiparametric MR imaging to understanding the tumor proliferation, hypoxia, and angiogenesis.[84]

There is an increasing interest in correlating prostate cancer genomics[85–87] with quantitative MR data. A recent study has shown that genomic profiling based on a biopsy-based 17-gene reverse transcriptase polymerase chain reaction assay may provide nonoverlapping information to multiparametric MR imaging that can result in an improved prostate cancer diagnosis.[88] Similarly, genetic markers such as phosphatase and tensin homolog gene can be used as a biomarker for prostate cancer presence. MR imaging can be used to identify and target the foci of cancer that carry the highest genomic risk.

MR-Guided Interventions and Follow-up

In addition to targeted biopsies, multiparametric MR imaging is also increasing being used to guide treatment and focal therapy. Focal therapy is an emerging paradigm and several different energies have been used under MR guidance including laser,[89–91] high-intensity focused ultrasound treatment,[92] and cryoablation.[93] Focal therapy aims to eradicate cancer while minimizing complications that can affect the quality of life. Focal therapy guided by multiparametric MR imaging has shown high success rates, with no reported mortality so far owing to these procedures, along with very good rates of avoiding incontinence and impotence. Therefore, these techniques are well-positioned to leverage the good soft tissue contrast and real-time temperature information from MR imaging to treat intermediate risk prostate cancers that were previously in risk of

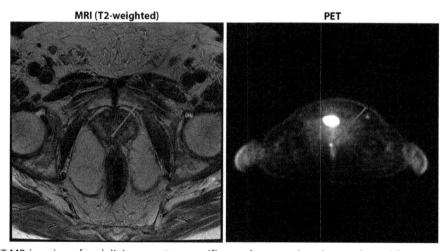

MRI (T2-weighted)　　　　**PET**

Fig. 6. PET-MR imaging of gadolinium prostate-specific membrane antigen in a patient with recurrent Gleason 3 + 3 prostate cancer (*red arrow*) after brachytherapy.

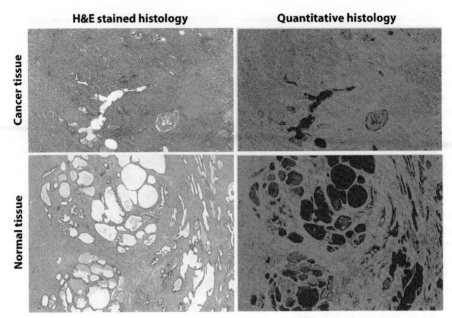

H&E stained histology   **Quantitative histology**

Cancer tissue

Normal tissue

Fig. 7. Quantitative histology performed on hematoxylin and eosin (H&E)–stained whole mount sections of the prostate tissue after radical prostatectomy to measure tissue composition (*green*, stroma; *red*, epithelium; *blue*, blue) in a 64-year-old patient with a prostate-specific antigen of 20.28 ng/mL. The tissue composition estimated by hybrid multidimensional MR imaging and quantitative histology showed good agreement for both Gleason 4 + 5 cancer (MR imaging: stroma = 50.3%, epithelium = 41.5%, lumen = 8.2%; histology: stroma = 46.0%, epithelium = 46.1%, lumen = 7.9%) and normal tissue (MR imaging: stroma = 46.4%, epithelium = 17.9%, lumen = 36.7%; Histology: stroma = 43.6%, epithelium = 24.2%, lumen = 32.2%).

undergoing more radical treatments such as radiotherapy or prostatectomy.[94] In addition, to the MR-guided therapy, multiparametric MR imaging can be used for active surveillance,[96] for tracking these procedures and following the long-term efficacy. However, the postprocedure changes and progression of disease at the ablation site are still not very well-studied. However, recent studies are starting to show that MR imaging can effectively be used to observe postablation changes in the prostate and can be a valuable tool for the follow-up of patients.[95] Therefore, in the future multiparametric MR imaging of the prostate will play a bigger role than just the diagnosis of prostate cancer.

SUMMARY

Prostate MR imaging has made huge advances since its earliest days using T2-weighted MR imaging only. The introduction of multiparametric approach and standardization based on PI-RADS v2 recommendations have improved the diagnosis of prostate cancer and led to its wider adoption. However, there remains a need for improvement before MR imaging becomes an accepted method for prostate cancer diagnosis and screening. In the future, we can expect to see the standardization of multiparametric MR imaging and an increased use

of quantitative multiparametric MR imaging, which will lead to more reproducible results and improved interpretation. The development of new acquisition techniques and use of artificial intelligence for image interpretation can lead to implementation of new clinical MR methods. Integration of other data (from modalities such as PET, clinical, genomics, and pathology) with multiparametric MR imaging can further enhance the potential of MR imaging.

REFERENCES

1. Siegel RL, Miller KD, Jemal A. Cancer statistics, 2016. CA Cancer J Clin 2016;66(1):7–30.
2. Cookson MM. Prostate cancer: screening and early detection. Cancer Control 2001;8(2):133–40.
3. Trpkov K, Yilmaz A, Bismar TA, et al. 'Insignificant' prostate cancer on prostatectomy and cystoprostatectomy: variation on a theme 'low-volume/low-grade' prostate cancer? BJU Int 2010;106(3):304–15.
4. Boccon-Gibod LM, Dumonceau O, Toublanc M, et al. Micro-focal prostate cancer: a comparison of biopsy and radical prostatectomy specimen features. Eur Urol 2005;48(6):895–9.
5. Gupta RT, Kauffman CR, Polascik TJ, et al. The state of prostate MRI in 2013. Oncology 2013;27(4):262.
6. Moldovan PC, Van den Broeck T, Sylvester R, et al. What is the negative predictive value of

multiparametric magnetic resonance imaging in excluding prostate cancer at biopsy? A systematic review and meta-analysis from the European Association of Urology Prostate Cancer Guidelines Panel. Eur Urol 2017;72(2):250–66.

7. Baur AD, Maxeiner A, Franiel T, et al. Evaluation of the prostate imaging reporting and data system for the detection of prostate cancer by the results of targeted biopsy of the prostate. Invest Radiol 2014; 49(6):411–20.

8. Weinreb JC, Barentsz JO, Choyke PL, et al. PI-RADS prostate imaging – reporting and data system: 2015, version 2. Eur Urol 2016;69(1):16–40.

9. Ahmed HU, El-Shater Bosaily A, Brown LC, et al. Diagnostic accuracy of multi-parametric MRI and TRUS biopsy in prostate cancer (PROMIS): a paired validating confirmatory study. Lancet 2017; 389(10071):815–22.

10. Kasivisvanathan V, Rannikko AS, Borghi M, et al. MRI-targeted or standard biopsy for prostate-cancer diagnosis. N Engl J Med 2018;378(19):1767–77.

11. Pahwa S, Schiltz NK, Ponsky LE, et al. Cost-effectiveness of MR imaging–guided strategies for detection of prostate cancer in biopsy-naive men. Radiology 2017;285(1):157–66.

12. Kitzing YX, Prando A, Varol C, et al. Benign conditions that mimic prostate carcinoma: MR imaging features with histopathologic correlation. Radiographics 2016;36(1):162–75.

13. Niaf E, Lartizien C, Bratan F, et al. Prostate focal peripheral zone lesions: characterization at multiparametric MR imaging—influence of a computer-aided diagnosis system. Radiology 2014;271(3):761–9.

14. Turkbey B, McKinney YL, Trivedi H, et al. Multiparametric 3T prostate magnetic resonance imaging to detect cancer: histopathological correlation using prostatectomy specimens processed in customized magnetic resonance imaging based molds. J Urol 2011;186(5):1818–24.

15. Vilanova JC, Barceló-Vidal C, Comet J, et al. Usefulness of prebiopsy multifunctional and morphologic MRI combined with free-to-total prostate-specific antigen ratio in the detection of prostate cancer. AJR Am J Roentgenol 2011;196(6):W715–22.

16. Rosenkrantz AB, Deng F-M, Kim S, et al. Prostate cancer: multiparametric MRI for index lesion localization– a multiple-reader study. AJR Am J Roentgenol 2012;199(4):830–7.

17. Greer MD, Brown AM, Shih JH, et al. Accuracy and agreement of PIRADSv2 for prostate cancer mpMRI: a multireader study. J Magn Reson Imaging 2017; 45(2):579–85.

18. Foltz WD, Chopra S, Chung P, et al. Clinical prostate T2 quantification using magnetization-prepared spiral imaging. Magn Reson Med 2010;64(4):1155–61.

19. Liney GP, Turnbull LW, Lowry M, et al. In vivo quantification of citrate concentration and water T2 relaxation time of the pathologic prostate gland using 1H MRS and MRI. Magn Reson Imaging 1997; 15(10):1177–86.

20. Hoang Dinh A, Souchon R, Melodelima C, et al. Characterization of prostate cancer using T2 mapping at 3 T: a multi-scanner study. Diagn Interv Imaging 2015;96(4):365–72.

21. Gibbs P, Tozer DJ, Liney GP, et al. Comparison of quantitative T2 mapping and diffusion-weighted imaging in the normal and pathologic prostate. Magn Reson Med 2001;46(6):1054–8.

22. Liu W, Turkbey B, Sénégas J, et al. Accelerated T(2) mapping for characterization of prostate cancer. Magn Reson Med 2011;65(5):1400–6.

23. Turkbey B, Merino MJ, Shih JH, et al. Is apparent diffusion coefficient associated with clinical risk scores for prostate cancers that are visible on 3-T MR images? Radiology 2011;258(2):488–95.

24. Wu L-M, Xu J-R, Gu H-Y, et al. Usefulness of diffusion-weighted magnetic resonance imaging in the diagnosis of prostate cancer. Acad Radiol 2012;19(10):1215–24.

25. Isebaert S, Van den Bergh L, Haustermans K, et al. Multiparametric MRI for prostate cancer localization in correlation to whole-mount histopathology. J Magn Reson Imaging 2013;37(6):1392–401.

26. de Rooij M, Hamoen EH, Fütterer JJ, et al. Accuracy of multiparametric MRI for prostate cancer detection: a meta-analysis. AJR Am J Roentgenol 2014; 202(2):343–51.

27. Kozlowski P, Chang SD, Jones EC, et al. Combined diffusion-weighted and dynamic contrast-enhanced MRI for prostate cancer diagnosis—Correlation with biopsy and histopathology. J Magn Reson Imaging 2006;24(1):108–13.

28. Othman AE, Falkner F, Weiss J, et al. Effect of temporal resolution on diagnostic performance of dynamic contrast-enhanced magnetic resonance imaging of the prostate. Invest Radiol 2016;51(5): 290–6.

29. Barentsz JO, Richenberg J, Clements R, et al. ESUR prostate MR guidelines 2012. Eur Radiol 2012;22(4): 746–57.

30. Esses SJ, Taneja SS, Rosenkrantz AB. Imaging facilities' adherence to PI-RADS v2 minimum technical standards for the performance of prostate MRI. Acad Radiol 2018;25(2):188–95.

31. Peng Y, Jiang Y, Antic T, et al. Apparent diffusion coefficient for prostate cancer imaging: impact of B values. AJR Am J Roentgenol 2014;202(3): W247–53.

32. Lemberskiy G, Rosenkrantz AB, Veraart J, et al. Time-dependent diffusion in prostate cancer. Invest Radiol 2017;52(7):405–11.

33. Bourne R, Panagiotaki E. Limitations and prospects for diffusion-weighted MRI of the prostate. Diagnostics (Basel) 2016;6(2):21.

34. Nolan P, Chatterjee A, Sun C, et al. Effect of echo times on prostate cancer detection on T2-weighted images. Paper presented at: The Cancer Imaging and Intervention Conference: Our multi-disciplinary approach. Houston (TX), April 5-8, 2018.

35. Chatterjee A, He D, Fan X, et al. Performance of ultrafast DCE-MRI for diagnosis of prostate cancer. Acad Radiol 2018;25(3):349–58.

36. Muller BG, Shih JH, Sankineni S, et al. Prostate cancer: interobserver agreement and accuracy with the revised prostate imaging reporting and data system at multiparametric MR imaging. Radiology 2015; 277(3):741–50.

37. Rosenkrantz AB, Zhang B, Ben-Eliezer N, et al. T2-weighted prostate MRI at 7 Tesla using a simplified external transmit-receive coil array: correlation with radical prostatectomy findings in two prostate cancer patients. J Magn Reson Imaging 2015;41(1): 226–32.

38. Turkbey B, Pinto PA, Mani H, et al. Prostate cancer: value of multiparametric MR imaging at 3 T for detection—histopathologic correlation. Radiology 2010;255(1):89–99.

39. Hagberg GE, Scheffler K. Effect of r1 and r2 relaxivity of gadolinium-based contrast agents on the T1-weighted MR signal at increasing magnetic field strengths. Contrast Media Mol Imaging 2013;8(6): 456–65.

40. Hardy CJ, Giaquinto RO, Piel JE, et al. 128-channel body MRI with a flexible high-density receiver-coil array. J Magn Reson Imaging 2008;28(5):1219–25.

41. Storås TH, Gjesdal K-I, Gadmar ØB, et al. Prostate magnetic resonance imaging: multiexponential T2 decay in prostate tissue. J Magn Reson Imaging 2008;28(5):1166–72.

42. Shinmoto H, Oshio K, Tanimoto A, et al. Biexponential apparent diffusion coefficients in prostate cancer. Magn Reson Imaging 2009;27(3):355–9.

43. Bihan DL, Breton E, Lallemand D, et al. Separation of diffusion and perfusion in intravoxel incoherent motion MR imaging. Radiology 1988;168(2):497–505.

44. Jensen JH, Helpern JA, Ramani A, et al. Diffusional kurtosis imaging: the quantification of non-Gaussian water diffusion by means of magnetic resonance imaging. Magn Reson Med 2005;53(6):1432–40.

45. Bennett KM, Schmainda KM, Bennett R, et al. Characterization of continuously distributed cortical water diffusion rates with a stretched-exponential model. Magn Reson Med 2003;50(4):727–34.

46. Chatterjee A, Devaraj A, Matthew M, et al. Performance of T2 maps in detection of prostate cancer. Acad Radiol 2018. [Epub ahead of print].

47. Tofts PS, Brix G, Buckley DL, et al. Estimating kinetic parameters from dynamic contrast-enhanced t1-weighted MRI of a diffusable tracer: standardized quantities and symbols. J Magn Reson Imaging 1999;10(3):223–32.

48. Fan X, Medved M, River JN, et al. New model for analysis of dynamic contrast-enhanced MRI data distinguishes metastatic from nonmetastatic transplanted rodent prostate tumors. Magn Reson Med 2004;51(3):487–94.

49. Kuhl CK, Bruhn R, Krämer N, et al. Abbreviated biparametric prostate MR imaging in men with elevated prostate-specific antigen. Radiology 2017;285(2):493–505.

50. Fascelli M, Rais-Bahrami S, Sankineni S, et al. Combined biparametric prostate magnetic resonance imaging and prostate-specific antigen in the detection of prostate cancer: a validation study in a biopsy-naive patient population. Urology 2016;88: 125–34.

51. Scialpi M, D'Andrea A, Martorana E, et al. Biparametric MRI of the prostate. Turk J Urol 2017;43(4): 401–9.

52. Ma D, Gulani V, Seiberlich N, et al. Magnetic resonance fingerprinting. Nature 2013;495(7440):187–92.

53. Yu AC, Badve C, Ponsky LE, et al. Development of a combined MR fingerprinting and diffusion examination for prostate cancer. Radiology 2017;283(3): 729–38.

54. Gleason DF. Classification of prostatic carcinomas. Cancer Chemother Rep 1966;50(3):125–8.

55. Langer DL, van der Kwast TH, Evans AJ, et al. Prostate tissue composition and MR measurements: investigating the relationships between ADC, T2, K(trans), v(e), and corresponding histologic features. Radiology 2010;255(2):485–94.

56. Kobus T, van der Laak JA, Maas MC, et al. Contribution of histopathologic tissue composition to quantitative MR spectroscopy and diffusion-weighted imaging of the prostate. Radiology 2015;278(3): 801–11.

57. Zhao M, Myint E, Watson G, et al. Comparison of conventional histology and diffusion weighted microimaging for estimation of epithelial, stromal, and acinar volumes in prostate tissue. In Proceedings of the 21st Annual Meeting of ISMRM. Salt Lake City (UT), April 20-26, 2013.

58. Chatterjee A, Watson G, Myint E, et al. Changes in epithelium, stroma, and lumen space correlate more strongly with Gleason pattern and are stronger predictors of prostate ADC changes than cellularity metrics. Radiology 2015;277(3):751–62.

59. Panagiotaki E, Chan RW, Dikaios N, et al. Microstructural characterization of normal and malignant human prostate tissue with vascular, extracellular and restricted diffusion for cytometry in tumours magnetic resonance imaging. Invest Radiol 2015; 50(4):218–27.

60. Sabouri S, Chang SD, Savdie R, et al. Luminal water imaging: a new MR imaging T2 mapping technique for prostate cancer diagnosis. Radiology 2017; 284(2):451–9.

61. Chatterjee A, Bourne R, Wang S, et al. Diagnosis of prostate cancer with noninvasive estimation of prostate tissue composition by using hybrid multidimensional MR imaging: a feasibility study. Radiology 2018;287(3):864–73.

62. Bourne RM, Kurniawan N, Cowin G, et al. Microscopic diffusivity compartmentation in formalin-fixed prostate tissue. Magn Reson Med 2012;68(2):614–20.

63. Bourne R, Kurniawan N, Cowin G, et al. 16 T diffusion microimaging of fixed prostate tissue: preliminary findings. Magn Reson Med 2011;66(1):244–7.

64. Kanda T, Ishii K, Kawaguchi H, et al. High signal intensity in the dentate nucleus and globus pallidus on unenhanced T1-weighted MR images: relationship with increasing cumulative dose of a gadolinium-based contrast material. Radiology 2014;270(3):834–41.

65. Robert P, Frenzel T, Factor C, et al. Methodological aspects for preclinical evaluation of gadolinium presence in brain tissue: critical appraisal and suggestions for harmonization—a joint initiative. Invest Radiol 2018;53(9):499–517.

66. Runge VM, Heverhagen JT. Advocating the development of next-generation high-relaxivity gadolinium chelates for clinical magnetic resonance. Invest Radiol 2018;53(7):381–9.

67. He D, Chatterjee A, Fan X, et al. Feasibility of dynamic contrast enhanced MRI using low dose Gadolinium: comparative performance with standard dose in prostate cancer diagnosis. Invest Radiol 2018;53(10):609–15.

68. Huang B, Liang CH, Liu HJ, et al. Low-dose contrast-enhanced magnetic resonance imaging of brain metastases at 3.0 T using high-relaxivity contrast agents. Acta Radiol 2010;51(1):78–84.

69. Boehm-Sturm P, Haeckel A, Hauptmann R, et al. Low-molecular-weight iron chelates may be an alternative to gadolinium-based contrast agents for T1-weighted contrast-enhanced MR imaging. Radiology 2018;286(2):537–46.

70. Mustafi D, Ward J, Dougherty U, et al. X-ray fluorescence microscopy demonstrates preferential accumulation of a vanadium-based magnetic resonance imaging contrast agent in murine colonic tumors. Mol Imaging 2015;14:14.

71. Litjens G, Debats O, Barentsz J, et al. Computer-aided detection of prostate cancer in MRI. IEEE Trans Med Imaging 2014;33(5):1083–92.

72. Vos PC, Hambrock T, Hulsbergen - van de Kaa CA, et al. Computerized analysis of prostate lesions in the peripheral zone using dynamic contrast enhanced MRI. Med Phys 2008;35(3):888–99.

73. Firjani A, Khalifa F, Elnakib A, et al. A novel image-based approach for early detection of prostate cancer. Paper presented at: 2012 19th IEEE International Conference on Image Processing (ICIP 2012). Orlando (FL), September 30 - October 3, 2012.

74. Chatterjee A, He D, Fan X, et al. Diagnosis of prostate cancer using risk maps derived from quantitative multi-parametric MRI. SAR 2018 Annual Scientific Meeting and Educational Course. Scottsdale (AZ), March 4-9, 2018.

75. Wang X, Yang W, Weinreb J, et al. Searching for prostate cancer by fully automated magnetic resonance imaging classification: deep learning versus non-deep learning. Sci Rep 2017;7(1):15415.

76. Le MH, Chen J, Wang L, et al. Automated diagnosis of prostate cancer in multi-parametric MRI based on multimodal convolutional neural networks. Phys Med Biol 2017;62(16):6497–514.

77. Peng Y, Jiang Y, Yang C, et al. Quantitative analysis of multiparametric prostate MR images: differentiation between prostate cancer and normal tissue and correlation with Gleason score—a computer-aided diagnosis development study. Radiology 2013;267(3):787–96.

78. Mustafi D, Gleber S-C, Ward J, et al. IV administered gadodiamide enters the lumen of the prostatic glands: x-ray fluorescence microscopy examination of a mouse model. AJR Am J Roentgenol 2015; 205(3):W313–9.

79. Bourne R, Power C, Chatterjee A, et al. Distinctive water diffusion properties of epithelia may be the key to better cancer imaging techniques. Paper presented at: Sydney Cancer Conference. Sydney, November 27-28, 2014.

80. Wetter A, Lipponer C, Nensa F, et al. Simultaneous 18F choline positron emission tomography/magnetic resonance imaging of the prostate: initial results. Invest Radiol 2013;48(5):256–62.

81. de Perrot T, Rager O, Scheffler M, et al. Potential of hybrid (1)(8)F-fluorocholine PET/MRI for prostate cancer imaging. Eur J Nucl Med Mol Imaging 2014;41(9):1744–55.

82. Mehralivand S, Shih JH, Rais-Bahrami S, et al. A magnetic resonance imaging–based prediction model for prostate biopsy risk stratification. JAMA Oncol 2018;4(5):678–85.

83. Li J, Weng Z, Xu H, et al. Support Vector Machines (SVM) classification of prostate cancer Gleason score in central gland using multiparametric magnetic resonance images: a cross-validated study. Eur J Radiol 2018;98:61 7.

84. Ma T, Yang S, Jing H, et al. Apparent diffusion coefficients in prostate cancer: correlation with molecular markers Ki-67, HIF-1alpha and VEGF. NMR Biomed 2018;31(3):9.

85. Rubin MA, Demichelis F. The Genomics of Prostate Cancer: emerging understanding with technologic advances. Mod Pathol 2018;31(S1):166.

86. VanderWeele DJ, Turkbey B, Sowalsky AG. Precision management of localized prostate cancer. Expert Rev Precis Med Drug Dev 2016;1(6): 505 15.

87. VanderWeele DJ, McCann S, Fan X, et al. Radiogenomics of prostate cancer: association between quantitative multiparametric MRI features and PTEN. J Clin Oncol 2015;33(7_suppl): 126.

88. Leapman MS, Westphalen AC, Ameli N, et al. Association between a 17-gene genomic prostate score and multi-parametric prostate MRI in men with low and intermediate risk prostate cancer (PCa). PLoS One 2017;12(10):e0185535.

89. Oto A, Sethi I, Karczmar G, et al. MR imaging–guided focal laser ablation for prostate cancer: phase I trial. Radiology 2013;267(3):932–40.

90. Eggener SE, Yousuf A, Watson S, et al. Phase II evaluation of magnetic resonance imaging guided focal laser ablation of prostate cancer. J Urol 2016;196(6): 1670–5.

91. Mehralivand S, George A, Hoang A, et al. MP26-10 Magnetic resonance imaging guided focal laser therapy of prostate cancer: follow up results from a single center phase I trial. J Urol 2018;199(4): e339–40.

92. Schulman AA, Tay KJ, Robertson CN, et al. High-intensity focused ultrasound for focal therapy: reality or pitfall? Curr Opin Urol 2017;27(2):138–48.

93. Ellis DS, Manny TB Jr, Rewcastle JC. Focal cryosurgery followed by penile rehabilitation as primary treatment for localized prostate cancer: initial results. Urology 2007;70(6 Suppl):9–15.

94. Walser EM, Sze TF, Ross JR, et al. MRI-guided prostate interventions. AJR Am J Roentgenol 2016; 207(4):755–63.

95. Westin C, Chatterjee A, Ku E, et al. MRI findings following MRI guided focal laser ablation of prostate cancer. AJR Am J Roentgenol 2018;211(3):595–604.

96. Bloom JB, Gold SA, Hale GR, et al. "Super-active surveillance": MRI ultrasound fusion biopsy and ablation for less invasive management of prostate cancer. Gland Surgery 2018;7:166–87.

MR Imaging–Guided Focal Therapies of Prostate Cancer

Melvy Sarah Mathew, MD*, Aytekin Oto, MD, MBA

KEYWORDS

- Cryotherapy • Laser ablation • HIFU • High-intensity focused ultrasound • MR imaging guidance
- Multiparametric MR imaging

KEY POINTS

- A greater number of small-volume, low-risk, and intermediate-risk prostate cancers are being detected.
- Multiparametric MR imaging serves as a valuable method of assessing the prostate gland for cancer in patients with high clinical suspicion of malignancy.
- Once detected, a suspected cancerous lesion in the prostate gland can be subsequently targeted for focal therapy using MR imaging for guidance.
- Early data relating to the use of MR imaging–guided focal therapies, including cryotherapy, high-intensity focused ultrasound, and focal laser ablation, have been promising.

BACKGROUND

Prostate cancer is a major cause of death among men, preceded only by lung cancer in the United States.[1] There has been an increase in the number of prostate cancer cases, localized and low-grade tumors in particular, leading to an interest in the development of alternative treatment methods with fewer complications.[2] The growing number of cases of prostate cancer diagnosed can be attributed in part to a greater reliance on prostate-specific antigen (PSA) as a harbinger of malignancy as well as the adoption of an overall lower clinical threshold for the performance of prostate tissue sampling.[2] Although the US Preventive Services Task Force (USPSTF) advised against the use of PSA as a screening mechanism for certain patients, that is, men of 70 years of age or older, the USPSTF recently updated stance recommends that clinicians conduct periodic checks of serum PSA levels in patients between the ages of 55 and 69.[3] Elevated PSA levels and abnormal digital rectal examinations represent the 2 major criteria currently used in the determination of a patient's need for prostate biopsy.

DIAGNOSIS AND TREATMENT OF PROSTATE CANCER

The traditional method of acquiring tissue samples of the prostate in a patient suspected of having cancer is to pursue a 12-core biopsy of the gland using a transrectal sonographic approach.[4] This conventional transrectal ultrasound (TRUS)-guided biopsy, however, has several disadvantages. Among these is the failure of a TRUS biopsy to consistently reach the apex of the prostate or the anterior aspect of the gland.[5] This leads to undersampling of these areas and missing anterior and apical cancers. In addition, there may be difficulty in the reliable detection of prostate cancer using sonography.[6] For these reasons, it is not

Dr M.S. Mathew has a research grant from Guerbet. Dr A. Oto has research grants from Philips, Profound, and Guerbet. He is on the Medical Advisory Board for Profound.
Department of Radiology, University of Chicago, 5841 South Maryland Avenue, Chicago, IL 60637, USA
* Corresponding author.
E-mail address: mmathew@radiology.bsd.uchicago.edu

Magn Reson Imaging Clin N Am 27 (2019) 131–138
https://doi.org/10.1016/j.mric.2018.08.004
1064-9689/19/© 2018 Elsevier Inc. All rights reserved.

entirely surprising that the rate of false-negative results after a TRUS-guided biopsy is high: up to 47% of patients may have an undetected prostate cancer after sampling.[4] Another problem with random biopsy is the unreliable Gleason score yielded by these biopsies. In approximately 30% of cases, the Gleason score obtained on random biopsy is upgraded on repeat tissue sampling or after prostatectomy.[7,8]

A more reliable method of detecting and diagnosing prostate cancer is multiparametric MR imaging. Prostate cancer has characteristic MR imaging features, including hypointense signal on T2-weighted imaging, low apparent diffusion coefficient (ADC) signal (restricted diffusion), and early arterial enhancement with subsequent washout on dynamic contrast-enhanced imaging.[9] MR imaging has been increasingly used for identification of targets for biopsy, and targeted biopsy is rapidly emerging as an alternative and more superior diagnostic paradigm.[9–11] Depending on the experience level of the radiologist reading the MR imaging examination, the accuracy of detection of prostate cancer can range between 70% and 90%.[9]

Once a suspicious site is identified on multiparametric MR imaging, MR imaging can be used either directly or indirectly to guide future biopsy of the prostate gland. With the direct method, tissue sampling is done in-bore while the patient is positioned within the scanner. When MR imaging is used in an indirect manner to perform a biopsy of the prostate gland, it is most often achieved through the use of an MR imaging/ultrasound fusion computer platform. In this scenario, the patient's earlier diagnostic MR images are able to be fused with real-time sonographic images and serve to guide the trajectory of the core biopsy needle during the procedure. The targeted biopsy paradigm has allowed for a more reliable and accurate mapping of cancer within the prostate gland and improved characterization of cancer aggressiveness at the time of diagnosis.

There are several therapy options currently available to patients diagnosed with prostate cancer, including whole-gland treatment, active surveillance, and, the latest approach, focal therapy. The primary aim of focal therapy is to selectively direct treatment to the index or largest in size cancerous prostatic lesion, while in the process avoiding inadvertent damage to critical locoregional anatomic structures. Among these are the neurovascular bundles, the adjacent urethra and urethral sphincter, the urinary bladder, and the rectum. Focally directed and less-invasive treatment approaches are advantageous, particularly in comparison to whole-gland treatment options,

such as a radical prostatectomy, where a greater incidence of post-prostatectomy complications, such as impotence and urinary continence, has been encountered.[12,13] In addition to clinical factors and patient and physician preference, other criteria used in the determination of whether an individual with localized prostate cancer is a satisfactory candidate for focal treatment are Gleason score of 6 or 7, a PSA level measuring less than 15 ng/mL, and a clinical stage of T1c to T2a, as defined by an international consensus group.[14]

PROS AND CONS OF FOCAL THERAPY

Focal therapy is an established paradigm in the treatment of several different cancers, including breast, kidney, thyroid, colon, lung, and liver. Its main advantage in the management of prostate cancer is its association with fewer complications while eradicating the cancer. Focal therapy for prostate cancer is a minimally invasive treatment that can be performed under conscious sedation or with spinal anesthesia without the need to admit patients overnight. Patients can return to their normal life immediately after the procedure. Another advantage of focal therapy is that it does not close the door to potential future whole-gland therapies. One of the main disadvantages of focal therapy is the multifocality of prostate cancer. Prostate cancer is multifocal 80% of the time[15] and focal therapy can only address the index lesion, which is typically the focus with the highest Gleason score and with the largest volume.[16] There is growing evidence that the index lesion determines the prognosis of the patient and, therefore, it may be adequate to ablate the index lesion.[17] Nevertheless, the main goal of focal therapy should be to treat patients with intermediate-risk prostate cancer who otherwise would need whole-gland therapy instead of treating patients with low-risk cancer who could benefit from active surveillance.

MR IMAGING–GUIDED FOCAL TREATMENTS

The most commonly used and studied methods of focal therapy for prostate cancer are cryotherapy, high-intensity focused ultrasound (HIFU), and laser ablation. These treatments offer patients alternatives to prostatectomy or radiation therapy and have been found efficacious in treating localized prostate cancer in a comparatively less-invasive manner. Patients undergoing MR imaging–guided tissue-sparing treatments, such as cryotherapy, HIFU, and focal laser ablation, are not entirely spared from the possibility of experiencing adverse side effects, among which are injury to the urethra, nerve damage, and bowel injury. Preventative measures, however, discussed in greater detail later, are taken during the course of all of these treatment procedures and aid in reducing such untoward sequelae.

Cryotherapy

Consisting of a freezing method used to achieve cellular disruption, cryotherapy is an increasingly used treatment method for prostate cancer. Using a transperineal approach, needles are placed in the prostate and the gland is cooled using argon probes.[18] Thermocouples monitor the patient's body temperature and a transurethral Foley catheter is placed in an effort to prevent urinary complications, including urethral sloughing and incontinence. Saline instilled into the perirectal space has a protective effect on the rectum.[18] Additionally, thermosensors are placed at several anatomic sites, among them the external anal sphincter, the prostate apex, and the neurovascular bundles.[19]

Cryotherapy causes cell apoptosis through the formation of ice crystals at the target site. As a result of the directed cold temperatures, there are cellular dehydration and destruction.[20] Several treatment variables have been found to contribute to a more successful post-therapy outcome: the lowest temperature reached during treatment (a temperature measuring $<-40°C$ is ideal), the rate at which cooling occurs during the freezing step, the length of time during which the freezing occurs, the velocity at which thawing takes place, the number of freeze-thaw cycles used (more extensive tissue damage is typically seen with the incorporation of a double freeze-thaw cycle), and whether there are enlarged vessels present.[21] During the cooling phase, argon gas is used, and helium gas is used in the thawing phase.[19]

Use of multiparametric MR imaging for guidance when performing cryotherapy has proved more beneficial than using the traditional method of TRUS imaging.[2,20] In the latter case, real-time evaluation during treatment may be impeded by the reflection of sound waves adjacent to the ultrasound probe, leading to an inaccurate assessment of the zone of treatment. Additionally, the ice ball formed during cryotherapy is better visualized on MR imaging than on sonography. Typical findings on follow-up MR imaging after cryotherapy include the appearance of hypovascularity and focal signal void at the site of treatment. See **Fig. 1** for an example of a postprocedural MR imaging appearance of the prostate after cryotherapy of a discrete cancerous lesion.

Research investigations have shown promising results for the treatment of focal prostate cancer with cryotherapy. Among 73 recipients of hemigland cryotherapy in a study led by Bahn and colleagues,[21] only a single patient developed ipsilateral recurrent cancer; in addition, none of the patients who received treatment developed post-therapy urinary incontinence. Another investigation directed by Onik and colleagues[22] found that 45 of 48 patients treated with locoregional cryoablation demonstrated stable PSA values and no evidence of cancer post-treatment. Although there remains a need for additional randomized clinical trials comparing cryotherapy to other regional therapies, early findings support cryotherapy as a promising treatment method for individuals with focal prostatic malignancy.

High-Intensity Focused Ultrasound

Using high-frequency sonographic waves, HIFU can successfully treat a cancerous focus in the prostate gland. A patient undergoing HIFU treatment receives either general or spinal anesthesia for the procedure. A spherical ultrasound transducer is used and the energy from the resultant ultrasound waves is applied to the region of interest in the prostate gland.[23,24] In this manner,

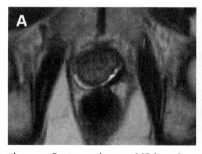
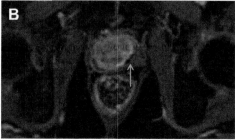

Fig. 1. Cryotherapy. Post-cryotherapy MR imaging of a 72-year-old man with a history of a left midgland peripheral zone prostate adenocarcinoma demonstrates asymmetric focal volume loss at the site of treatment. (A) T2-weighted imaging shows ill-defined or amorphous dark signal in the area of treatment in the left midgland. (B) Postcontrast imaging of the prostate gland in the axial plane at the midgland level demonstrates thin linear hypointense signal (arrow) at the treatment site without evidence of focal nodular enhancement.

coagulative necrosis and cell death are achieved at the site of the cancer. Heat is applied to the cancerous focus for a few seconds (typically 3 seconds), and this is followed by a cooling period of approximately 6 seconds.[24] After HIFU therapy, there are corresponding expected signal changes on MR imaging and the zone of treatment may appear cystic with correlating increased T2 signal intensity and regional hypovascularity on contrast-enhanced imaging. See **Figs. 2** and **3** for examples depicting MR imaging findings related to HIFU treatment of regional prostate cancer.

In a study led by Ahmed and colleagues,[25] HIFU was delivered to a group of individuals with histories of low-risk and intermediate-risk prostate cancers. Up to 95% of the patients who were studied reported preserved urinary incontinence after 1 year. Persistent cancer, however, was seen in more than 20% of the men who were rebiopsied.[25] In addition, although 31 of the 35 patients

assessed stated that erectile function for intercourse was overall acceptable, the scores associated with orgasmic function and overall erectile satisfaction were significantly below baseline.[25] Continued follow-up is necessary to better understand long-term treatment outcomes after HIFU therapy.[25,26]

Focal Laser Ablation

Another increasingly used MR imaging–directed method of treating regional prostate cancer is laser ablation. Focal laser therapy consists of the delivery of thermal energy or high-energy photons to the region of interest. Tumor necrosis ensues as a result of this method of rapid heating. The soft tissues of the prostate gland are relatively hypovascular and this in conjunction with its inherent optical absorption rate makes prostatic tissue particularly responsive to laser ablation.[27] At the

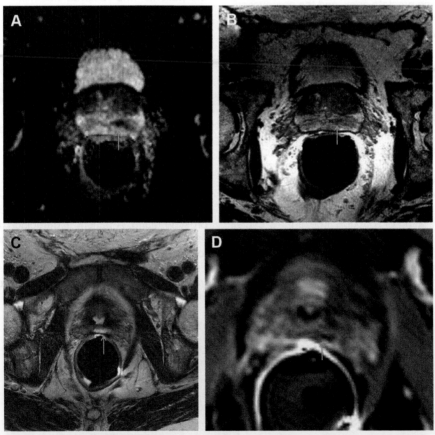

Fig. 2. HIFU treatment. MR imaging of a 61-year-old patient pre-HIFU and post-HIFU treatment of a left-sided Gleason 6 prostate cancer located in the peripheral zone of the medial left midgland/base (*arrows*). (*A*) The peripheral zone cancerous focus in the left midgland/base demonstrates low ADC signal on pretherapy imaging. (*B*) The lesion shows corresponding T2 hypointense signal. (*C*) After HIFU therapy, focal cystic change is seen in the medial left midgland/base, including at site of preexisting cancerous lesion. (*D*) On post-treatment contrast-enhanced MR imaging, there is localized nonenhancement in the region of the patient's original left-sided prostate cancer.

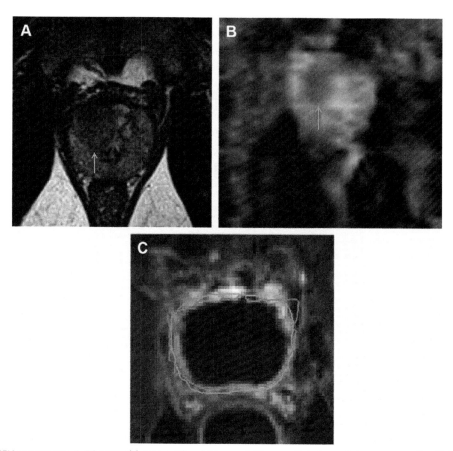

Fig. 3. HIFU treatment. A 56-year-old man with a history of Gleason 3 + 4 prostate cancer and a PSA value of 8.1 ng/mL underwent HIFU therapy for a right-sided transition zone cancer evident on MR imaging (*arrows*). (*A*) A rounded T2 hypointense lesion is identified in the right transition zone of the gland. (*B*) The lesion demonstrates restricted diffusion with corresponding decreased ADC signal visualized. (*C*) Post-treatment dynamic MR imaging after the administration of intravenous contrast shows expected avascularity of the gland. The green/yellow lines are indicative of the region of interest, the prostate gland.

start of the procedure and using MR imaging for guidance, optical fibers are placed in the prostate gland using a transperineal route. The efficacy of locoregional laser treatment is dependent on the depth of photon dispersal and the amount of heat energy distributed. It is helpful to reach a minimum temperature of 60°C to better ensure tumor destruction. Fluoroptic or MR-directed thermometry is used to assess the effects of treatment on the rectum and other critical anatomic structures. In addition to its ability to target a lesion exactly, focal laser ablation has several other benefits, including its ability to assess therapy effects in a real-time fashion and at a low cost. Additionally, laser fibers used in the procedure are MR imaging compatible. There is also no distortion of the electromagnetic field by the optical fibers; thus, image degradation or MR imaging artifacts at the treatment site do not pose a problem.[20] Prefocal and postfocal laser ablation findings on MR imaging are shown in **Fig. 4**.

Several research investigations have demonstrated the clinical efficacy of focal laser ablation in treating regional prostate malignancy. At the University of Chicago, a phase I trial led by Oto and colleagues[28] was conducted in 2013 to evaluate the feasibility of focal laser ablation in the treatment of low-risk prostate cancer; postablation biopsy of the treatment zone demonstrated no evidence of malignancy in 7 of the 9 patients included in the study. In 2016, a phase II trial at the institution also deemed focal laser ablation a safe form of treatment; patients assessed 1 year after therapy were found to have satisfactory morbidity rates and clinical outcomes.[29] Raz and colleagues[30] conducted a feasibility study in 2010 confirming that regional laser ablation is a successful method of treatment of prostate cancer; 2 patients underwent laser ablation treatment with no immediate post-treatment complications seen and no injury to the adjacent rectum or neurovascular bundles identified on MR imaging

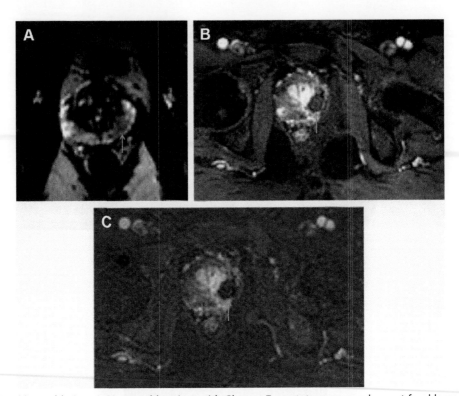

Fig. 4. Focal laser ablation. A 60-year-old patient with Gleason 7 prostate cancer underwent focal laser ablation for a lesion located in the left apex (*arrows*). Prophylactic antibiotics were administered to the patient prior to and after the procedure. Treatment was done using moderate-degree conscious sedation. A laser ablation template was placed on the patient's perineal surface and a lesion on MR imaging suspicious for prostate cancer was successfully localized. After the administration of lidocaine for local anesthetic, MR-compatible needles were directed into the area of the aforementioned lesion. After confirmation of needle location, ablation was performed. (*A*) A T2 hypointense cancerous focus is seen in the peripheral zone of the left apex. (*B, C*) After localized laser ablation, regional hypoenhancement is apparent in the left apex/midgland on unsubtracted and subtracted postcontrast imaging sequences, respectively.

performed 2 weeks after the procedure. In a phase I trial directed by Natarajan and colleagues,[31] 8 men were treated with directed laser ablation for intermediate-risk prostate cancer, with 5 of the patients determined cancer-free in the treatment area at their 6-month follow-up evaluation; in addition, the patients' sexual function and urinary habits were essentially preserved. Lindner and colleagues[32] conducted a phase I trial in which 12 patients harboring low-risk prostate cancers underwent focal laser therapy; post-treatment analysis performed after 3 months to 6 months demonstrated that more than half of the patients' rebiopsy results were negative for cancer in the region of treatment, and the primary complaint reported by most patients was simply perineal irritation. Another investigation led by Lepor and colleagues[33] followed 25 men who had undergone focal laser ablation, and no residual prostate cancer was detected in the post-treatment zones on rebiopsy performed 3 months later; an overall decrease in the patients' PSA values was also appreciated.

SUMMARY

Focal therapies, including cryotherapy, HIFU treatment, and regional laser ablation, are viable treatment options for men with intermediate-risk prostate cancer. By directing treatment to the site of interest, the adverse effects of the more traditional radical treatment options, such as prostatectomy or whole-gland brachytherapy and external beam radiation therapy, may be avoided. Fewer post-treatment urinary side effects, for instance, have been reported after locoregional cryotherapy and HIFU.[21,25]

Multiparametric MR imaging is the imaging modality of choice when performing focal therapies for locoregional prostatic tumor due to its accuracy in the initial detection of index lesions and its allowance for real-time monitoring during the course of treatment.[34] Treatment directed to the index lesion, or largest-volume or dominant tumoral focus, has been found to dictate the overall prognosis of the patient's disease process[17] and thus its reliable identification on MR imaging is vital. During the therapy process, the monitoring of temperatures in the adjacent soft tissues can help confirm that appropriate therapeutic levels are being reached. Additionally, real-time temperature checks can aid in avoiding inadvertent damage to nontarget anatomic structures, such as the urethra, urethral sphincter, bladder, and bowel.

Although continued scientific inquiry is required, current data regarding the efficacy of focal therapy options in the treatment of localized, low-risk, and intermediate-risk prostate cancer have been highly encouraging. Positive oncologic outcomes with an accompanying decreased incidence of untoward side effects have been observed. Additional longitudinal studies will help to clarify the long-term effects of focal treatments targeting prostate cancer.

REFERENCES

1. National Cancer Institute (surveillance, epidemiology, and end results program). "Cancer stat facts: common cancer sites." Available at: https://seer.cancer.gov/statfacts/html/common.html. Source: estimated new cancer cases and deaths for 2018. Web. Accessed May 18, 2018.

2. Wu X, Zhang F, Chen R, et al. Recent advances in imaging-guided interventions for prostate cancer. Cancer Lett 2014;349(2):114–9.

3. United States Preventive Services Task Force (USPSTF), Grossman DC, Curry SJ, Owens DK, et al. Screening for prostate cancer: U.S. Preventive Services Task Force (USPSTF) recommendations statement. JAMA 2018;319(18):1901–13.

4. Le JD, Huang J, Marks LS. Targeted prostate biopsy: value of multiparametric magnetic resonance imaging in detection of localized cancer. Asian J Androl 2014;16(4):522–9.

5. Stephenson SK. Screening & detection advances in MRI-guided prostate biopsy. Urol Clin North Am 2014;41(2):315–26.

6. Peltier A, Aoun F, Lemort M, et al. MRI-targeted biopsies versus systematic transrectal ultrasound-guided biopsies for the diagnosis of localized prostate cancer in biopsy naïve men. Biomed Res Int 2015;2015:571708.

7. Cicione A, Cantiello F, De Nunzio C, et al. Needle biopsy size and pathological Gleason Score diagnosis: no evidence for a link. Can Urol Assoc J 2013;7(9–10):E567–71.

8. Cohen MS, Hanley RS, Kurteva T, et al. Comparing Gleason prostate biopsy and Gleason prostatectomy grading system: The Lahey Clinic Medial Center experience and an international meta-analysis. Eur Urol 2008;54:371–81.

9. Boonsirikamchai P, Choi S, Frank SJ, et al. MR imaging of prostate cancer in radiation oncology: what radiologists need to know. Radiographics 2013;33: 741–61.

10. Ahmed HU, Bosaily AE, Brown LC, et al. Diagnostic accuracy of multiparametric MRI and TRUS biopsy in prostate cancer (PROMIS): a paired validating confirmatory study. Lancet 2017;389(10071): 815–22.

11. Kasivisvanathan V, Rannikko AS, Borghi M, et al. MRI-targeted or standard biopsy for prostate-cancer diagnosis. N Engl J Med 2018;378:1767–77.

12. Wilt TJ, Brawer MK, Jones KM, et al. Radical prostatectomy versus observation for localized prostate cancer. N Engl J Med 2012;367:203–13.

13. Valerio M, Ahmed HU, Emberton M, et al. The role of focal therapy in the management of localised prostate cancer: a systematic review. Eur Urol 2014; 66(4):732–51.

14. Harvey CJ, Pilcher J, Richenberg J, et al. Applications of transrectal ultrasound in prostate cancer. Br J Radiol 2012;85(Spec Iss 1):S3–17.

15. Le JD, Tan N, Shkolyar E, et al. Multifocality and prostate cancer detection by multiparametric magnetic resonance imaging: correlation with whole-mount histopathology. Eur Urol 2015;67(3):569–76.

16. Tan N, Margolis DJ, Lu DY, et al. Characteristics of detected and missed prostate cancer foci on 3-T multiparametric MRI using an endorectal coil correlated with whole-mount thin-section histopathology. AJR Am J Roentgenol 2015;205(1):W87–92.

17. Rosenkrantz AB, Deng F, Kim S. Prostate cancer: multiparametric MRI for index lesion localization—a multiple-reader study. AJR Am J Roentgenol 2012; 199:830–7.

18. Bozzini G, Colin P, Nevoux P, et al. Focal therapy of prostate cancer: energies and procedures. Urol Oncol 2013;31(2):155–67.

19. Jácome-Pita FX, Sánchez-Salas R, Cathelineau X, et al. Focal therapy in prostate cancer: the current situation. Ecancermedicalscience 2014;8:435.

20. Da Rosa MR, Trachtenberg J, Chopra R, et al. Early experience in MRI-guided therapies of prostate cancer: HIFU, laser and photodynamic treatment. Cancer Imaging 2011;11(1A):S3–8.

21. Bahn D, de Castro Abreu AL, Gill IS, et al. Focal cryotherapy for clinically unilateral, low-intermediate-risk prostate cancer in 73 men with a median follow-up of 3.7 years. Eur Urol 2012;62(1): 55–63.

22. Onik G, Vaughan D, Lotenfoe R, et al. The "male lumpectomy": focal therapy for prostate cancer using cryoablation results in 48 patients with at least 2-year follow-up. Urol Oncol 2008;26:500–5.

23. Ghai S, Louis AS, Van Vilet M, et al. Real-time MRI-guided focused ultrasound for focal therapy of locally confined low-risk prostate cancer: feasibility and preliminary outcomes. AJR Am J Roentgenol 2015;205:W177–84.

24. Marien A, Gill I, Ukimura O, et al. Target ablation—image-guided therapy in prostate cancer. Urol Oncol 2014;32(6):912–23.

25. Ahmed HU, Hindley RG, Dickinson L, et al. Focal therapy for localised unifocal and multifocal prostate cancer: a prospective developmental study. Lancet Oncol 2012;13(6):622–32.

26. Dickinson L, Ahmed HU, Kirkham AP, et al. A multi-centre prospective development study evaluating focal therapy using high intensity focused ultrasound for localised prostate cancer: the INDEX study. Contemp Clin Trials 2013;36(1):68–80.

27. Wenger H, Yousuf A, Oto A, et al. Laser ablation as focal therapy for prostate cancer. Curr Opin Urol 2014;24(3):236–40.

28. Oto A, Sethi I, Karczmar G, et al. MR imaging-guided focal laser ablation for prostate cancer: phase I trial. Radiology 2013;267(3):932–40.

29. Eggener SE, Yousuf A, Watson S, et al. Phase II evaluation of magnetic resonance imaging-guided focal laser ablation of prostate cancer. J Urol 2016;196(6):1670–5.

30. Raz O, Haider MA, Davidson ST, et al. Real-time magnetic resonance imaging-guided focal laser therapy in patients with low-risk prostate cancer. Eur Urol 2010;58:173–7.

31. Natarajan S, Raman S, Priester AM, et al. Focal laser ablation of prostate cancer: phase I clinical trial. J Urol 2016;196(1):68–75.

32. Lindner U, Weersink RA, Haider MA, et al. Image-guided photothermal focal therapy for localized prostate cancer: phase I trial. J Urol 2009;182(4):1371–7.

33. Lepor H, Llukani E, Sperling D, et al. Complications, recovery, and early functional outcomes and oncologic control following in-bore focal laser ablation of prostate cancer. Eur Urol 2015;68(6):924–6.

34. Yacoub JH, Oto A, Miller FH. MR imaging of the prostate. Radiol Clin North Am 2014;52(4):811–37.

MR Imaging of the Penis and Urethra

Ersan Altun, MD[1]

KEYWORDS

• Penis • Urethra • MR imaging

KEY POINTS

- The use of appropriate MR imaging technique is critical for the assessment of penis, and male and female urethra because the demonstration of critical structures such as the tunica albuginea or walls of the urethra highly depend on the employment of appropriate imaging MR technique, including high-resolution T2-weighted turbo spin echo sequences.
- Penile fracture is characterized by discontinuation of normal low T2 signal intensity of tunica albuginea on high-resolution T2-weighted images with associated hematoma showing MR imaging signal, depending on the age of blood products.
- T staging of penile cancer and local extent of urethral carcinoma can be determined with MR imaging according to the extent of the disease on high-resolution T2-weighted images.
- MR imaging successfully demonstrates urethral diverticulum and its associated complications, and can differentiate the periurethral disease mimicking urethral diverticulum.

INTRODUCTION

Ultrasound examination is the initial and most of the time the primary modality for the evaluation of penis.[1,2] However, it is limited owing to limited field of view (FOV), operator dependence, and low soft tissue contrast resolution.[1,2] Therefore, MR imaging has been increasingly used as a problem-solving adjunct after an initial ultrasound study.[1,2] Additionally, MR imaging is the best cross-sectional imaging modality for the assessment of urethra and periurethral disease owing to its high soft contrast resolution.[3,4] MR imaging also provides larger FOV for better evaluation of the extent of the disease process, varying ages of the blood products, and critical anatomic structures such as the tunica albuginea.[1–3]

The most common disease processes of the penis and urethra and their MR imaging findings are reviewed in this article.

MR IMAGING TECHNIQUE
Imaging Technique of the Penis and Male Urethra

MR imaging is performed with the patient in a supine and feet first position on the table either at 1.5 T or 3.0 T magnets. The penis and scrotum should be elevated with a towel located under these structures between the upper thighs. The dorsiflexed penis should be taped against the anterior abdominal wall to prevent any motion. This positioning also enables a good view of anatomy of the penis because the penis is seen at its full length without any curves or folding. Another towel is also used to cover the penis and scrotum before the placement of phased array coil or coils, covering the whole pelvis and lower abdomen.

The examination is usually performed when the penis is in a flaccid state. It is possible to use intracavernosal prostaglandin E1 injections to enable imaging of the erect penis[1,2,5,6]; however, this

The author has nothing to disclose.
Department of Radiology, The University of North Carolina at Chapel Hill, 101 Manning Drive, Chapel Hill, NC 27514, USA
[1] Also holds a degree of Associate Professorship of Radiology in Turkey.
E-mail address: ersan_altun@med.unc.edu

Magn Reson Imaging Clin N Am 27 (2019) 139–150
https://doi.org/10.1016/j.mric.2018.09.006

usually slows the workflow and necessitates more rigorous workup and screening, we do not perform it at our institution routinely. Additionally, the use of prostaglandin E1 is contraindicated in patients with penile prosthesis and conditions predisposing priapism.[1,2,5]

The examination includes 2 portions, including (i) imaging of the penis with sequences having high resolution and (ii) imaging of the whole pelvis extending from the iliac bifurcation to the inferior border of the scrotum with sequences having standard routine resolution. The details of the imaging technique is given in **Table 1**.

High-resolution imaging of the penis should be performed with high-resolution T2-weighted turbo spin echo (TSE) sequences in the axial, coronal, and sagittal planes with a small FOV (16 cm) and thin sections (4 mm). Two planes of fat-suppressed T2-weighted TSE with similar FOV and slice thickness are also acquired.

Standard resolution imaging of the pelvis should be performed with axial, coronal and sagittal T2-weighted single shot echo train spin echo sequences, axial fat-suppressed T2-weighted single shot echo train spin echo sequences, axial 2-dimensional or 3-dimensional T1-weighted dual gradient echo (GE) sequence, axial diffusion-weighted imaging and precontrast T1-weighted fat-suppressed 3-dimensional GE imaging.

Postgadolinium imaging should be performed with fat-suppressed 3-dimensional GE sequence in the axial, coronal, and sagittal planes covering the whole pelvis followed by small FOV axial and sagittal T1-weighted TSE sequences.

It is safe to image modern penile implants except 2 types of prostheses—the OmniPhase and Dura-Phase (Dacomed, Minneapolis, MN), which should not be imaged with MR imaging owing to the implants' potential tendency to deflect.[2]

Imaging Technique of the Female Urethra

Imaging technique of the female urethra again requires the use of axial, coronal ,and sagittal high-resolution T2-weighted TSE sequences with a small FOV and thin sections as well as 2 planes of fat-suppressed T2-weighted TSE sequences with a similar FOV and slice thickness that are acquired similarly, focused on the female urethra.[4,7] Standard resolution pelvic MR imaging with postgadolinium imaging can be performed similarly to the protocol described for the penile and male urethra MR imaging. The details of the imaging technique is given in **Table 1**.

Table 1
Pelvic MR imaging protocol for the evaluation of penis and urethra

Sequence	Plane	TR	TE	Flip Angle	Thickness/Gap	FOV	Matrix
Localizer	3-Plane	—	—	—	—	—	—
SS-ETSE	Coronal	1500[a]	85	170	6 mm/20%	350–400	192 × 256
SS-ETSE	Axial	1500[a]	85	170	6 mm/20%	350–400	192 × 256
SS-ETSE	Sagittal	1500[a]	85	170	6 mm/20%	350	192 × 256
SS-ETSE fat suppressed	Axial	1500[a]	85	170	8–10 mm/20%	350–400	192 × 256
T1 SGE in/out of phase	Axial	170	2.2/4.4	70	7 mm/20%	350–400	192 × 320
T2 3D TSE	Axial	1200	120	150	1.5 mm/—	250	256 × 256
T2 TSE	Axial/coronal/sagittal	5000	80	90	4 mm/—	230	256 × 256
T2 TSE fat suppressed	Coronal/sagittal	5000	89	90	4 mm/—	230	256 × 256
Diffusion-weighted imaging	Axial	4500	88	90	4 mm/—	270	128 × 128
T1 3D GE FS pre	Axial	3.8	1.7	10	3 mm/—	350–400	160 × 256
Postgadolinium sequences							
T1 3D GE fat suppressed[b]	Axial/coronal/sagittal	3.8	1.7	10	3 mm/—	350–400	160 × 256

Abbreviations: 3D GE, 3-dimensional gradient echo; FOV, field of view; SGE, spoiled gradient echo; SS-ETSE, single shot echo train spin echo; TE, echo time; TR, repetition time.
[a] TR between slice acquisitions.
[b] Optional: T1 TSE fat-suppressed images could also be acquired in 2 planes including axial and sagittal planes.

MR Imaging Anatomy of the Penis and Urethra

The midline corpus spongiosum and paired corpora cavernosa demonstrate similar high T2 signal and intermediate T1 signal, and are covered by tunica albuginea, showing low signal intensity on both T2- and T1-weighted images.[1,2,5,6] On postgadolinium T1-weighted sequences, the corpora cavernosa and corpus spongiosum show enhancement with progressive centripedal filling although the corpus spongiosum shows earlier enhancement.[2]

The male urethra runs from the bladder neck to the external meatus and is divided into the anterior and posterior urethra by the urogenital diaphragm, which contains the external sphincter and Cowper glands on each side.[3,8] The posterior urethra including the prostatic and membranous urethra extends from the bladder neck to the inferior border of the urogenital diaphragm.[3,8] The proximal prostatic urethra is located between the transitional zone and central zone of the prostate and is surrounded by the peripheral zone more distally. The membranous urethra is a short segment of the urethra passing through the urogenital diaphragm, which is a ringlike, T2 hypointense structure surrounding the urethra.[3] The anterior urethra extends from the inferior border of the urogenital diaphragm to the external meatus including the penile and bulbar urethra.[3] The penoscrotal junction is the boundary separating the penile and bulbar urethra.[3] The uroepithelium lines the prostatic urethra whereas pseudostratified columnar epithelium lines the membranous, bulbar, and penile urethra to the level of fossa navicularis, which is lined by nonkeratizing squamous epithelium. The male urethra is seen as a low signal intensity structure owing to its musculature and walls on T2-weighted images, and is surrounded by the high signal intensity corpus spongiosum.

The female urethra is short, measuring approximately 4 cm, and extends from the bladder neck to the external meatus through the urogenital diaphragm.[3,4,7] The proximal third of the urethra is lined by urothelium and the distal two-thirds is lined by stratified squamous epithelium. Paraurethral glands of Skene also open into the urethra, which can only be visualized when they are dilated or associated with cysts.[4] The female urethra shows a target-like appearance with low T2 signal intensity on T2-weighted images and progressive enhancement on postgadolinium sequences.[3,4] The target-like appearance of the female urethra is secondary to the presence of 4 concentric rings of tissue, namely, (i) the low outer signal layer corresponding with striated muscle, (ii) middle layer of high signal intensity corresponding with the submucosa, (iii) the inner layer of low signal intensity corresponding with the lamina propria and mucosa, and (iv) the central layer of high signal intensity corresponding with urine and secretions in the lumen.[3,4]

DISEASE PROCESSES OF THE PENIS
Trauma

Penile fracture is characterized by disruption of the tunica albuginea, suggestive of a rupture of the corpus cavernosum, and is usually associated with a hematoma.[1,2,5,6] The most common pathologic mechanism leading to the fracture is blunt trauma resulting from lateral motion of the erect penis during sexual intercourse.[2] The discontinuation of the low T2 signal intensity of the tunica albuginea is seen on high-resolution T2-weighted images with an associated hematoma showing an MR imaging signal depending on the age of blood products (**Fig. 1**).[1,2,5,6] The hematoma is more commonly acute (1–2 days) or subacute (7–28 days) demonstrating intermediate T1 signal and low T2 signal in the acute period, and high T1 signal and low or high T2 signal in the subacute period. The hematoma can involve the corpora cavernosa or corpus spongiosum and/or superficial soft tissues of the penis and adjacent scrotum. The typical management of a penile fracture is surgical.[2] The urethra should also be evaluated on MR imaging and, if there is suspicion of urethral injury, further assessment with retrograde urethrography is usually performed.

A penile contusion should be differentiated from penile fracture because its management is conservative (**Fig. 2**).[2,5,6] A penile contusion is usually characterized by the presence of mildly low T2 signal with associated corresponding T1 signal secondary to signal of small hematoma located in the corpora cavernosa and corpus spongiosum without evidence of rupture of tunica albuginea.[2]

Infection

Penile involvement in Fournier gangrene is rare and characterized by necrotizing soft tissue infection involving the penile superficial or deep fascial planes and can be seen as part of the extensive disseminated perineal Fournier gangrene.[2] The etiologic factors are variable and include epididymorchitis, scrotal cellulitis, urinary tract infections, pressure ulcers, inflammatory bowel disease complicated by perianal fistulizing disease, and perirectal and gluteal abscesses.[2] Computed tomography scanning has significant advantages over MR imaging in the diagnosis of Fournier

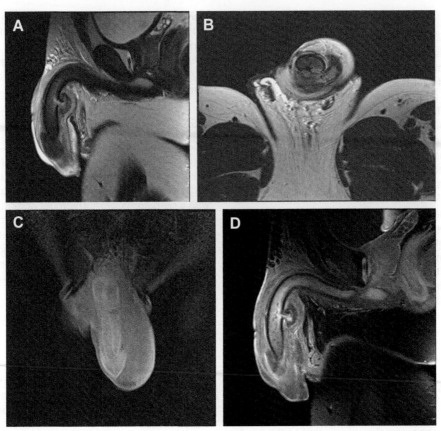

Fig. 1. Sagittal (*A*) and axial (*B*) T2-weighted high-resolution turbo spin echo, coronal T1-weighted fat-suppressed 3-dimensional gradient echo (GE) (*C*), and sagittal T1-weighted postgadolinium fat-suppressed 2-dimensional GE (*D*) images demonstrating penile fracture. The disruption of the tunica albuginea of the corpus cavernosum is evident with an associated small hematoma and contrast extravasation on the left side posteriorly.

gangrene owing to its higher sensitivity to demonstrate soft tissue gas and therefore should be the modality of choice for the assessment of suspected Fournier gangrene.[2] MR imaging findings of Fournier gangrene should also be recognized, because some patients with atypical clinical findings or another suspected diagnosis can be referred to MR imaging or MR imaging could be performed for the better delineation of anatomy. MR imaging findings in Fournier gangrene include prominent high T2 and low T1 signal of the soft tissues owing to edema and inflammation with associated increased enhancement on postgadolinium images. The fascial planes demonstrate thickening, and soft tissue gas shows susceptibility artifact, which is most prominent on in-phase T1-weighted GE sequences, decreasing in intensity on out-of-phase T1-weighted GE sequences. Additionally, abscesses can be seen as fluid collections showing rim enhancement and diffusion restriction, sometimes with air–fluid levels.

Penile abscess can also be seen as a complication of penile prosthesis placement or owing to a direct extension of the adjacent infectious process.

Inflammation

Peyronie disease likely results from chronic penile trauma, and has typically 2 phases: (i) an acute inflammatory phase and (ii) a chronic fibrotic phase. Peyronie disease is a chronic inflammatory condition and characterized by the presence of typically palpable plaques of the tunica albuginea showing low T1 and T2 signal and enhancement on postgadolinium T1-weighted images.[1,2,5,6] These plaques can rarely form in the cavernosal bodies. Ultrasound examination is the initial modality used for this assessment; however, MR imaging is more helpful for surgical planning owing to the more accurate evaluation of plaque location and thickness, as well as disease extent.

Primary Penile Cancer

Squamous cell cancer is the most common penile cancer, comprising 95% of all penile

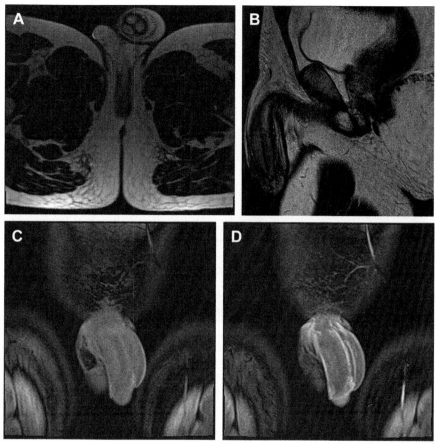

Fig. 2. Axial (*A*) and sagittal (*B*) high-resolution T2-weighted TSE, coronal T1-weighted precontrast (*C*) and post-gadolinium (*D*) fat-suppressed 3-dimensional gradient echo images demonstrating soft tissue edema of the penis without evidence of tunica albuginea disruption. These findings are suggestive of soft tissue injury and contusion without penile fracture.

malignancies.[1,2,5] Sarcomas can also be seen in the penis and constitute 5% of all penile malignancies including leiomyosarcoma, rhabdomyosarcoma, and Kaposi sarcoma.[2]

Squamous cell carcinoma is usually seen in the glans and prepuce. Well-known risk factors include old age, an uncircumcised penis, inflammatory conditions such as phimosis or lichen sclerosus, and human papillomavirus 16 and 18.[1,2,5] Squamous cell carcinoma is usually seen as an infiltrative mass and MR imaging is essential to determine the extent of the disease and to assess the invasion of the corpora cavernosa and corpus spongiousum/urethra.[1,2,5] The tumor demonstrates low T1 and T2 signal with irregular and ill-defined borders with postgadolinium enhancement, which is usually heterogeneous (**Figs. 3** and **4**).[1,2,5,9–11] The tumor usually demonstrates diffusion restriction on diffusion-weighted imaging (see **Fig. 6**). The evaluation of inguinal and pelvic lymph nodes is critical for the assessment of local lymphatic involvement, which is usually bilateral and is the principal prognostic sign.[1,2,5,9–11]

Sarcomas are usually characterized as irregular, large, heterogeneous locally invasive mass lesions showing heterogeneous low T1 signal, high T2 signal, diffusion restriction, and heterogeneous enhancement.[2]

Penile Metastases

Penile metastases are rare; however, they can be seen particularly with primary malignancies of the urogenital system, most commonly the prostate and bladder cancer.[2] These neoplasms also appear as single or multiple tumors in the corpora cavernosa and corpus spongiosum showing low T1 and T2 signal with associated diffusion restriction on diffusion-weighted imaging, and variable postgadolinium enhancement.[2]

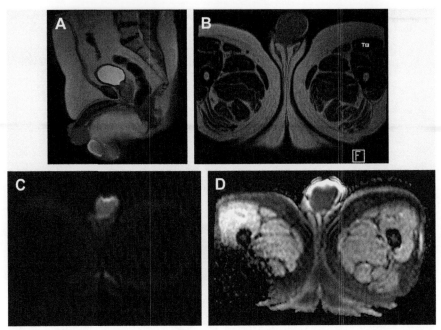

Fig. 3. Sagittal T2-weighted single shot echo train spin echo (*A*), axial T2-weighted high-resolution turbo spin echo (*B*), and axial diffusion-weighted image (*C*) with associated apparent diffusion coefficient map (*D*) demonstrate squamous cell carcinoma of the distal penis. The lesion invades both the corpus cavernosum and corpus spongiosum. The lesion shows low T2 signal with an associated diffusion restriction.

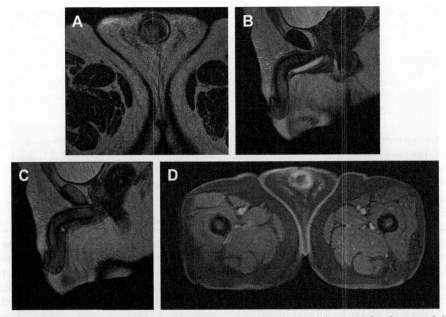

Fig. 4. Axial (*A*) and sagittal (*B*, *C*) T2-weighted turbo spin echo, and axial T1-weighted postgadolinium fat-suppressed 3-dimensional gradient echo (*D*) images demonstrate squamous cell carcinoma involving the distal and midportions of the penis. The lesion shows low T2 signal and heterogeneous enhancement. The lesion invades the corpora cavernosa and corpus spongiosum and causes obstruction of the urethra, which is dilated and fluid filled.

DISEASES PROCESSES OF THE URETHRA
Primary Urethral Carcinoma

Urethral carcinomas in men mostly occur in the bulbous or membranous portions of the urethra, although less commonly they can occur in the fossa navicularis.[2,3] Chronic infectious or inflammatory processes with or without associated strictures are the predisposing factors.[2,3] These tumors are mostly squamous cell cancers, mostly involving the urethra other than prostatic urethra. Urothelial cell carcinomas and adenocarcinomas can also occur occasionally and urothelial cell carcinoma typically affects the prostatic urethra.[2,3]

Urethral carcinoma is also a very rare malignancy in women. Predisposing factors include urinary tract infections, urethral diverticulum, human papilloma infection, and chronic inflammatory and tumoral conditions such as caruncles, polyps, and adenomas.[3,4,7] Squamous cell carcinoma is also the most common type and mostly involves the distal urethra and external urethral meatus; the less common transitional cell adenocarcinomas and adenocarcinomas typically involve the more proximal urethra.

Depending on the location of the tumor, superficial and deep pelvic lymph nodes could be involved. The penile urethra in men and distal urethra in women drain into the superficial and deep inguinal lymph nodes, whereas the bulbar, membranous, and prostatic urethra in men and proximal urethra in women drain into deep pelvic lymph node chains including obturator, internal, and external iliac chains.[3,4]

In male patients, these tumors are centered at the corpus spongiosum and around the urethra, demonstrating low T1 and T2 signals with associated diffusion restriction and mild postgadolinium enhancement.[2,3] MR imaging is particularly helpful for the demonstration of involvement of the tunica albuginea or septa of the corpus cavernosum on T2-weighted images in male patients.[2,3]

In female patients, these tumors again show a low T1 signal, but increased T2 signal owing to low signal intensity of the background urethra.[3,4] The normal target-like appearance of the female urethra could be disrupted.[3,4] The extent of the tumor and invasion of the adjacent perineal tissues and vagina are best demonstrated with high-resolution T2-weighted images.

Secondary Urethral Carcinoma

These result from direct extension of the malignancies involving the bladder, prostate, cervix, vagina, uterus, and anus (**Fig. 5**). Hematogenous spread to the urethra is rare, but melanoma is the most common primary malignancy causing hematogenous urethral metastasis.[4]

Urethral Diverticulum

Urethral diverticulum occurs in 1% to 6% of women and is rare in men.[3,4,7,12] The diverticulum is more commonly seen between third and fifth decades and most commonly arises from the posterolateral wall of the midurethra, usually at the level of symphysis pubis.[3,4,7,8,12]

Congenital urethral diverticulum is rare and more commonly seen males.[4] Acquired urethral diverticula accounts for the great majority of urethral diverticula. According to the widely accepted underlying pathophysiologic mechanism, the diverticulum develops secondary to the rupture of a chronically obstructed and inflamed periurethral gland into the urethral lumen, and shows later epithelization.[3,4,12] Common infectious organisms causing the infection of these glands include Escherichia coli and, less frequently, gonococci and Chlamydia species.[3,4,12] Additionally, inflammation of these glands could be due to birth trauma or urethral instrumentation.

Although the typical clinical presentation is the triad of dysuria, dyspareunia, and postvoid dribbling, nonspecific symptoms including lower urinary tract symptoms, incontinence, urinary retention, and those related to urinary tract infection are seen in most patients.[3,4,12] Physical examination is usually not helpful to narrow the differential and is not helpful to differentiate urethral carcinoma or mimicking vaginal wall lesions.[4]

One of the critical features of diverticulum that should be determined on MR imaging include its exact location, which can be described according to clock face template on axial T2-weighted images; this classification is helpful for surgical planning.[3,4,12] Additionally, more than 1 diverticulum could be present and each diverticulum should be identified separately. The diverticulum may have a narrow or wide neck or could be unilocular versus multilocular with multiple septations. The diverticulum could be an oval simple diverticulum although U shaped or circumferential diverticula can also be seen (**Figs. 6 and 7**).

The simple diverticula demonstrate high T2 signal and low T1 signal. More complex diverticula demonstrate heterogeneous T1 signal with areas of high signal intensity on T1-weighted images with associated corresponding low T2 signal on T2-weighted images.[3,4,12] Septations, layering debris, and a fluid–fluid levels can be seen in complex diverticula, which could also be infected.[3,4,12]

Calculus formation, infection, and malignancy development are the 3 main complications of

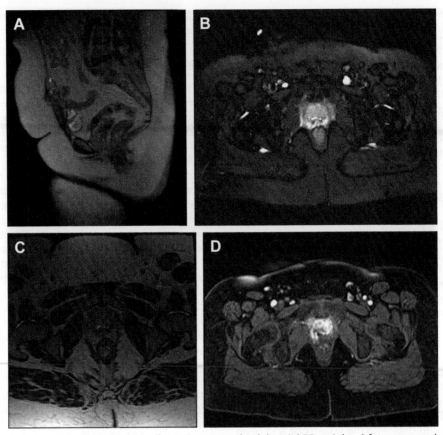

Fig. 5. Sagittal T2-weighted single shot echo train spine echo (*A*), axial T2-weighted fat-suppressed single shot echo train spin echo (*B*), axial T2-weighted high-resolution T2-weighted turbo spin echo (*C*), and T1-weighted postgadolinium fat-suppressed 3-dimensional gradient echo (*D*) images demonstrate recurrent transitional cell carcinoma arising from the urethra. The tumor shows high T2 signal on fat-suppressed images and intermediate T2 signal on non–fat-suppressed images. The lesion shows prominent heterogeneous enhancement and invades the vagina and abuts the rectum.

urethral diverticulum.[3,4,12] Calculi demonstrate low T1 and T2 signal in the diverticula.[4] The presence of very high T2 signal in the diverticulum compared with urine and areas of high T1 signal compared with urine could be a sign of infection in the appropriate clinical setting.[4] The most feared complication of urethral diverticulum is the development of malignancy inside the diverticulum, although this is very rare.[4] Although squamous cell carcinoma is the most common malignancy arising from the normal female urethra, adenocarcinoma is the most common malignancy (60%) seen in the urethral diverticulum.[4] Urothelial carcinoma is seen in 30% and squamous cell carcinoma is seen in 10% of patients with a urethral diverticulum.[4] The mass arising from the urethral diverticulum is seen as enhancing soft tissue, usually with irregular contours with possible infiltrative potential to the surrounding tissues.

Periurethral Cystic Lesions

Periurethral cysts are seen in females and the most common ones include Gartner duct cyst, Bartholin gland cyst, Skene duct cyst, and Mullerian cyst. These periurethral cystic lesions do not demonstrate any communication with the urethra and should be differentiated from urethral diverticula.

Gartner duct cyst

Gartner duct cysts arise from the residual mesonephric duct remnants (Wolffian) ducts and are also secretory retention cysts.[4] Typically, these cysts are located along the anterolateral vaginal wall above the level of inferior border of the symphysis pubis. These cysts are usually unilocular and demonstrate high T2 signal. However, depending on the presence of protein, mucus content, and sometimes blood products, these

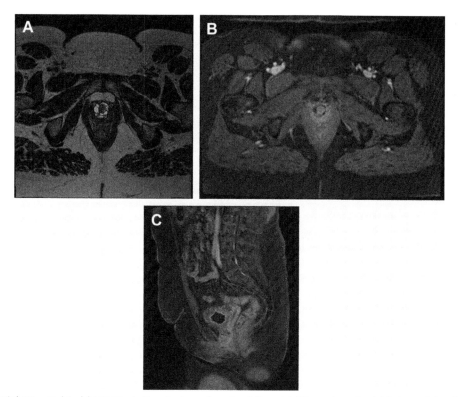

Fig. 6. Axial T2-weighted high-resolution turbo spin echo (*A*), axial (*B*), and sagittal (*C*) T1-weighted fat-suppressed 3-dimensional gradient echo images show a circumferential diverticulum containing septations surrounding the urethra.

cysts may demonstrate a low T2 signal and a high T1 signal.[4] The cyst wall also may show mild enhancement on postgadolinium images (**Fig. 8**).

Skene duct cyst

Skene duct cysts also result from the inflammatory ductal obstruction of the paraurethral Skene glands. They are located on both

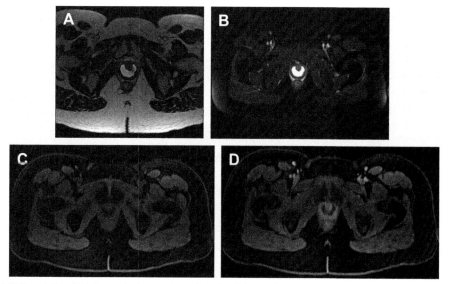

Fig. 7. Axial T2-weighted high-resolution turbo spin echo (*A*), axial T2-weighted fat-suppressed single shot echo train spin echo (*B*), and axial T1-weighted fat-suppressed precontrast (*C*) and postgadolinium (*D*) 3-dimensional gradient echo images show a semicircular urethral diverticulum surrounding the urethra.

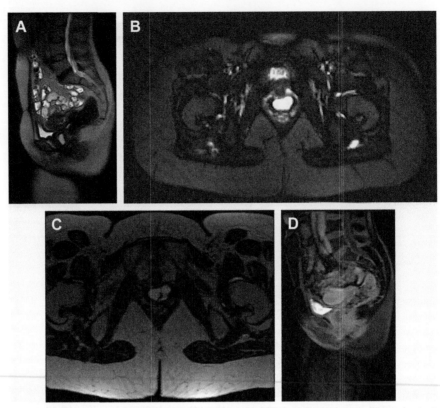

Fig. 8. Sagittal non–fat-suppressed (*A*) and axial fat-suppressed (*B*) T2-weighted single shot echo train spin echo, axial T2-weighted high-resolution turbo spin echo (*C*), and sagittal fat-suppressed T1-weighted postgadolinium 3-dimensional gradient echo (*D*) images demonstrate a Gartner's duct cyst located along the anterior vaginal wall without enhancement. Note the presence of nonenhancing septations in the cyst.

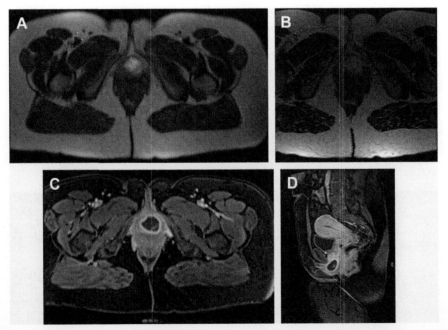

Fig. 9. Axial T2-weighted single shot echo train spin echo (*A*), axial T2-weighted high-resolution turbo spin echo (*B*), and axial (*C*) and sagittal (*D*) T1-weighted fat-suppressed postgadolinium 3-dimensional gradient echo images demonstrate a Skene gland abscess located at the level of urethra with prominent peripheral enhancement

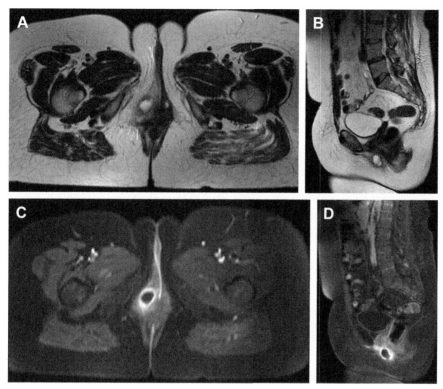

Fig. 10. Axial (*A*) and sagittal (*B*) T2-weighted turbo spin echo images, and axial (*C*) and sagittal (*D*) T1-weighted fat-suppressed postgadolinium 3-dimensional gradient echo images demonstrate a right sided Bartholin gland abscess with associated thick peripheral wall enhancement and surrounding inflammatory changes. There is also a tiny left-sided Bartholin gland cyst.

sides of the external urethral meatus inferior to the symphysis pubis.[4] These cysts also demonstrate high T2 signal with variable T1 signal depending on the protein/mucin content and mild peripheral wall enhancement on postgadolinium sequences (**Fig. 9**).[4]

Bartholin gland cyst

Bartholin gland cysts develop secondary to ductal obstruction owing to chronic inflammation and infection of the Bartholin glands, which are located at the posterolateral wall of the inferior third of the vagina, at or below the level of symphysis pubis (**Fig. 10**).[4] These cysts are usually unilocular and demonstrate high T2 signal with a variable T1 signal, depending on the protein and mucin content.[4] These cysts usually demonstrate mild to moderate peripheral wall enhancement. If the cyst is multilocular and shows heterogeneous T1 and T2 signals with intense wall enhancement and associated pericystic soft tissue edema and inflammation, infection should be suspected and this can easily be confirmed clinically.

Other periurethral cystic lesions

Additionally, perineal endometriosis and injected collagen can also cause development of periurethral cysts. Epidermal inclusion cysts can also be seen in this region.[4]

SUMMARY

MR imaging is the best imaging modality for the evaluation of penis and urethra and can consistently demonstrate and characterize the disease processes and determine their extent, which is critical for therapeutic approach including surgical planning.

REFERENCES

1. Shenoy-Bangle A, Perez-Johnston R, Singh A. Penile imaging. Radiol Clin North Am 2012;50: 1167–81.

2. Parker RA, Menias CO, Quazi R, et al. MR imaging of the penis and scrotum. Radiographics 2015;35:1033–50.

3. Ryu J, Kim B. MR imaging of the male and female urethra. Radiographics 2001;21:1169–85.

4. Chaudhari VV, Patel M, Douek M, et al. MR imaging and US of female urethral and periurethral disease. Radiographics 2010;30:1857–74.

5. Kirkham A. MRI of the penis. Br J Radiol 2012;85:S86–93.

6. Kirkham APS, Illing RO, Minhas S, et al. MR imaging of nonmalignant penile lesions. Radiographics 2008;28:837–53.

7. Dwarkasing RS, Dinkelaar W, Hop WCJ, et al. MRI evaluation of urethral diverticula and differential diagnosis in symptomatic women. Am J Roentgenol 2011;197:676–82.

8. Kawashima A, Sandler CM, Wasserman NF, et al. Imaging of urethral disease: a pictorial review. Radiographics 2004;24:S195–216.

9. Kochhar R, Taylor B, Sangar V. Imaging in primary penile cancer: current status and future directions. Eur Radiol 2010;20:36–47.

10. Suh CH, Baheti AD, Tirumani SH, et al. Multimodality imaging of penile cancer: what radiologists need to know. Abdom Imaging 2015;40:424–35.

11. Lucchesi FR, Reis RB, Faria EF, et al. Incremental value of MRI for preoperative penile cancer staging. J Magn Reson 2017;45:118–24.

12. Chou C-P, Levenson RB, Elyases KM, et al. Imaging of female urethral diverticulum: an update. Radiographics 2008;28:1917–30.

MR Imaging of the Testicular and Extratesticular Tumors
When Do We Need?

Mahan Mathur, MD[a],*, Michael Spektor, MD[b]

KEYWORDS

- Testicle • Extratesticular • Paratesticular • Germ cell tumor • MR imaging

KEY POINTS

- Scrotal MR imaging provides valuable information when clinical and/or ultrasound evaluations are inconclusive.
- Specific advantages include more accurate lesion localization and characterization.
- Distinction between testicular and paratesticular location is crucial for management and prognosis.
- Certain imaging features on MR imaging help in differentiating benign versus malignant lesions, as well as in distinguishing between specific malignant histologies.
- MR imaging is accurate in local staging of testicular neoplasms.

INTRODUCTION

Imaging evaluation for suspected scrotal pathology should commence with ultrasound (US), owing to its low cost, widespread availability, lack of ionizing radiation, and its high sensitivity in the detection of scrotal masses.[1,2] However, MR imaging provides valuable information if US and/or clinical examination findings are equivocal or incongruent.[2,3] One study of 26 patients who underwent MR imaging after an inconclusive US, reported that MR imaging provided additional and correct information in 23/26 patients (82.1%).[3] In another study of 34 patients with an inconclusive clinical and US evaluation, the leading MR imaging diagnosis was correct in 31/34 patients (91% vs 29% for the leading correct diagnosis on the inconclusive US), improving management for both the urologist and urologic oncologist.[4] This study also reported that the use of MR imaging in this setting yielded cost savings for the referring physician (ranging from $530 to $730 per patient) and the patient ($3833 per patient originally scheduled for surgery).[4]

Specific advantages of MR imaging in the setting of a suspected scrotal neoplasm include accurate lesion localization and characterization.[5] Accurate lesion location as intratesticular or paratesticular is critical, as the latter is most often benign and can obviate the need for a radical orchiectomy.[5,6] Owing to its wider field of view, several studies have shown MR imaging to be excellent in this setting, particularly when the scrotum is markedly enlarged.[2,7,8] The inherent soft tissue resolution capabilities of MR imaging enable accurate identification of lesions containing blood, fat, and/or fibrous tissue and allow for the detection of subtle enhancement that may be missed on US, leading to more accurate characterization of intra- and paratesticular masses.[9]

Disclosure Statement: The authors have nothing to disclose.
[a] Section of Body Imaging, Diagnostic Radiology Residency Program, Yale School of Medicine, 20 York Street, PO Box 208042, New Haven, CT 06520-8042, USA; [b] Section of Body Imaging, Yale School of Medicine, 20 York Street, PO Box 208042, New Haven, CT 06520-8042, USA
* Corresponding author.
E-mail address: mahan.mathur@gmail.com

Magn Reson Imaging Clin N Am 27 (2019) 151–171
https://doi.org/10.1016/j.mric.2018.08.006

MR imaging has also been shown to be accurate in the local staging of testicular neoplasms, which is of particular importance in patients considered for organ-sparing surgery.[5,10–12]

Following a review of normal MR imaging scrotal anatomy and imaging technique, the following review will elucidate specific indications in which MR imaging is useful in the evaluation of intra- and extratesticular tumors. For extratesticular masses, this includes accurate lesion localization and characterization. For intratesticular masses, this includes distinguishing benign masses and pseudotumors from malignant neoplasms, differentiating between germ cell tumors (GCTs) (seminomas vs nonseminomatous tumors) and between GCTs and nongerm cell tumors, and evaluating local spread of disease.

NORMAL ANATOMY AND IMAGING TECHNIQUE

Normal adult testes are well-defined ovoid structures that demonstrate hyperintense T2 signal and low to intermediate T1 signal[13] (**Fig. 1A, B**). After administration of intravenous contrast, both testes demonstrate moderate homogenous enhancement with a gradual increase in signal on dynamic contrast-enhanced imaging[14,15] (**Fig. 1C**). On diffusion weighted imaging (DWI), normal testicle parenchyma is homogenously hyperintense[13] (**Fig. 1D**).

The tunica albuginea manifests as a thin hypointense band on all imaging sequences and is indistinguishable from the visceral layer of the tunica vaginalis[13] (see **Fig. 1A, B**). The visceral and parietal layers of the tunica vaginalis may be separated by a variable amount of T2 hyperintense fluid.[13] The mediastinum testis appears as T1 and T2 hypointense band extending along the long axis of the testicle (this is better seen on the T2-weighted sequences owing to the inherent hyperintense T2 parenchymal signal)[14] (**Fig. 1E**). The rete testis may manifest as T2 hypointense bands or thin enhancing bands on T1 postcontrast sequences, extending from the mediastinum testis to the tunica albuginea.[13,14]

The epididymis is T2 hypointense and T1 isointense with respect to the testicular parenchyma.[14] On postcontrast sequences, the epididymis is hyperintense with respect to the testicular parenchyma[14] (**Fig. 2**). The scrotal wall is typically hypointense on both T1- and T2-weighted sequences.[14]

'The biological effects of the magnetic field in the MR environment on spermatogenesis are not clearly understood.[16] One study concluded that a 30-minute exposure to a 1.5 Tesla (T) static magnetic field resulted in some deleterious effects on spermatogenesis in mice.[17] Another study noted that MR imaging at high specific absorption rates (mean 0.72 W/kg, average imaging time 23 minutes) resulted in statistically significant increase in average scrotal temperature (up to 3.0°C).[18] However, these temperatures were noted to be below the level known to affect spermatogenesis in humans.[18] Therefore, as with any imaging study,

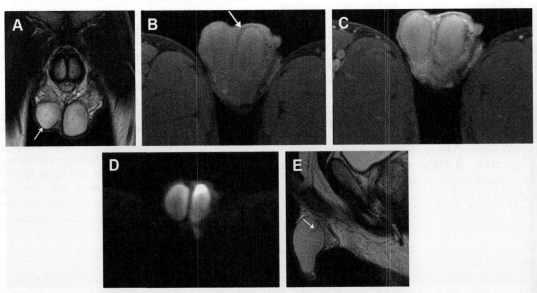

Fig. 1. Normal testicular appearance on MR imaging. Testes demonstrate homogenous hyperintense T2 signal (*A*), intermediate T1 signal (*B*), moderate homogeneous enhancement (*C*), and hyperintense signal on diffusion weighted imaging (*D*). Tunica albuginea manifests as a low T1 and T2 signal structure enveloping the testes (*arrows*). Mediastinum testis appears as a low signal band extending along the long axis of the testicle, as pointed with an *arrow* on the sagittal T2 image (*E*).

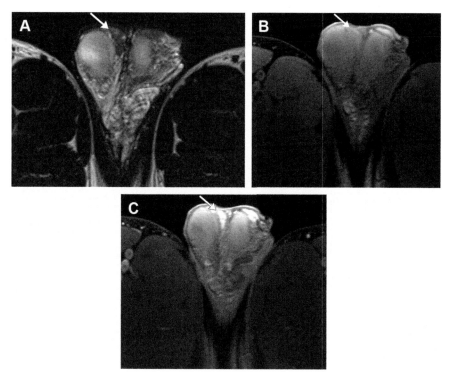

Fig. 2. Normal epididymis. The epididymis is T2 hypointense and T1 isointense with respect to the testicular parenchyma (*arrows* in *A* and *B*). After administering contrast the epididymis is hyperintense with respect to the testicular parenchyma (*arrow* in *C*).

it is imperative to weigh the risks and benefits before proceeding with the MR examination.[16]

All MR examinations of the scrotum are monitored by the radiologist to ensure adequate coverage. The patient is placed supine with feet first in the MR imaging unit. The penis should be raised, covered in gauze, and taped to the lower abdominal wall. In order to elevate the scrotum, a folded towel is placed between the upper thighs. An additional towel is placed over the scrotum and penis with the coil placed on top of the second towel.[5] Either a circular surface coil or a phased-array multichannel coil can be used.[5] Scrotal MR examinations at the authors' institution are performed on either a 1.5- or a 3.0-T magnet system, with the latter allowing for higher signal-to-noise ratio

A sample MR imaging protocol is provided in **Table 1**. After obtaining localizer sequences, small field-of-view T2-weighted turbo spin echo (TSE) sequences with thin sections are performed in the axial, coronal, and sagittal planes. Subsequently, a T2-weighted TSE fat-saturated sequence is performed through the scrotum in order to detect subtle regions of T2 hyperintensity and to depict fluid collections and edema. The use of fat saturation is also helpful in detecting macroscopic fat. By default, this is performed in the sagittal plane, although axial and/or coronal images may be used if the findings are better depicted in these planes. Thereafter, the authors routinely perform axial T1-weighted dual-echo spoiled gradient echo (GRE, both in phase and out of phase) sequences to detect microscopic lipid and/or blood products. Some institutions perform additional T1-weighted TSE images in one or multiple planes due to their higher spatial resolution and increased signal-to-noise ratio.

Axial T1-weighted fat-saturated 3-dimensional (3D) volumetric GRE sequences are subsequently performed, both before and after the administration of a gadolinium-based contrast agent, in order to detect enhancement (with the postcontrast images performed 1 minute following contrast injection). Obtaining 3D volumetric GRE sequences allows for rapid imaging acquisition with an isotropic data set that can be reconstructed with equal resolution in additional planes if needed. In order to fully appreciate the extent of the pathologic process, the authors routinely perform an additional large field-of-view T1-weighted fat-saturated 3D volumetric GRE sequence extending from the inferior aspect of the kidneys to the scrotum. Postprocessed subtraction images

Table 1
Sample protocol for scrotal MR imaging

Imaging Plane and Sequence	Section Thickness (mm)	Gap (mm)	Matrix Size	TR/TE (msec)
Sagittal, axial, and coronal localizers	10	15	128 x 256	15/5
Sagittal, axial, and coronal T2W turbo spin-echo (TSE)	3	0.3	192 x 256	4420/126
Sagittal T2W TSE fat-saturated[a]	3	0.3	256 x 179	4660/143
Axial T1W dual-echo spoiled GRE (in phase and out of phase)	8	10	256 x 190	TR = 212 TE (in phase) = 5.2 TE (out of phase) = 2.3
Axial unenhanced and contrast-enhanced T1W fat-saturated 3D volume GRE	1.1	0	256 x 256	5.6/2.7
Axial contrast-enhanced T1W fat-saturated 3D volume GRE (large field-of-view)	3	0	256 x 135	5.0/2.4
Axial DWI (ADC generated using the highest b value)	3	0.5	116 x 116	4300/63; b value of 50, 400, and 800 s/mm^2

Abbreviations: ADC, apparent diffusion coefficient; GRE, gradient echo; T1W, T1-weighted; T2W, T2-weighted; TE, echo time; TR, repetition time.

[a] Default plane is sagittal although this should be monitored and performed in the plane that best depicts the pathology.

(precontrast images subtracted from contrast-enhanced images) are provided and are particularly useful for lesions that demonstrate inherent hyperintense T1 signal.

Several studies have investigated the use of dynamic contrast-enhanced (DCE) sequences in scrotal MR imaging. A study in 2013 concluded that DCE MR imaging may be used to differentiate malignant from benign intratesticular masses, with the former demonstrating rapid enhancement and gradual washout and the latter exhibiting similar initial imaging features (although time to peak enhancement was delayed) followed by either a plateau or a slower increase in enhancement.[15] More recently, one study concluded that DCE may be used to distinguish between benign and malignant nonpalpable intratesticular tumors and reported some DCE parameters that may differentiate seminomas from Leydig cell tumors.[19] A sample protocol for DCE imaging provided by the European Society of Urogenital Radiology is provided in **Table 2**.[5]

Some studies have also demonstrated the utility of DWI in scrotal MR imaging, reporting lower apparent diffusion coefficient (ADC) values in seminomas versus nonseminomatous tumors, a finding that may aid in their differentiation.[20,21] Several studies have also shown that the use of high b value DWI, when combined with conventional MR sequences, is associated with increased accuracy in characterizing scrotal masses and detecting nonpalpable cryptorchidism over using DWI or conventional MR sequences alone.[22,23] A study in 2014 reported lower ADC values in the ipsilateral testicular parenchyma of patients with varicoceles compared with healthy control volunteers, concluding that this may be used as a diagnostic indicator of fibrosis.[24] At the authors' institution, DWI images are performed in the axial plane with an eco planar diffusion pulse sequence using b values of 50, 400, and 800 s/mm^2. ADC maps, generated on the MR console using the highest b value, are provided for assessment.

IMAGING FINDINGS/PATHOLOGY
Extratesticular Masses

- Lesion localization and characterization:

Although US remains the first-line imaging modality in compartmentalizing scrotal masses, MR

Table 2
Sample protocol for DCE imaging provided by the European Society of Urogenital Radiology

Imaging Plane and Sequence	Thickness	Contrast Timing	Imaging Duration
Coronal 3D fast field-echo sequence	4 mm with 2 mm overlapping sections	Bolus injection (1–2 mL/s)	• 15 s after bolus injection, obtain 5–7 consecutive imaging sets, each of 50–60 s duration • Imaging acquisitions continued for 8 min to evaluate washout

imaging may be helpful if findings are inconclusive.[5] This problem can arise when the relationship of the lesion to the hyperechoic tunica albuginea on sonography is difficult to establish.[7] In addition, MR imaging provides for wider field-of-view imaging, allowing complete assessment of lesions that may only be partially imaged using US.[9]

Several studies have demonstrated the utility of MR imaging in localizing scrotal masses and delineating their relationship to surrounding structures.[7,25] In one study, all 23 scrotal lesions (20 intratesticular, 3 extratesticular) were correctly localized by MR imaging.[8] In another recent study, MR imaging demonstrated high accuracy in distinguishing intra- and extratesticular masses, appropriately localizing all 80 scrotal lesions (28 intratesticular and 52 extratesticular).[7]

The superior soft tissue resolution characteristics of MR imaging, in conjunction with lesion location and morphology, may also aid in the characterization of extratesticular scrotal masses.[2] For aggressive paratesticular neoplasms, MR imaging can depict the local extent of disease and detect the presence or absence of metastases.[5] Diffusion-weighted imaging may also be of utility with one study reporting hypointense DWI signal with increased ADC ($1.72 \pm 0.60 \times 10-3$ mm^2/s) favoring benignity in paratesticular lesions.[23]

Accurate localization and characterization are imperative because most extratesticular lesions are either benign or mimic neoplasms, obviating the need for radical orchiectomy.[7,25] Examples of benign lesions include epididymal cystic lesions (cysts or spermatoceles), tunica albuginea cysts, inflammatory conditions (epididymitis), fluid collections (hydroceles, pyoceles), varicoceles, polyorchidism, or hernias.[7,25] Primary solid paratesticular tumors are uncommon and can range from benign lesions, such as lipoma, adenomatoid tumor, fibrous pseudotumor, and cellular angiofibroma, to malignant neoplasms, such as spermatic cord sarcoma and metastases (Table 3).[25]

Paratesticular lipomas are the most common benign extratesticular masses, often arising in the spermatic cord.[26] Although most lipomas are hyperechoic on US, the echotexture can be variable, likely related to the number of internal interfaces.[26,27] MR findings are diagnostic, demonstrating a nonenhancing mass with identical signal intensity to fat on T1- and T2-weighted images[14] (Fig. 3). Chemical shift artifact will be present at any water-fat interfaces associated with the lipoma.[14]

Adenomatoid tumors are the second most common extratesticular masses, often arising from the epididymal tail.[14,25] Lesions are typically unilateral and occur more frequently on the left side.[28] Adenomatoid tumors are often diagnosed between the ages of 20 and 50 years, and while most often an incidental finding, they may alternatively manifest as a painless testicular mass.[26] In approximately 30% of patients, adenomatoid tumors can present with pain.[25] Although both US and MR imaging findings are nonspecific, MR imaging can be more definitive about the paratesticular location of the mass allowing for a more confident diagnosis. Adenomatoid tumors have been reported to be T2 hypointense with respect to the testicular parenchyma.[29] Postcontrast imaging appearance may be hypo- or hypervascular, possibly related to the amount of associated granulation tissue[14,29] (Fig. 4).

Although uncommon, fibrous pseudotumors (FPTs) are the third most common extratesticular masses, following lipomas and adenomatoid tumors.[14] In one case series, FPTs were found in 7/114 paratesticular tumors (0.061%).[30] This lesion is not a true neoplasm, but rather represent a benign fibrous proliferation of paratesticular tissue, most often occurring in the tunica vaginalis, followed by the epididymis, spermatic cord, and tunica albuginea.[2,31] Clinically, FPTs manifest as a firm nodule or diffuse nodular thickening of the scrotum with an antecedent history of trauma or infection found in 30% of patients.[25,32] MR

Table 3
Clinical and MR imaging features of extratesticular masses

Extratesticular Mass	Clinical Features	MR Imaging Appearance
Lipoma	• Most common benign extratesticular mass	• Nonenhancing mass that follows signal of macroscopic fat on all sequences
Adenomatoid tumor	• 2nd most common extratesticular mass • Often arises in epididymal tail	• Often T2 hypointense with variable enhancement
Fibrous pseudotumor	• 3rd most common extratesticular mass • Represents a fibrous proliferation of paratesticular tissue	• Markedly hypointense T1 and T2 signal with variable enhancement
Cellular angiofibroma	• Rare, mesenchymal neoplasm composed of spindle-shaped cells, collagen-rich myxoid stroma, and small- to medium-sized blood vessels	• Heterogenously T2 hyperintense with heterogenous enhancement • Intratumoral fat reported in 24%–56% of cases
Sarcoma	• Most common malignant mass of the spermatic cord • Frequency: rhabdomyosarcoma > liposarcoma > leiomyosarcoma	• Heterogenous, with regions of necrosis and hemorrhage • Presence of fat suggests liposarcoma
Metastases	• Rare and seen with the following primary sites of disease: prostate gland, kidney, stomach, colon, carcinoid tumor of the ileum), and pancreas	• Nonspecific • High index of suspicion needed in the setting of primary disease elsewhere

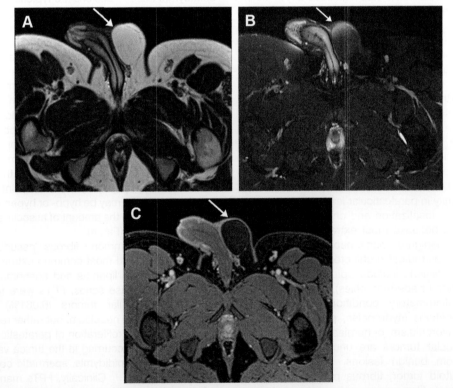

Fig. 3. Paratesticular lipoma. Axial T2-weighted (*A*), T2-weighted with fat saturation (*B*), and T1-weighted post contrast (*C*) images demonstrate a nonenhancing left paratesticular mass (*arrows*) that follows fat signal on all sequences, consistent with a lipoma.

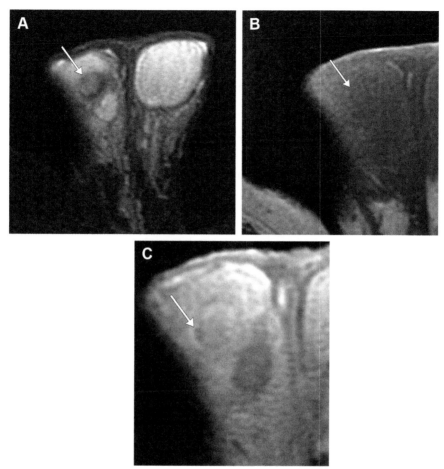

Fig. 4. Adenomatoid tumor. Axial T2-weighted with fat saturation (*A*), axial T1-weighted before and after contrast images (*B, C*) demonstrate an enhancing T2 hypo and T1 isointense right paratesticular mass (*arrows*).

imaging can allow for accurate paratesticular localization as well as characterization, with FPTs often demonstrating markedly hypointense T1 and T2 signal with variable enhancement on postcontrast imaging sequences[33] (**Fig. 5**).

Cellular angiofibroma is a rare, benign neoplasm, composed of spindle-shaped cells, a collagen-rich myxoid stroma, and small- to medium-sized blood vessels.[34] The presence of intratumoral fat has been reported in 24% to 56% of cases.[35,36] It is usually found in patients during the fifth to eighth decade of life and most often arises in the inguinal region, followed by the scrotum and perineum.[34] Clinically, patients

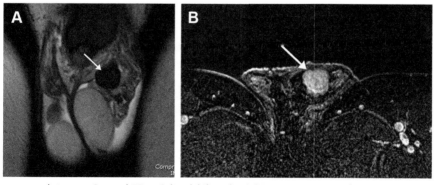

Fig. 5. Fibrous pseudotumor. Coronal T2-weighted (*A*) and axial T1 postcontrast subtraction (*B*) images demonstrate a markedly T2 hypointense and avidly enhancing left paratesticular mass (*arrows*).

present with a painless, slow-growing scrotal mass with one study reporting a size range of 3.0 to 25.0 cm (mean 7.9, median 7.0 cm).[35] Although MR imaging findings are nonspecific, they have been noted to follow the histologic appearance of this neoplasm. Owing to its myxoid stroma and numerous vessels, cellular angiofibromas demonstrate heterogeneously hyperintense T2 signal with heterogeneous enhancement on post-contrast imaging[34,35] (Fig. 6). If present, intratumoral fat can also be detected on MR imaging.[37] On DWI, cellular angiofibromas demonstrate no area of restricted diffusion.[34,38]

Sarcomas are the most common malignant masses of the spermatic cord.[14] Histologic subtypes include rhabdomyosarcoma, liposarcoma, leiomyosarcoma, malignant fibrous histiocytoma, fibrosarcoma, and undifferentiated sarcoma.[14] Of these, rhabdomyosarcoma is the most common (40% of cases), followed by liposarcoma and leiomyosarcoma.[25] Although most spermatic cord sarcomas occur in older patients, rhabdomyosarcoma frequently occurs in children and young adults.[25] Sarcomas most often manifest as a painless and hard inguinal/scrotal mass, although malignant fibrous histiocytoma has been reported to present with pain.[25,39] MR imaging is useful for preoperative planning and confirming the relationship of the mass to adjacent structures (such as the testicle and vasculature).[9] Although most sarcomas have a nonspecific appearance, demonstrating heterogeneous enhancement with variable amounts of internal hemorrhage and necrosis, MR imaging may detect the presence of fat within the lesion suggesting the diagnosis of liposarcoma[25] (Fig. 7).

Paratesticular metastases are rare, with less than 8% of epididymal neoplasms representing metastases.[25] The most common primary tumor sites associated with metastases to this region are (in decreasing order of frequency) prostate gland, kidney, stomach, colon, carcinoid tumor of the ileum, and pancreas.[25]

Intratesticular Masses

- Differentiating benign masses and pseudotumors from malignant masses:

MR imaging of the scrotum has been shown to accurately differentiate benign from malignant intratesticular masses in cases where US and/or clinical findings are inconclusive.[3,4,40] Preoperative diagnosis of benign intratesticular lesions avoids unnecessary radical orchiectomy, with alternative treatment strategies such as follow-up, biopsy, tumor enucleation, or testis-sparing surgery potentially justified.[5] Examples of such lesions include intratesticular hematoma, tubular ectasia of the rete testis, epidermoid cyst, and segmental (or diffuse) testicular infarction.

One study of 34 patients reported an MR accuracy rate of 91% in distinguishing benign from malignant testicular lesions after inconclusive clinical and US evaluations.[4] In a study of 17 cases of tumors or pseudotumors in whom an MR imaging was performed after an inconclusive US, 15/17 were reliably characterized with the negative predictive value of characterizing a benign lesion on MR imaging reported as 100%.[3] Another group demonstrated high sensitivity (100%), specificity (87.5%), and accuracy (96.4%) in differentiating benign from malignant intratesticular masses using MR imaging.[40]

Absence of contrast enhancement within intratesticular masses has been described as the most sensitive sign for predicting benignity.[40] However, in cases where benign lesions enhance (eg, in inflammatory conditions such as epididymo-orchitis), DCE and DWI imaging may be useful for further characterization.[15,23,41] The

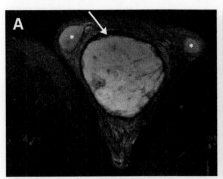
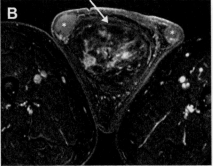

Fig. 6. Cellular angiofibroma. Axial T2-weighted fat-suppressed (A) and axial T1-weighted postcontrast subtraction (B) images demonstrate a large, heterogeneously T2 hyperintense mass with heterogeneous enhancement (arrows). The right and left testes are partially imaged and are separate from the neoplasm (asterisks).

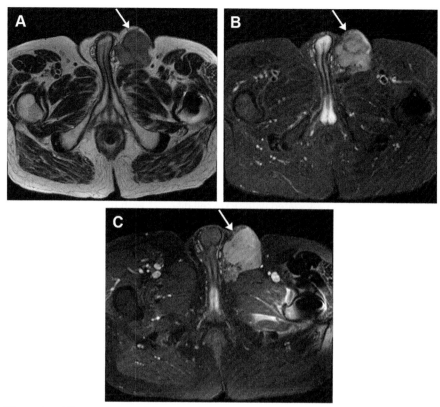

Fig. 7. Dedifferentiated liposarcoma. Axial T2-weighted (*A*), axial T2-weighted with fat suppression (*B*), and axial T1-weighted postcontrast (*C*) images demonstrate a mildly T2 hyperintense and avidly enhancing lobulated left paratesticular mass (*arrows*).

DCE features of benign lesions in one study were reported as strong enhancement with a late peak followed by either a plateau or a gradual increase in signal intensity.[15] Benign lesions have been reported to demonstrate no restricted diffusion with higher ADC values than malignant intratesticular masses. Using a cut-off value equal or less than $0.99 \times 10-3$ mm²/s, one study showed high sensitivity (93.3%), specificity (90.0%), positive predictive value (87.5%), and negative predictive value (94.7%) in characterizing malignant intratesticular masses.[41] Another study reported a mean ADC value of $1.56 \pm 0.85 \times 10-3$ mm²/s for benign intratesticular lesions (**Table 4**).[23]

Tubular ectasia of the rete testis (TERT) is a relatively common, benign nonneoplastic condition more commonly seen in patients older than 55 years, which is characterized by dilatation of the mediastinal tubules due to complete or partial obliteration of the efferent ducts.[13] Findings are often bilateral and can be associated with spermatoceles.[13] Although US findings are often characteristic, MR imaging may be of value if the appearance is atypical. On MR imaging, this manifests as a nonenhancing T2 hyperintense

multicystic masslike structure centered in the mediastinum testis. The hyperintense T2 signal coupled with the lack of enhancement differentiate TERT from an intratesticular neoplasm (**Fig. 8**).

Although epidermoid cysts account for 1% to 2% of all intratesticular masses, they are the most common benign tumors originating in the testicle.[42] The histogenesis remains unclear with proposed mechanisms including monodermal development of a teratoma or squamous metaplasia of surface mesothelium.[26] Epidermoid cysts are composed of multiple concentric layers of keratinizing, squamous epithelium with a well-defined outer fibrous wall. Although findings on US can be highly suggestive, a hypovascular neoplasm could be considered, particularly if the concentric layers are not evident on sonography. This differentiation is critical, because confident preoperative diagnosis of an epidermoid cyst may obviate the need for an orchiectomy, with surgeons often opting for testis-sparing techniques such an enucleation. MR imaging findings will often mirror these layers, with a "bulls-eye" or targetoid appearance composed of a hyperintense mid-zone on T1- and

Table 4
Clinical and MR imaging features of intratesticular masses

Intratesticular Mass	Clinical Features	MR Imaging Appearance
Tubular ectasia of the rete testis	• Dilatation of mediastinal tubules due to obliteration of the efferent ducts • Often bilateral and associated with spermatoceles	• Nonenhancing T2 hyperintense multicystic masslike structure centered in mediastinum testis
Epidermoid cyst	• Most common benign intratesticular tumor	• "Bulls-eye" or targetoid appearance • No internal enhancement
Segmental testicular infarction	• Often idiopathic, although has been associated with sickle cell disease, polycythemia vera, and vasculitis • Predilection for superior pole of testes	• Triangular or wedge-shaped mass with its apex pointing toward the rete testis • Variable T1 and T2 signal, peripheral rim enhancement without internal enhancement
Hematoma	• Most often seen with blunt trauma • 10%–15% may be associated with underlying tumor • Spontaneous hemorrhage is rare	• Avascular mass with variable T1 and T2 signal dependent on age of blood products
Seminoma	• Presents as a painless scrotal mass, most commonly in 4th decade of life	• Multinodular with homogeneous hypointense T2 and isointense T1 signal • Enhancing T2 hypointense bands may be present
Nonseminomatous tumor	• Presents as a painless scrotal mass, most commonly in 3rd decade of life • Histologically diverse: choriocarcinoma, yolk sac tumors, embryonal cell carcinoma, teratoma, and mixed	• Heterogeneous T1 and T2 signal with heterogeneous enhancement, necrosis, and hemorrhage
Leydig cell tumor	• Most common sex cord-stromal tumor • Hormonal manifestations reported in 10%–20% of patients (most common is gynecomastia)	• Limited data: well-defined T2 hypointense mass with marked rapid wash-in and prolonged washout
Sertoli cell tumor	• 2nd most common sex cord-stromal tumors • Hormonal manifestations reported in 25% of patients	• Limited data with variable T2 signal and enhancement characteristics
Primary testicular lymphoma	• Most common primary testicular malignancy above the age of 60 years and most common bilateral testicular tumor • Poor prognosis	• Hypointense T1 and T2 signal with low-level enhancement • Infiltrative with propensity to invade epididymis and/or spermatic cord

T2-weighted imaging interposed between outer and inner layers of hypointense signal.[43,44] The outer hypointense layer is thought to reflect a combination of the fibrous wall and adjacent keratin, whereas the inner hypointense layer reflects dense debris and calcification.[43] The hyperintense layer in between has been shown to correspond to desquamated cellular debris containing high water and lipid content.[43] Although the T1- and T2-weighted MR findings can be variable (without the aforementioned concentric appearance), the lack of internal contrast enhancement confirms the benignity of the lesion.[2,43]

Segmental testicular infarction is a rare condition, most commonly seen in men aged 20 to 40 years.[42] Although often idiopathic, several predisposing factors have been described, including epididymo-orchitis, trauma, hematologica

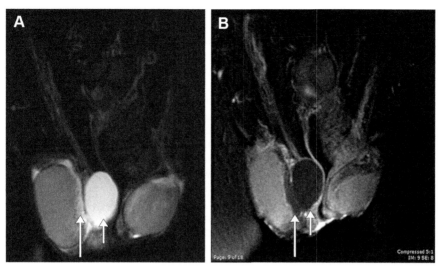

Fig. 8. Tubular ectasia of the rete testis. Coronal T2-weighted fat suppressed (*A*) and coronal T1-weighted post-contrast (*B*) images demonstrate a T2 hyperintense multicystic and nonenhancing masslike structure centered in the mediastinum testis (*long arrows*). Incidentally noted is a large right-sided epididymal cyst (*short arrows*).

conditions (such as sickle cell disease or polycythemia vera), and vasculitis (such as hypersensitivity angiitis).[45–48] Patients most often present with acute scrotal pain.[42] On US, segmental infarcts may be difficult to distinguish from a hypovascular neoplasm, the differentiation of which is critical because the former is treated conservatively.[42] On MR, segmental testicular infarction often manifests as a triangular or wedge-shaped mass with its apex pointing toward the rete testis.[2] Both the T1 and T2 signal can be variable, with hyperintense T1 foci indicating hemorrhagic infarction.[49] No internal vascularity is present on postcontrast imaging with peripheral rim enhancement described in up to 90% of patients[50] (**Fig. 9**). There is a predilection for the superior aspect of

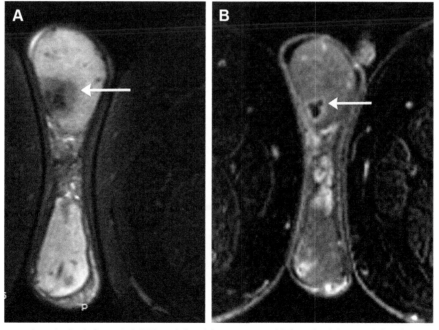

Fig. 9. Segmental testicular infarct. Axial T2-weighted fat suppressed (*A*) and axial T1-weighted postcontrast subtraction (*B*) images demonstrate an avascular and peripherally located testicular lesion that has heterogeneous, although predominantly hypointense, T2 signal with peripheral enhancement (*arrows*).

the testes due to the lack of significant collateral vasculature in this location[50] (**Fig. 10**).

Intratesticular hematomas most commonly occur after blunt trauma.[9] Spontaneous hemorrhage is exceedingly rare with only a few reports described in the literature.[51] Although US findings suggest a hematoma, it may be challenging to make a definitive diagnosis, particularly if the clinical history of trauma is unclear. In addition, 10% to 15% of testicular tumors have been found to manifest after scrotal trauma.[52] MR imaging is useful in these settings with hematoma manifesting as an avascular mass with variable T1 and T2 signal depending on the age of the collection. Subacute hematomas demonstrate hyperintense T1 signal due to the presence of methemoglobin, whereas chronic hematomas may demonstrate a T2 hypointense hemosiderin ring[53] (**Fig. 11**).

- Differentiating GCTs (seminomas from nonseminomatous tumors):

Although testicular neoplasms represent approximately 1% of all solid tumors in men, they are the most common solid malignancy between the ages of 15 and 35 years.[54] These are further categorized into GCTs, which comprise 95% of testicular neoplasms, and nongerm cell tumors (NGCTs).[2]

Patients most commonly present with a palpable painless scrotal mass, although up to 10% of patients may present with acute testicular pain.[55]

GCTs are divided into pure seminomas or nonseminomatous tumors, the incidence of which is evenly distributed.[6] Nonseminomatous GCTs include choriocarcinoma, yolk sac tumors, embryonal cell carcinoma, and teratoma, with lesions often reflecting a mixture of the aforementioned histologic subtypes.[14] The average age at presentation differs amongst the 2 subtypes of GCTs, with seminomas presenting relatively later in life (fourth decade vs third decade in NSGCTs).[56] In general, seminomas are less aggressive and more sensitive to radiation and chemotherapy, portending a better prognosis than NSGCTs.[55] Tumor markers, such as beta human chorionic gonadotropin, alpha fetoprotein, and lactate dehydrogenase may be elevated with GCTs and can be used to monitor treatment response and in detection of recurrent disease.[57]

MR imaging has shown promise in distinguishing seminomas from nonseminomatous tumors.[6,21,58] Based on T2-weighted and contrast-enhanced appearances, one study correctly differentiated seminomas from nonseminomatous tumors in 19/21 (91%) intratesticular lesions.[6] This distinction is critical in the setting of widespread or life-threatening

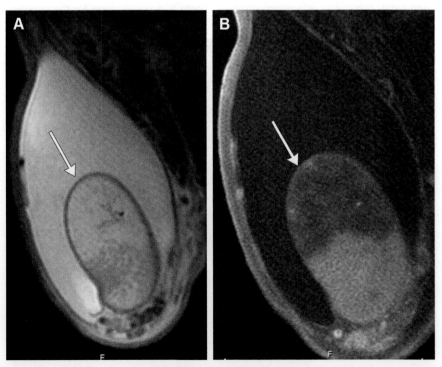

Fig. 10. Focal upper pole infarction. Sagittal T2-weighted (*A*) and sagittal T1-weighted postcontrast (*B*) images demonstrate a large, peripheral, avascular region at the superior testicular pole consistent with a focal infarct (*arrows*).

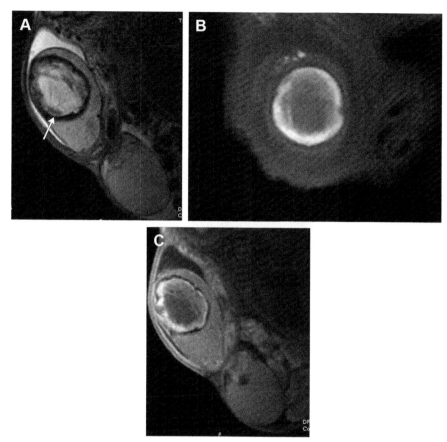

Fig. 11. Intratesticular hematoma. Sagittal T2-weighted (*A*) and T1-weighted before and after contrast (*B*, *C*) images demonstrate a round, avascular, and hemorrhagic testicular lesion with a T2 hypointense hemosiderin ring (*arrow*).

metastatic disease where chemotherapy may be administered to ensure clinical improvement before orchiectomy.[10] In addition, this differentiation allows for appropriate treatment planning because patients with pure seminomas undergo radiation therapy, whereas those with nonseminomatous neoplasms undergo retroperitoneal lymph node dissection and chemotherapy.[58]

The reported MR findings of seminomas and nonseminomatous tumors correlate to their histologic appearance.[2,58] On pathology, pure seminomas are homogonous, solid masses with lobulated borders.[2,58] Internally, they are composed of nests of uniform tumors cells with clear cytoplasm separated by fibrous bands containing lymphocytes and plasma cells.[2,58] The presence of hemorrhage and/or necrosis is uncommon.[58] Nonseminomatous tumors demonstrate a more heterogeneous internal architecture owing to their diverse histologic features as well as regions of necrosis and hemorrhage, with the latter due to invasion of blood vessels.[2,58]

On MR imaging, seminomas manifest as multinodular masses with homogenously hypointense T2 and isointense T1 signal[2,58] (**Fig. 12**). Several studies have observed the additional presence of T2 hypointense bandlike structures that enhance more than the tumor itself, a finding which corresponds to the fibrous septations seen on histology.[2,58] One study in 2007 used these 2 imaging features to correctly diagnosis 9/10 seminomas on preoperative imaging.[6] In 2010, another study used these features to correctly characterize 13/28 intratesticular masses as seminomas on preoperative MR imaging.[40] Nonseminomatous tumors demonstrate a more heterogeneous appearance on T1- and T2-weighted imaging with regions of necrosis and hemorrhage[6] (**Fig. 13**). The presence of a fibrous pseudocapsule manifesting as a T2 hypointense halo surrounding the tumor has been reported more often with nonseminomatous tumors.[2] Postcontrast sequences demonstrate the presence of heterogeneous enhancement.[6] Diffusion-weighted imaging may provide an additional noninvasive

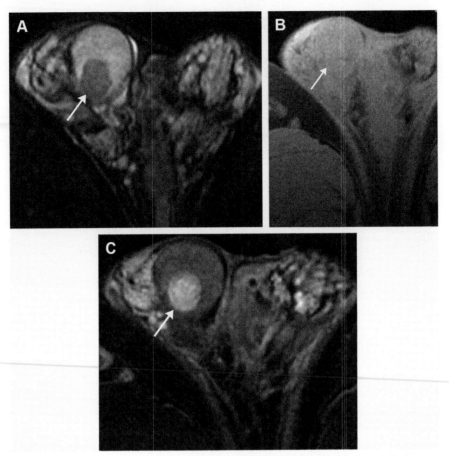

Fig. 12. Seminoma. Axial T2-weighted fat-suppressed (*A*) and axial T1-weighted before and after contrast (*B, C*) images demonstrate a lobulated right testicular mass that manifests characteristic homogeneous T2 hypointense and T1 isointense signals with homogenous enhancement (*arrows*).

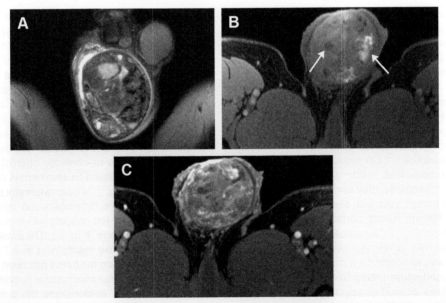

Fig. 13. Nonseminomatous tumor. Axial T2-weighted (*A*) and axial T1-weighted before and after contrast (*B, C*) images demonstrate a very heterogeneous right testicular mass with areas of necrosis and hemorrhage (*arrows* in *B*).

means to distinguish seminomas from nonseminomatous tumors with several recent studies reporting lower ADC values in the former.[20,21] One study in 2015 found lower ADC values in seminomas ($0.59 \times 10-3$ mm^2/s $\pm$ 0.009) versus nonseminomatous germ cell tumors ($0.90 \times 10-3$ mm^2/s $\pm$ 0.33, P = .01), with an optimal ADC cut-off value of $0.68 \times 10-3$ mm^2/s.[21]

- Differentiating testicular germ cell neoplasms from nongerm cell neoplasms:

Nongerm cell tumors comprise a wide histologic range of neoplasms, most of which represent sex cord-stromal tumors. Sex cord-stromal tumors account for 4% of all testicular malignancies in adults, although this increases to 8% in the pediatric population.[59,60] Leydig cell tumor is the most common histologic subtype, followed by Sertoli cell tumor and granulosa cell tumor.[61] Gonadoblastoma is an additional uncommon category of NGCT, which is histologically composed of germ cells, immature Sertoli or granulosa cells, as well as round deposits of basement membrane with occasional calcifications.[61] If not excised, 50% will progress to dysgerminoma/seminoma and 8% to a nonseminomatous tumor subtype.[62] Other rare NGCT categories include ovarian epithelial-type tumors (these arise from the testis/paratestis with histologic features of ovarian surface epithelial tumors), juvenile xanthogranuloma, hemangioma, and hematolymphoid tumors (including diffuse large B-cell lymphoma [DLBCL]).[61]

Leydig cell tumors arise from the male gonadal interstitium and account for 1% to 3% of all testicular neoplasms.[14] Clinical presentation can occur at any age, although is usually seen in adults with the median age in 2 series ranging from 40 to 50.[63,64] Hormonal manifestations, resulting in virilizing or feminizing symptoms, have been reported in 20% to 30% of cases.[59,65] These include gynecomastia (most common), as well as loss of libido, erectile dysfunction, impotence, and infertility.[63] Precocious puberty may be seen when Leydig cell tumors occur in children.[59] A minority of these tumors are malignant, with one study of 70,120 cases of testicular cancer in the National Cancer Database reporting 250 (0.3%) malignant Leydig cell tumors. The following features have been correlated with malignant potential: large size (>5 cm), infiltrative borders, cytologic atypia, increased number of mitotic figures, vascular invasion, and necrosis.[61]

Sertoli cell tumors account for 1% of testicular neoplasms, with patients most commonly presenting between the ages of 35 and 50 years (mean age 45 years).[66,67] One specific subtype (large cell calcifying subtype) has been reported to present at a younger age (mean age of 21 years) and can be seen bilaterally in 20% of cases (with this feature often reported in patients with Carney syndrome).[68,69] Hormonal manifestations, such as gynecomastia, may occur in 25% of cases.[69] Most tumors are benign with metastases seen in 6% to 15% of patients.[14,69] Features that suggest malignancy are similar to those seen in Leydig cell tumors, with one study reporting 11/14 malignant lesions to have a size greater than 5 cm.[69,70]

Although primary testicular lymphoma is uncommon, it is the most common testicular malignancy above the age of 60 years and is the most common bilateral testicular neoplasm with reported prevalence of synchronous involvement approaching 20%.[14] It accounts for 1% of all non-Hodgkin lymphomas, with DLBCL being the most common subtype.[14] In one study, DLBCL was found in 33/35 patients with histologically confirmed lymphoma.[71] Patients most commonly present with painless testicular enlargement, although 25% may present with systemic symptoms such as weight loss and anorexia.[26,72] Primary testicular lymphoma is an aggressive tumor with a propensity for local invasion to the epididymis, spermatic cord, or scrotal skin, and metastases occurring in the central nervous system and lung.[72] Overall prognosis is poor with high relapse rates and a medial survival of 12 to 24 months.[73] In one study of 373 patients with primary testicular lymphoma, 56 (15%) demonstrated central nervous system relapse and/or progressive disease.[74]

Several studies have proposed MR imaging features that aid in differentiating GCTs from NGCTs, although it should be noted that definitive characterization remains difficult.[14] This distinction allows for preoperative prognostication and treatment planning, particularly with increased consideration for testis-sparing surgery for sex cord-stromal tumors in certain clinical settings.[75,76]

Leydig cell tumors have been reported to exhibit isointense and hypointense signal on T1- and T2-weighted images relative to normal testicle parenchyma, with marked homogenous enhancement on postcontrast sequences[77] (**Fig. 14**). One study of 44 patients reported an accuracy of 93% in differentiating seminomas from Leydig cell tumors, with imaging features of the latter including well-defined margins, markedly hypointese T2 signal and homogenous enhancement with marked, rapid wash-in followed by prolonged washout.[78] Findings of internal hyperintense T2 signal (corresponding on pathology to central scars) as well as a T2 hyperintense rim (which corresponded to a fibrous rim) have also been reported.[77]

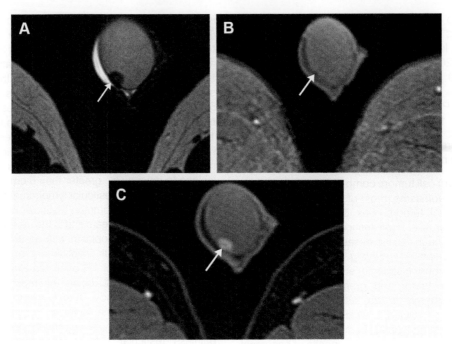

Fig. 14. Leydig cell tumor. Axial T2-weighted (*A*) and axial T1-weighted before (*B*) and after contrast images (*C*) demonstrate a T2 hypointense testicular lesion that is isointense on T1 imaging and exhibits marked homogeneous enhancement (*arrows*).

There are more limited data on the MR imaging appearance of Sertoli cell tumors. Two studies each reported a lesion with hypointense T2 signal and homogenous, rapid contrast enhancement followed by rapid washout.[15,79] Another study reported multiple intermediate T1 and hyperintense T2 signal nodules with rim enhancement.[80] Sertoli cell tumors have also been reported to demonstrate less restricted diffusion than GCTs.[23]

Primary testicular lymphoma has been described as a homogenous mass with hypointense T1 and T2 signal and low-level enhancement, although heterogeneous and nodular masses with variable T1 and T2 signal have also been reported.[14,81,82] Several studies have described an infiltrative, although nondestructive, mass with extension to the epididymis and/or spermatic cord, a finding that helps to differentiate it from seminomas[26,82] (**Fig. 15**). Unlike nonseminomatous GCTs, primary testicular lymphoma is usually more homogenous in appearance.[83] The presence of bilateral intratesticular masses with concomitant involvement of the epididymis in a patient older than 60 years should raise the possibility of lymphoma.[14]

- Local staging of testicular neoplasms:

Accurate preoperative imaging of intratesticular masses to assess local extent of disease is critical in patients for whom organ-sparing surgery is

considered. These indications include the following: tumor in a solitary testicle, small tumor (<20 mm) confined to one testis with normal preoperative testosterone levels, bilateral synchronous testicular tumors, and metachronous

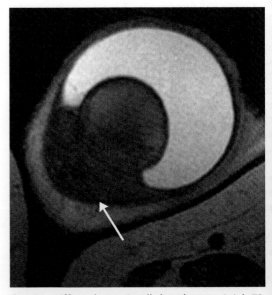

Fig. 15. Diffuse large B-cell lymphoma. Axial T2-weighted image demonstrates a low signal mass infiltrating the entire testicle with extension into the epididymis (*arrow*).

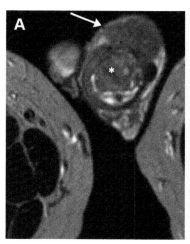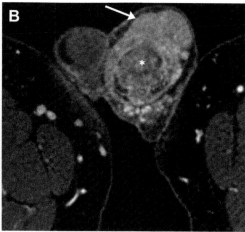

Fig. 16. Sex cord-stromal with epididymal involvement. Axial T2-weighted (*A*) and axial T1-weighted postcontrast (*B*) images demonstrate a heterogeneous left testicular mass (*asterisks* in *A, B*) extending into epididymis (*arrows*).

contralateral testicular tumors with normal preoperative testosterone levels.[11,12,84]

MR imaging of the scrotum has been shown to be highly accurate in the local staging of testicular neoplasms. One study reported an overall MR imaging accuracy rate of 92.8% in assessing the local extent of malignant testicular tumors.[40] In this study, the presence of an intact hypointense tunica layer correctly staged 12/13 (92%) T1 lesions, whereas localized interruption of the tunica was seen in 11/12 (92%) T2 lesions.[40] All T3 (3/3) neoplasms were accurately staged, manifesting as a contrast-enhanced component infiltrating into the spermatic cord[40] (**Fig. 16**). In addition, MR imaging can accurately delineate tumor dimensions, assess for involvement of the rete testis, and potentially detect a tumor pseudocapsule, with the latter finding reported to facilitate tumor enucleation when organ-sparing surgery is considered.[5,12] In one study from 2010, the presence of a tumor pseudocapsule, manifesting as a hypointense halo and histologically corresponding to a fibrous capsule, was found in 9/28 intratesticular neoplasms.[40]

Although not routinely used in the assessment of retroperitoneal lymphadenopathy due to longer examination times, higher costs, and limited availability, several studies have shown that MR imaging is comparable to computed tomography (CT) imaging in the detection of retroperitoneal lymph nodes.[85–87] One study reported that MR imaging, as interpreted by 2 attending radiologists with more than 10 years of experience, demonstrated a sensitivity of 97% for detecting retroperitoneal lymph nodes when compared with CT.[88] Continued advances in MR imaging, resulting in faster acquisition times, make MR imaging a reasonable option for staging and surveillance of testicular neoplasms, particularly given the concerns associated with ionizing radiation[89] (**Fig. 17**).

Both CT and MR imaging are limited in assessing disease in normal-sized lymph nodes and are unable to reliably differentiate reactive from malignant lymphadenopathy.[87] The use of lymphotropic nanoparticle-enhanced MR imaging (LNMRI) may overcome these limitations, having shown promise in evaluating lymph nodes in different neoplasms.[90,91] In one retrospective study of 18 patients, LNMRI yielded higher sensitivities, specificities, and accuracy rates for detecting malignant lymph nodes (88.2%, 92%, and 90.4%, respectively) versus using size criteria on MR imaging (70.5%, 68%, and 69%, respectively).[90] Although these results are encouraging, the role of LNMRI in testicular cancer remains unclear with prospective studies required for further clarification (**Tables 3** and **4**).

What the Referring Physician Needs to Know

Indications for scrotal MR imaging after an inconclusive clinical and/or US evaluation:

- Extratesticular masses:
  - Accurate localization and characterization
  - Preoperative planning
- Intratesticular masses:
  - Differentiating benign masses and pseudotumors from malignant masses
  - Differentiating seminomas from nonseminomatous tumors
  - Potentially distinguishing GCTs from non-germ cell neoplasms
  - Local staging of neoplasms
  - Preoperative planning if organ-sparing surgery is being considered

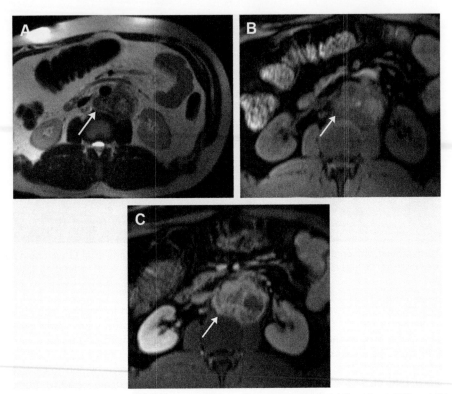

Fig. 17. Metastatic left-sided nonseminomatous neoplasm. Axial T2-weighted (A) and axial T1-weighted before and after contrast (B, C) images demonstrate heterogeneously enhancing retroperitoneal lymphadenopathy (arrows) associated with the known testicular neoplasm.

SUMMARY

An understanding of normal scrotal anatomy and MR imaging techniques is imperative before interpretation. The wider field of view and advanced soft tissue resolution properties of MR imaging allow it to accurately localize and characterize both intra- and extratesticular masses. In addition, MR imaging is important in local staging of intratesticular neoplasms as well as preoperative planning, particularly in patients in whom organ-sparing surgery is being considered. Application of established MR imaging techniques, such as DWI and DCE, to this region has demonstrated some potential in further characterizing both benign and malignant masses. Overall, MR imaging remains an underutilized technique in evaluating the scrotum, although it is valuable in certain settings, particularly when sonographic and/or clinical findings are inconclusive.

REFERENCES

1. Kühn AL, Scortegagna E, Nowitzki KM, et al. Ultrasonography of the scrotum in adults. Ultrasonography 2016;35(3):180.

2. Tsili AC, Giannakis D, Sylakos A, et al. MR imaging of scrotum. Magn Reson Imaging Clin North Am 2014;22(2):217–38.

3. Muglia V, Tucci S Jr, Elias J Jr, et al. Magnetic resonance imaging of scrotal diseases: when it makes the difference. Urology 2002;59(3):419–23.

4. Serra AD, Hricak H, Coakley FV, et al. Inconclusive clinical and ultrasound evaluation of the scrotum: impact of magnetic resonance imaging on patient management and cost. Urology 1998;51(6):1018–21.

5. Tsili AC, Bertolotto M, Turgut AT, et al. MRI of the scrotum: recommendations of the ESUR scrotal and penile imaging working group. Eur Radiol 2018;28(1):31–43.

6. Tsili AC, Tsampoulas C, Giannakopoulos X, et al. MRI in the histologic characterization of testicular neoplasms. Am J Roentgenol 2007;189(6):W331–7.

7. Mohrs OK, Thoms H, Egner T, et al. MRI of patients with suspected scrotal or testicular lesions: diagnostic value in daily practice. Am J Roentgenol 2012;199(3):609–15.

8. Thurnher S, Hricak H, Carroll PR, et al. Imaging the testis: comparison between MR imaging and US. Radiology 1988;167(3):631–6.

9. Mathur M, Mills I, Spektor M. Magnetic resonance imaging of the scrotum: pictorial review wit

ultrasound correlation. Abdom Radiol (NY) 2017; 42(7):1929–55.

10. Albers P, Albrecht W, Algaba F, et al. Guidelines on testicular cancer: 2015 update. Eur Urol 2015;68(6): 1054–68.

11. Heidenreich A, Weissbach L, Höltl W, et al. Organ sparing surgery for malignant germ cell tumor of the testis. J Urol 2001;166(6):2161–5.

12. Yossepowitch O, Baniel J. Role of organ-sparing surgery in germ cell tumors of the testis. Urology 2004; 63(3):421–7.

13. Bertolotto M, Cacciato F, Cazzagon M, et al. MR imaging of the scrotum. In: Manfredi R, Pozzi Mucelli R, editors. MRI of the Female and Male Pelvis. Cham: Springer International Publishing; 2015. p. 229–47.

14. Cassidy FH, Ishioka KM, McMahon CJ, et al. MR imaging of scrotal tumors and pseudotumors. Radiographics 2010;30(3):665–83.

15. Tsili AC, Argyropoulou MI, Astrakas LG, et al. Dynamic contrast-enhanced subtraction MRI for characterizing intratesticular mass lesions. Am J Roentgenol 2013;200(3):578–85.

16. Parker RA III, Menias CO, Quazi R, et al. MR imaging of the penis and scrotum. Radiographics 2015; 35(4):1033–50.

17. Narra VR, Howell RW, Goddu SM, et al. Effects of a 1.5-Tesla static magnetic field on spermatogenesis and embryogenesis in mice. Invest Radiol 1996; 31(9):586–90.

18. Shellock FG, Rothman B, Sarti D. Heating of the scrotum by high-field-strength MR imaging. AJR Am J Roentgenol 1990;154(6):1229–32.

19. Manganaro L, Saldari M, Pozza C, et al. Dynamic contrast-enhanced and diffusion-weighted MR imaging in the characterisation of small, non-palpable solid testicular tumours. Eur Radiol 2018;28(2):554–64.

20. Tsili AC, Ntorkou A, Astrakas L, et al. Diffusion-weighted magnetic resonance imaging in the characterization of testicular germ cell neoplasms: effect of ROI methods on apparent diffusion coefficient values and interobserver variability. Eur J Radiol 2017;89:1–6.

21. Tsili AC, Sylakos A, Ntorkou A, et al. Apparent diffusion coefficient values and dynamic contrast enhancement patterns in differentiating seminomas from nonseminomatous testicular neoplasms. Eur J Radiol 2015;84(7):1219–26.

22. Kantarci M, Doganay S, Yalcin A, et al. Diagnostic performance of diffusion-weighted MRI in the detection of nonpalpable undescended testes: comparison with conventional MRI and surgical findings. Am J Roentgenol 2010;195(4):W268–73.

23. Tsili AC, Argyropoulou MI, Giannakis D, et al. Diffusion-weighted MR imaging of normal and abnormal scrotum: preliminary results. Asian J Androl 2012; 14(4):649.

24. Karakas E, Karakas O, Cullu N, et al. Diffusion-weighted MRI of the testes in patients with varicocele: a preliminary study. Am J Roentgenol 2014; 202(2):324–8.

25. Akbar SA, Sayyed TA, Jafri SZ, et al. Multimodality imaging of paratesticular neoplasms and their rare mimics. Radiographics 2003;23(6):1461–76.

26. Woodward PJ, Sohaey R, O'Donoghue MJ, et al. From the archives of the AFIP: tumors and tumorlike lesions of the testis: radiologic-pathologic correlation. Radiographics 2002;22(1):189–216.

27. Gooding G. Sonography of the spermatic cord. Am J Roentgenol 1988;151(4):721–4.

28. Kim W, Rosen MA, Langer JE, et al. US–MR imaging correlation in pathologic conditions of the scrotum. Radiographics 2007;27(5):1239–53.

29. Patel MD, Silva AC. MRI of an adenomatoid tumor of the tunica albuginea. Am J Roentgenol 2004;182(2): 415–7.

30. Williams G, Banerjee R. Paratesticular tumours. BJU Int 1969;41(3):332–9.

31. Epstein J. Diseases of the spermatic cord and paratesticular tissue. Urologic pathology. Philadelphia: WB Saunders; 1989. p. 219–48.

32. Srigley J, Hartwick R. Tumors and cysts of the paratesticular region. Pathol Annu 1990;25:51–108.

33. Bulakci M, Tefik T, Kartal MG, et al. Imaging appearances of paratesticular fibrous pseudotumor. Pol J Radiol 2016;81:10.

34. Ntorkou AA, Tsili AC, Giannakis D, et al. Magnetic resonance imaging findings of cellular angiofibroma of the tunica vaginalis of the testis: a case report. J Med Case Rep 2016;10(1):71.

35. Iwasa Y, Fletcher CD. Cellular angiofibroma: clinicopathologic and immunohistochemical analysis of 51 cases. Am J Surg Pathol 2004;28(11):1426–35.

36. Laskin WB, Fetsch JF, Mostofi FK. Angiomyofibroblastomalike tumor of the male genital tract: analysis of 11 cases with comparison to female angiomyofibroblastoma and spindle cell lipoma. Am J Surg Pathol 1998;22(1):6–16.

37. Miyajima K, Hasegawa S, Oda Y, et al. Angiomyofibroblastoma-like tumor (cellular angiofibroma) in the male inguinal region. Radiat Med 2007;25(4): 173–7.

38. Maruyama M, Yoshizako T, Kitagaki H, et al. Magnetic resonance imaging features of angiomyofibroblastoma-like tumor of the scrotum with pathologic correlates. Clin Imaging 2012; 36(5):632–5.

39. Hyouchi N, Yamada T, Takeuchi S, et al. Malignant fibrous histiocytoma of spermatic cord: a case report. Hinyokika Kiyo 1996;42(6):469–71.

40. Tsili AC, Argyropoulou MI, Giannakis D, et al. MRI in the characterization and local staging of testicular neoplasms. Am J Roentgenol 2010;194(3): 682–9.

41. Algebally AM, Tantawy HI, Yousef RR, et al. Advantage of adding diffusion weighted imaging to routine MRI examinations in the diagnostics of scrotal lesions. Pol J Radiol 2015;80:442.

42. Aganovic L, Cassidy F. Imaging of the scrotum. Radiol Clin North Am 2012;50(6):1145–65.

43. Cho J-H, Chang JC, Park BH, et al. Sonographic and MR imaging findings of testicular epidermoid cysts. Am J Roentgenol 2002;178(3):743–8.

44. Langer J, Ramchandani P, Siegelman ES, et al. Epidermoid cysts of the testicle: sonographic and MR imaging features. AJR Am J Roentgenol 1999; 173(5):1295–9.

45. Baer HM, Gerber WL, Kendall AR, et al. Segmental infarct of the testis due to hypersensitivity angiitis. J Urol 1989;142(1):125–7.

46. Bird K, Rosenfield A. Testicular infarction secondary to acute inflammatory disease: demonstration by B-scan ultrasound. Radiology 1984;152(3):785–8.

47. Costa M, Calleja R, Ball RY, et al. Segmental testicular infarction. BJU Int 1999;83(4):525.

48. Gofrit ON, Rund D, Shapiro A, et al. Segmental testicular infarction due to sickle cell disease. J Urol 1998;160(3):835–6.

49. Baratelli G, Vischi S, Mandelli PG, et al. Segmental hemorrhagic infarction of testicle. J Urol 1996; 156(4):1442.

50. Fernandez-Perez GC, Tardáguila FM, Velasco M, et al. Radiologic findings of segmental testicular infarction. Am J Roentgenol 2005;184(5):1587–93.

51. Gaur S, Bhatt S, Derchi L, et al. Spontaneous intratesticular hemorrhage. J Ultrasound Med 2011; 30(1):101–4.

52. Tumeh S, Benson C, Richie J. Acute diseases of the scrotum. Semin Ultrasound CT MR 1991;12(2): 115–30.

53. Bhatt S, Dogra VS. Role of US in testicular and scrotal trauma. Radiographics 2008;28(6):1617–29.

54. Siegel RL, Miller KD, Jemal A. Cancer statistics, 2018. CA Cancer J Clin 2018;68(1):7–30.

55. Wagner BJ. Imaging of the male pelvis: scrotum. In: Hodler J, von Schulthess GK, Kubik-Huch RA, et al, editors. Diseases of the Abdomen and Pelvis 2014–2017. Milano: Springer; 2014.

56. Ulbright T, Amin M, Young R. Armed forces institute of pathology atlas of tumor pathology: tumors of the testis, adnexa, spermatic cord and scrotum. Washington, DC: AFIP Press; 1999.

57. Gilligan TD, Seidenfeld J, Basch EM, et al. American Society of Clinical Oncology Clinical Practice Guideline on uses of serum tumor markers in adult males with germ cell tumors. J Clin Oncol 2010;28(20): 3388–404.

58. Johnson J, Mattrey R, Phillipson J. Differentiation of seminomatous from nonseminomatous testicular tumors with MR imaging. AJR Am J Roentgenol 1990;154(3):539–43.

59. Dilworth JP, Farrow GM, Oesterling JE. Non-germ cell tumors of testis. Urology 1991;37(5):399–417.

60. Kim I, Young RH, Scully RE. Leydig cell tumors of the testis. A clinicopathological analysis of 40 cases and review of the literature. Am J Surg Pathol 1985;9(3): 177–92.

61. Idrees MT, Ulbright TM, Oliva E, et al. The World Health Organization 2016 classification of testicular non-germ cell tumours: a review and update from the International Society of Urological Pathology Testis Consultation Panel. Histopathology 2017; 70(4):513–21.

62. Scully RF. Gonadoblastoma. A review of 74 cases. Cancer 1970;25(6):1340–56.

63. Al-Agha OM, Axiotis CA. An in-depth look at Leydig cell tumor of the testis. Arch Pathol Lab Med 2007; 131(2):311–7.

64. Conkey D, Howard GC, Grigor KM, et al. Testicular sex cord–stromal tumours: the Edinburgh experience 1988–2002, and a review of the literature. Clin Oncol 2005;17(5):322–7.

65. Gabrilove J, Nicolis GL, Mitty HA, et al. Feminizing interstitial cell tumor of the testis: personal observations and a review of the literature. Cancer 1975; 35(4):1184–202.

66. Kaplan GW, Cromie WJ, Kelalis PP, et al. Gonadal stromal tumors: a report of the prepubertal testicular tumor registry. J Urol 1986;136(1):300–1.

67. Young R, Koelliker D, Scully RE. Sertoli cell tumors of the testis, not otherwise specified. A clinicopathologic analysis of 60 cases. J Urol 1999;161(3):1024–5.

68. Proppe KH, Scully RE. Large-cell calcifying Sertoli cell tumor of the testis. Am J Clin Pathol 1980; 74(5):607–19.

69. Young RH. Sex cord-stromal tumors of the ovary and testis: their similarities and differences with consideration of selected problems. Mod Pathol 2005; 18(S2):S81.

70. Nielsen K, Jacobsen GK. Malignant sertoli cell tumour of the testis. Apmis 1988;96(7-12):755–60.

71. Hasselblom S, Ridell B, Wedel H, et al. Testicular lymphoma a retrospective, population-based, clinical and immunohistochemical study. Acta Oncologica 2004;43(8):758–65.

72. Shahab N, Doll DC. Testicular lymphoma. Semin Oncol 1999;26(3):259–69.

73. Fonseca R, Habermann TM, Colgan JP, et al. Testicular lymphoma is associated with a high incidence of extranodal recurrence. Cancer 2000;88(1):154–61.

74. Zucca E, Conconi A, Mughal TI, et al. Patterns of outcome and prognostic factors in primary large-cell lymphoma of the testis in a survey by the International Extranodal Lymphoma Study Group. J Clin Oncol 2003;21(1):20–7.

75. Henderson CG, Ahmed AA, Sesterhenn I, et al. Enucleation for prepubertal leydig cell tumor. J Urol 2006;176(2):703–5.

76. Nicolai N, Necchi A, Raggi D, et al. Clinical outcome in testicular sex cord stromal tumors: testis sparing vs radical orchiectomy and management of advanced disease. Urology 2015;85(2):402–6.

77. Fernandez G, Tardáguila F, Rivas C, et al. MRI in the diagnosis of testicular Leydig cell tumour. Br J Radiol 2004;77(918):521–4.

78. Manganaro L, Vinci V, Pozza C, et al. A prospective study on contrast-enhanced magnetic resonance imaging of testicular lesions: distinctive features of Leydig cell tumours. Eur Radiol 2015;25(12):3586–95.

79. Reinges MT, Kaiser W, Miersch W, et al. Dynamic MRI of benign and malignant testicular lesions: preliminary observations. Eur Radiol 1995;5(6):615–22.

80. Drevelengas A, Kalaitzoglou I, Destouni E, et al. Bilateral Sertoli cell tumor of the testis: MRI and sonographic appearance. Eur Radiol 1999;9(9):1934.

81. Emura A, Kudo S, Mihara M, et al. Testicular malignant lymphoma; imaging and diagnosis. Radiat Med 1996;14(3):121–6.

82. Saito W, Amanuma M, Tanaka J, et al. A case of testicular malignant lymphoma with extension to the epididymis and spermatic cord. Magn Reson Med Sci 2002;1(1):59–63.

83. Castrodeza AV, Torres Nieto A, Mendo González M, et al. Diagnosis of a primary testicular lymphoma by echography and magnetic resonance imaging. Clin Transl Oncol 2006;8(6):456–8.

84. Albers P, Albrecht W, Algaba F, et al. Guidelines on testicular cancer. Eur Urol 2005;48(6):885–94.

85. Ellis JH, Bies JR, Kopecky KK, et al. Comparison of NMR and CT imaging in the evaluation of metastatic retroperitoneal lymphadenopathy from testicular carcinoma. J Comput Assist Tomogr 1984;8(4):709–19.

86. Hogeboom W, Hoekstra HJ, Mooyaart EL, et al. The role of magnetic resonance imaging and computed tomography in the treatment evaluation of retroperitoneal lymph-node metastases of non-seminomatous testicular tumors. Eur J Radiol 1991;13(1):31–6.

87. Sohaib SA, Koh D-M, Husband JE. The role of imaging in the diagnosis, staging, and management of testicular cancer. Am J Roentgenol 2008;191(2):387–95.

88. Sohaib S, Koh DM, Barbachano Y, et al. Prospective assessment of MRI for imaging retroperitoneal metastases from testicular germ cell tumours. Clin Radiol 2009;64(4):362–7.

89. Kreydin EI, Barrisford GW, Feldman AS, et al. Testicular cancer: what the radiologist needs to know. Am J Roentgenol 2013;200(6):1215–25.

90. Harisinghani MG, Saksena M, Ross RW, et al. A pilot study of lymphotrophic nanoparticle-enhanced magnetic resonance imaging technique in early stage testicular cancer: a new method for noninvasive lymph node evaluation. Urology 2005;66(5):1066–71.

91. Rockall AG, Sohaib SA, Harisinghani MG, et al. Diagnostic performance of nanoparticle-enhanced magnetic resonance imaging in the diagnosis of lymph node metastases in patients with endometrial and cervical cancer. J Clin Oncol 2005;23(12):2813–21.

Moving?

Make sure your subscription moves with you!

To notify us of your new address, find your **Clinics Account Number** (located on your mailing label above your name), and contact customer service at:

Email: journalscustomerservice-usa@elsevier.com

800-654-2452 (subscribers in the U.S. & Canada)
314-447-8871 (subscribers outside of the U.S. & Canada)

Fax number: 314-447-8029

Elsevier Health Sciences Division
Subscription Customer Service
3251 Riverport Lane
Maryland Heights, MO 63043

*To ensure uninterrupted delivery of your subscription, please notify us at least 4 weeks in advance of move.

Printed and bound by CPI Group (UK) Ltd, Croydon, CR0 4YY

08/05/2025

01864740-0002